KINESIOLOGY
for
OCCUPATIONAL THERAPY

KINESIOLOGY *for* OCCUPATIONAL THERAPY

Melinda Rybski, MS, OTR/L

Department of Occupational Therapy
The Ohio State University
Columbus, OH

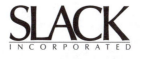

SLACK
INCORPORATED

An innovative information, education, and management company
6900 Grove Road • Thorofare, NJ 08086

Illustrator: Shelley Nickel

Printed in the United States.

Published by: SLACK Incorporated
                  6900 Grove Road
                  Thorofare, NJ 08086 USA
                  Telephone: 856-848-1000
                  Fax: 856-853-5991
                  www.slackbooks.com

Rybski, Melinda.
  Kinesiology for occupational therapy / Melinda Rybski.
     p. ; cm.
  Includes bibliographical references and index.
  ISBN 1-55642-491-4 (alk. paper)
  1. Kinesiology. 2. Human mechanics. 3. Musculoskeletal system. 4. Occupational therapy.
  [DNLM: 1. Kinesiology, Applied. 2. Movement--physiology. 3. Musculoskeletal Physiology. 4. Occupational Therapy. WE 103 R989k 2004] I. Title.
  QP303.R93 2004
  612.7'6--dc22
                            2003027462

Last digit is print number: 10 9 8 7 6 5 4 3 2

DEDICATION

This book is dedicated to the occupational therapy students of the future, to the occupational therapy practicing clinicians, and to the clients they serve.

Contents

Instructors: Kinesiology for Occupational Therapy Instructor's Manual is also available from SLACK Incorporated. Don't miss this important companion to Kinesiology for Occupational Therapy. To obtain the Instructor's Manual, please visit http://www.efacultylounge.com

ACKNOWLEDGMENTS

I wish to thank Amy, Debra, and John for encouraging me throughout this writing endeavor. Shelley Nickel was timely, skillful, and professional in her work as illustrator and I appreciate her time and efforts.

The occupational therapy faculty members at The Ohio State University, my teachers as well as my peers, demonstrated a long-established confidence in my abilities.

My parents taught me the wonder of life and the fun of curiosity. Most of all, I want to thank Tom, Katherine, and Greg for their patience and understanding, and I appreciate Ivy, who was my constant companion as I wrote this text.

ABOUT THE AUTHOR

Melinda Rybski, MS, OTR/L is a faculty member of the Occupational Therapy Division at The Ohio State University. Ms. Rybski graduated from The Ohio State University College of Allied Medical Professions with a bachelor of science in 1979, and in 1987 with a masters degree. She taught occupational therapy students for 18 years, with a primary focus on kinesiology, physical disabilities, and the practice of occupational therapy and Level I fieldwork. She has also taught or assisted with other occupational therapy courses including Application of Neurodevelopmental Construct, Practice of Occupational Therapy in the Hospital Setting, Interpersonal Dynamics and Task-Oriented Groups in Occupational Therapy, Occupational Therapy in Mental Health, Introduction to Alternative Research Methodologies, and Critical Phases of Life.

Her clinical experience includes inpatient rehabilitation, acute care, outpatient, and long-term care. She has also served on the Board of Trustees for the Ohio Occupational Therapy Association and is a book reviewer for several publishing companies.

PREFACE

This book is written for occupational therapists and occupational therapy students. The purpose of this book is to explore and explain how movement occurs from a musculoskeletal orientation. This text does not discuss the influence and contribution of the sensory system, nervous systems, volition, or cognition on the production of movement, although these are clearly vital parts of movement.

This text includes descriptions of how joints, muscles, and bones all interact to produce movement. General information about muscles and assessment of strength, as well as joints and assessment of joint motion, is contained in two chapters that will elucidate this idea of movement. There are 6 chapters devoted to how movement is produced at each joint (shoulder, elbow, wrist, hand, lower extremity, and posture).

In order to understand how movement is produced, kinesiology concepts are explained with regard to forces acting on the body and how these forces influence not only movement but ultimately our intervention with clients.

Since this book is written for occupational therapists, the first chapter briefly explains concepts particularly related to the profession of occupational therapy. Terminology is defined according to *Occupational Therapy Practice Framework: Domain and Process* as well as International Classification of Impairments, Disabilities, and Handicaps (ICIDH-2) terminology.

Once one understands how movement is produced and how to assess strength and joint motion, the next logical step is to learn about appropriate intervention. The last two chapters are devoted to two intervention frames of reference used in occupational therapy. Included in each of these chapters are goals relative to areas of focus that include the theoretic principles that underlie intervention.

Inside the back cover of the book you will find a copy of *Goniometry: An Interactive Tutorial* by Lynn Van Ost. This CD-ROM is included to help the reader more fully understand the principles of goniometry, which is a critical element of occupational therapy.

Conceptual Foundations

Occupational Therapy Concepts

Chapter 1

INTRODUCTION

"Occupational therapy enables people to do the day to day activities that are important to them despite impairments, activity limitations or participation restrictions or despite risks for these problems" (Moyers, 1999). By using these everyday activities, or *occupations*, increased functional performance that is meaningful to the client is the outcome of occupational therapy intervention.

Occupation is used to organize and define occupational therapy's domain of concern (AOTA, 1995a). Clients are individuals, groups, or populations served by occupational therapists. It is the *client's* designation of the meaning and importance of each occupation or activity that is the focus of intervention in occupational therapy.

Performance in areas of occupation refers to participation in activities of daily living, instrumental activities of daily living (such as care for others, health maintenance, or financial management), educational activities, work, play, leisure, and social participation (AOTA, 2002). Occupations will be defined by the client as part of an occupational profile in which the therapist gains an understanding of the client's history, interests, values, and priorities that forms the basis of intervention (Table 1-1).

OCCUPATIONAL PERFORMANCE

Occupational performance is the interaction of the client, context, and activity that enables successful engagement in the areas of occupation. The client's actual performance may be observed in the context in which it normally occurs so that performance skills and patterns can be clearly seen. Evaluation of occupational performance focuses on context, activity demands, and client factors that may hinder or facilitate participation in desired activities.

Contextual factors are those related to the physical environment, cultural and social systems, simulation of environmental conditions, and spiritual aspects of being (AOTA, 2002). This definition of contextual factors is very similar to that used in the International Classification of Functioning, Disability and Health (ICF) (World Health Organization [WHO], 1997) which defines *context* as the "complete background of a person's life and living." ICIDH-2 further clarified the use of the term *context* by separating it into environmental and personal factors. Environmental factors are those in the natural environment and in the human-made environment and include social attitudes, customs, rules, practices, institutions, and other individuals. Personal factors are those components that are not part of the health condition, including age, race, gender, educational background, experiences, personality and character style, aptitudes, other health conditions, fitness, lifestyle, habits, upbringing, coping styles, social background, profession, and past and current experience (WHO, 1997).

Occupational therapists also conceptualize occupational performance as being a function of activity demands and client factors. Activity demands are those variables directly related to purposeful activities in which the client engages. Whether the activity demands are too great for the client depends on the client's abilities and performance skills. Abilities are related to learning and involve cognition, and social-emotional and physical factors. Performance skills are observable and relate to successful participation in activities (Figure 1-1).

When intervention is directed toward improving physical factors related to body/structure and function (such as physiological function, neuromusculoskeletal, sensory, or perceptual areas) or motor skills (such as coordination, posture, and mobility), it is based on the understanding that these factors influence a client's ability to participate in life tasks that are important to him or her.

OCCUPATIONAL THERAPY INTERVENTION

Occupational therapy intervention is designed to "improve the occupational performance of persons who lack the ability to perform an action or activity considered necessary for their everyday lives" (AOTA, 1995b, p. 1019), as well as to achieve the outcomes of prevention of injury or disability, promotion of health, and quality of life (Moyers, 1999). In order to conceptualize this improvement in the occupational performance of our clients, Fisher (1998) uses four continua to evaluate the characteristics of any activity used in intervention (see Figure 1-1). The further to the right one moves, the more client-centered the intervention (Table 1-2). From this, Fisher identified four common intervention models.

Fisher's Models of Intervention

The first intervention model is that of *exercise*. This would be seen in rote exercise or practice activities that may have a purpose or goal, but often this originated with the practitioner and not the client. The task has little or no meaning to the client and the focus is on remediation of impairments at the client factor level.

Contrived occupation is "exercise with added purpose and occupation with a contrived component." There may be a purpose or a goal, but again, it originated with the practitioner so it is meaningless to the client. The focus is again on remediation of impairments. Contrived occupation can include exercise with added purpose, which is exercise that is embedded in an activity. Both the task objects and the potential purpose or meaning are contrived. An example is having the client place cones on a shelf, pretending they are glasses and he is putting dishes away. The cones have little relevance to actual tasks being simulated. Or another variation might be occupation with a contrived component where the

Table 1-1.

OVERVIEW OF OCCUPATIONAL THERAPY PROCESS

Occupational Profile

Who is the Client?

Why is the Client seeking services?

What areas of occupation are affected?

- ADL
- IADL
- Work
- Play
- Leisure
- Social Participation

Contexts

- Life experiences
- Values
- Interests
- Previous patterns of engagement
- Meanings of patterns

Client's occupational history

Client's priorities and targeted outcomes

Intervention Plan

Plan that includes:

- Objective and measurable goals with timeframe
- Theory and evidence
- Create or promote (health promotion)
- Establish or restore

(Remediation/biomechanical/NDT/ cognitive-perceptual)

- Maintain
- Modify (Rehabilitation: adaptation/ compensation
- Prevent (disability prevention)

Mechanisms for delivery:

- Who will deliver....role delineation
- Types of intervention
- Frequency, duration
- Outcome measures
- D/c needs and plans
- Recommendations or referrals

Outcome Measures

Select outcome measures

- Occupational performance
- Client satisfaction
- Adaptation
- Health and wellness
- Prevention
- Quality of life

Analysis of Occupational Performance

- Performance skills (motor, process, communication/ interaction)
- Performance patterns habits, routines, roles
- Factors (context, activity demands, client)

Type of Intervention

Therapeutic use of self

Use of occupations or activities

- Occupation-based
- Purposeful activity
- Preparatory

Consultation

Education

Measure and Use Outcomes

- Compare goal achievement to targeted outcomes
- Assess outcome results

---

objects are real but the task has no purpose. For example, pounding nails into a board to pretend to be building a birdhouse. The purpose and meaning are contrived.

Therapeutic occupation is when the client actively participates in occupation. The client identifies the task as purposeful and meaningful and the performance of the task is naturalistic and contextual. Real objects are used in natural environments. The focus is on remediation of impairments in the context of occupation.

The final intervention model is *adaptive* or *compensatory occupation*. This type of intervention occurs with the client's active participation in occupations chosen by the client, which are purposeful and meaningful, naturalistic and contextual. The intervention is focused on improved occupational performance and is not directed toward remediation of impairments. Intervention may include assistive devices, teaching alternative or compensatory strategies, or modification of physical and social environments.

Occupational therapy intervention that is primarily in the therapeutic occupation or compensatory adaptive models is more client-centered and provides meaningful and functional outcomes for the client.

Remediation Approach

Therapeutic occupation as defined by Fisher is considered a *remediation approach*. Remediation approaches are selected when there is an expectation for reduction in the limitations in client factors that influence performance in areas of occupation. It may involve learning new skills, slowing the decline in abilities, or in maintaining or improving quality of life (Moyers, 1999). Examples of remediation techniques might be the use of enabling activities, sensorimotor techniques, graded exercises, physical agent modalities, or manual techniques (Moyers, 1999). Arts, crafts, games, sports, exercise, and daily activities may also be used to improve the function of a specific body structure or function and each of these therapeutic methods would be tailored to each individual to fit the capacities and goals of that person.

If the remediation is to be considered successful and to be considered occupational therapy, the intervention will need to occur in a natural context. Moyers (1999) adds "simply expecting improvements in impairments to automatically produce change in level of disablement without addressing performance in occupa-

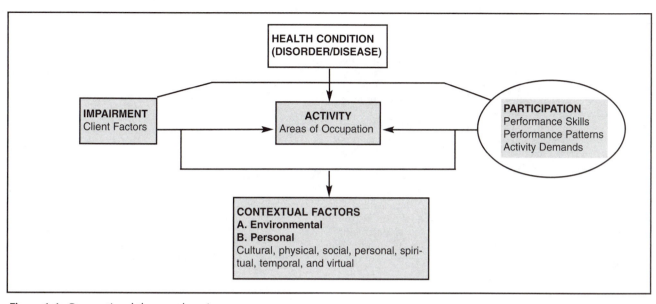

Figure 1-1. Occupational therapy domain.

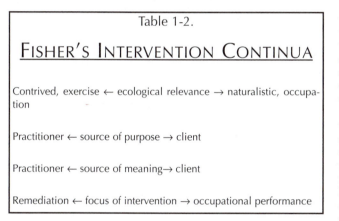

tions within the intervention plan is inappropriate" (p. 276). Intervention that concentrates on client factors must also be contextually meaningful and occur in a natural environment to avoid being rote exercise or contrived occupation. The biomechanical approach used in occupational therapy intervention is the remediation approach discussed in this text since this approach is most beneficial in intervention for clients with decreased strength, endurance, and range of motion (ROM).

Compensation and Adaptation Approach

Compensation and adaptation intervention is used when there is little expectation for change in client factors and subsequent performance skills. This approach may be selected when there is limited time for intervention or when the client or family prefers this approach to remedial techniques, seeing compensation and adaptation as providing more immediate success in performance of the areas of occupation (Moyers, 1999). Compensation and adaptation approaches are often referred to as the *rehabilitation approach* (Pedretti, 1996; Rybski, 1990) and this approach concentrates not on the client factors but instead on performance in areas of occupation. An assumption of this approach is that the performance of the activity or task that the person sees as important is the focus of

the intervention (Rybski, 1990). Techniques used in this approach include changing the task, altering the task method, adapting the task object, changing the context, family and caregiver education, and environmental adaptation. Disability prevention may be considered part of this approach in that education of the client and caregivers is vital in preventing further disease or disability, especially in those who already have impairments or limitations.

The rehabilitation approach is discussed in this text as an intervention strategy for use with those clients with movement impairments preventing full participation in occupations for which remediation is not possible. Both biomechanical and rehabilitation interventions are used extensively in occupational therapy and require knowledge of the structure and function of the body, knowledge about specific diagnostic categories and procedural reasoning, and knowledge about specific individual clients, their activities, roles, and values.

OVERVIEW OF THIS TEXT

This text is comprised of three distinct sections. Section I is designed to provide background information, knowledge, and facts that will be applied to later sections. The chapters in this foundational section pertain to basic concepts about movement, factors that influence ROM, and those factors that influence strength. Terminology is explained that will be used throughout the text and the relationships between body structures and functional movement are introduced. Assessment of joint movement and strength is included in this section. This section is provided to enable greater understanding of body structure and function as a basis of movement necessary for performance in areas of occupation.

Section II discusses how the general principles introduced in Section I apply to specific joints. How is joint motion produced at the wrist? What bones and muscles are involved? Is this a stable joint? These chapters that focus on specific joints relate structural anatomy with functional motion. Readers are encouraged to palpate the anatomical structures (muscles and bones) and to see and feel how these structures work together to produce joint movement. Most joints are actually made up of multiple articulations; each articulation contributes to the overall motion produced at that joint, so these articulations are discussed separately and as contributors to joint motion. Not every structure of the joint is included or discussed in detail; only those structures that most influence movement or stability are included. A summary chart describing joint movements, the plane and axis in which the movement occurs, normal limiting factors in movement production, the specific "end feel" per motion, and the muscles producing the motion is provided in the Appendices for each joint to recapitulate information presented in the chapter. Detailed descriptions of muscles are provided so that students can clearly see how muscle orientation affects muscle action. It is not always clear how one muscle can have multiple and seemingly incongruent muscle actions without seeing how a muscle acts at different joints. A clear understanding of normal joint movement is essential to occupational therapy practice and is the basis of the biomechanical intervention approach. Knowing how a normal joint should move is the essence of assessment. Specific factors that are relevant to the assessment of individual joints are discussed and specific joint pathology is provided as an overview of possible limitations in function related to specific structures and disease processes or trauma (see Appendices).

Section III of this text provides two different intervention strategies that could be used if there are activity limitations or participation restrictions due primarily to musculoskeletal or motor impairments. Remediation via the biomechanical approach and adaptation/compensation via the rehabilitation approach are the primary intervention strategies discussed. For each approach, intervention principles are provided and explained, as are examples of goal statements and specific methods that could be used to implement the intervention selected.

SUMMARY

1. Occupational therapy uses occupation, or the everyday things that people do, as the basis of intervention.
2. Intervention can be classified as remediation (change in the existing condition) or compensation/adaptation (alter the way or the place in which tasks are performed).
3. Remediation approaches focus on client factors (specifically physical abilities and motor skills) and often reflect the short-term goals of intervention. The assumption with this approach is that changes in the these factors will permit improvement in the areas of performance.
4. Adaptation/compensation approaches focus on functional areas or areas of occupation. The emphasis is in improvements in work, play, or self-care skills and resumption of roles and health.

REFERENCES

American Occupational Therapy Association. (1995a). Position paper: Occupation. *Am J Occup Ther*, *49*(10), 1015-1018.

American Occupational Therapy Association. (1995b). Position paper: Occupational performance: Occupational therapy's definition of function. *Am J Occup Ther*, *49*(10), 1019-1020.

American Occupational Therapy Association. (2002). Occupational therapy practice framework. *Am J Occup Ther*, *56*(6), 609-639.

Fisher, A. G. (1998). Uniting practice and theory in an occupational framework: 1998 Eleanor Clarke Slagle lecture. *Am J Occup Ther*, *52*(7), 509-521.

Moyers, P. A. (1999). The guide to occupational therapy practice. *Am J Occup Ther*, *53*(3), 247-321.

Pedretti, L. W. (1996). *Occupational therapy: Practice skills for physical dysfunction* (4th ed.). St. Louis, MO: Mosby.

Rybski, M. F. Occupational Therapy Practice in Ohio, presentation at the American Occupational Therapy Association annual conference, Cincinnati, Ohio, June 1990.

World Health Organization (1997). *International classification of impairments, activities, and participation: A manual of dimensions of disablement and functioning* (Beta-1 draft for the field trials). Geneva: World Health Organization.

BIBLIOGRAPHY

American Occupational Therapy Association. (1993). Core values and attitudes of occupational therapy practice. *Am J Occup Ther*, *47*(12), 1085-1086.

American Occupational Therapy Association. (1994a). Uniform terminology for occupational therapy (3rd ed.). *Am J Occup Ther*, *48*(11), 1047-1054.

American Occupational Therapy Association. (1994b). The philosophical base of occupational therapy. *Am J Occup Ther*, *49*(10), 1026.

American Occupational Therapy Association. (1997). Statement: Fundamental concepts of occupational therapy: Occupation, purposeful activity and function. *Am J Occup Ther*, *51*(10), 864-866.

Chisholm, D., Dolhi, C., & Schreiber, J. (2000). Creating occupation-based opportunities in a medical model clinical practice setting. *O.T. Practice*, pp ce1-7.

Dutton, R. (1995). *Clinical reasoning in physical disabilities*. Baltimore: Williams and Wilkins.

Kielhofner, G. (1992). *Conceptual foundations of occupational therapy*. Philadelphia: F. A. Davis Co.

Kielhofner, G. (1983). *Health through occupations: Theory and practice in occupational therapy*. Philadelphia: F. A. Davis Co.

Marrelli, T. M., & Krulish, L. H. (1999). *Home care therapy: Quality, documentation and reimbursement*. Boca Grande, FL: Marrelli and Associates, Inc.

Neistadt, M. E., & Seymour, S. G. (1995). Treatment activity preferences of occupational therapists in adult physical dysfunction settings. *Am J Occup Ther*, *49*(5), 437-443.

Trombly, C. A. (Ed.). (1995). *Occupational therapy for physical dysfunction* (4th ed.). Baltimore: Williams and Wilkins.

Trombly, C. A. (1995). Occupation: Purposefulness and meaningfulness as therapeutic mechanisms: 1995 Eleanor Clarke Slagle lecture. *Am J Occup Ther*, *49*(10), 960- 970.

Kinesiology Concepts

Chapter 2

It is important to take a moment to appreciate the complexity of movement and the integration of functions that are necessary at many levels to enable successful participation in everyday activities.

A person wants to move. This desire to move sets off a series of physiological responses to produce efficient volitional movement:

- Spinal reflexes that underlie reciprocal movements need to be able to respond quickly to stimuli.
- Sensory afferent tracts need to be intact to receive sensory input through intact skin and deep receptors in order to guide movement.
- Perceptual processes must be intact in order to interpret the sensory information.
- Motor efferent tracts need to be intact to send messages to muscle fibers.
- The brain stem must mediate tonic patterned responses of trunk and limb in relation to the head.
- Basal ganglia facilitate adjustments of head in relation to body and aid in balance and automatic motor plans.
- The cerebellum is concerned with speed, smoothness, force, and accuracy of movement.
- The association cortex plans movement.
- The motor cortex executes movement and controls recruitment of motor units.
- Movement is completed due to normal elasticity in tissues, contractile capacity of muscle fibers, freely moveable joints in which the motion is occurring, and stabilization of other joints.
- The person needs motivation to move volitionally, which is reflective of mood, interest, and emotion.
- Cognition is required to maintain interest, use of prior motor learning and experiences, and use of judgment, concentration, and memory (Trombly, 1995).

A more simplified definition of *movement* is the observable behavioral response that will result in the displacement of one or more limb segments of the body. This definition includes aspects of movement that can be described by watching a person move, as well as those factors that influence movement that are not visible.

The science of movement, *kinesiology*, is the study of the forces and of the active and passive structures that are involved in human movement (Table 2-1). By understanding these forces and their impact on the body, occupational therapy intervention can be directed towards the optimal occupational performance in our clients, and also in preventing injury by recommending appropriate positioning of the body and location of objects in relation to the body.

According to Gench, Hinson, and Harvey (1995), a further refinement in the science of movement includes two subsections of kinesiology—*anatomy* and *mechanics*. Anatomy is the understanding of the production of movement by muscles of the body. Mechanics is the study of forces; when applied to the living human body, it is most often referred to as *biomechanics*. Biomechanics deals with forces related to the body and their effect on body movement, size, shape, and structure, which may be due to internal or external force. This is a description of the forces rather than of the movement itself.

Biomechanics can be further subdivided into two areas. *Statics* includes equilibrium and is the study of systems at rest or those moving at a constant speed. An understanding of equilibrium and statics is helpful in identifying stresses on anatomical structures (Smith, Weiss, & Lehmkuhl, 1996). *Dynamics* is concerned with movement.

Within dynamics, *kinematics* is the science of motion of bodies in space, concerned with issues of displacement, velocity, and acceleration with respect to time. Considerations of how fast, how high, and how far can be thought of as the "observational geometry of motion" (Durwood, Baer, & Rowe, 1999). *Kinetics* is the study of forces acting in and on the body producing stability or mobility. These forces cannot be seen. Studying kinetics is helpful in identifying which muscles are the strongest, as well as which aspects of movement are most prone to injury (Hamil & Knutzen, 1995). To understand normal human movement, principles of both static and dynamic biomechanics are important.

STATIC BIOMECHANICS

Equilibrium

Equilibrium has to do with two or more forces that enable a body or object to remain at rest or to move at a constant speed. Forces act in pairs and there will be no movement or equilibrium without the pairing of forces. If a force is greater than the resistance offered by an object, then movement will occur. If a force is not applied to an object that is moving, then the object will continue to move at a constant speed unless acted upon by an another force. The definition of equilibrium clarifies this summation of forces.

The sum of all forces that are applied to the object must be zero for the object to be in equilibrium. Multiple forces act upon the body at all times. Forces are internal, external, observable, and indiscernible. It is important to realize, for example, that gravity exerts a constant force on all objects. This force of gravity has an effect on both equilibrium and on movement and is summarized in Newton's First Law, which states: "a body will remain at rest or will continue in motion unless acted upon by an external force that brings about a change in the existing state".

Inertia is the body's reluctance to change what it is doing. Inertia is evident when one tries to push a wheelchair; the hardest part of pushing a wheelchair is when you first push it because you need to overcome inertia before acceleration can occur. Once the wheelchair is set in motion, it will continue until another force stops the motion. The other force may be another object or it can be friction or gravity. Greene and Roberts (1999) provided this example of Newton's First Law:

> *Bernice Richards has quadriplegia and minimal control of the muscles balancing her trunk. She directs her electric wheelchair through the main thoroughfare of a shopping mall, and a child darts in front of her. As she stops the chair, Bernice continues moving forward, stopped only by her chest and pelvic seatbelts. In Bernice's situation, when she stopped quickly, she and her wheelchair traveled together. An outside force (friction) slowed the chair, but Bernice's body continued moving forward. The force of friction on the chair did not affect Bernice's body. A separate, outside force, provided by the seatbelts, stopped her body from continuing forward. (p. 32)*

The above example also describes whiplash, which occurs when an automobile is hit from behind. The body moves forward while the head lags behind. The stretching of the neck and head muscles occurs with the resultant and rapid flexion of the head.

Another example of Newton's First Law, provided by McGinnis (1999), is when you throw a ball in the air from one hand to another. If you resolve the motion into horizontal and vertical components, gravity is an external force for the vertical component in pulling the ball toward the ground. In this case, Newton's First Law does not apply. However, since the force of the air in which the ball travels horizontally exerts a minimal force, this horizontal motion of the ball provides an example of Newton's First Law. "This means that the horizontal velocity of the ball will not change from the time it leaves your hand until it contacts your other hand or another object" (McGinnis, 1999). The reason that this example is relevant to occupational therapists is that muscle actions are also resolved into vertical and horizontal components, and understanding the forces acting on these aspects of muscle activity provides information about joint movement.

Newton's First Law can be interpreted in several ways:
1. If an object is at rest and no external forces act on it, the object remains at rest. If you don't push a person in a wheelchair and no other forces act on the wheelchair, the person in the wheelchair will not move.
2. If an object is in motion and no external forces act on it, the object will continue moving at the constant velocity in a straight line. If gravity and other external forces didn't act on a wheelchair moving on a straight path with no changes in horizontal alignment, then the wheelchair could continue indefinitely.
3. If an object is at rest and external forces do act on it, the object remains at rest only if the resultant of the external forces is zero (the net external force is zero). If a person pushes on a wheelchair and the weight of the person is equal to the force applied, the resultant of the two forces will be zero and no movement will occur. If the person pushing on the wheelchair applies a force greater than that of the weight of the person, then movement occurs.
4. If an object is in motion and external forces do act on it, the object will continue moving at constant velocity in a straight line only if the net external force is zero (McGinnis, 1999).

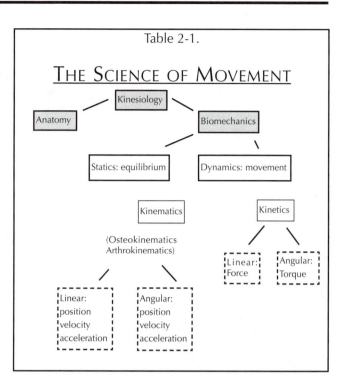

Table 2-1.

THE SCIENCE OF MOVEMENT

DYNAMIC BIOMECHANICS: KINEMATICS

Kinematics looks at aspects of movement like acceleration, velocity, and associated forces with respect to time (Loth & Wadsworth, 1998). The description of movement can represent displacement within a body's position in space, or with a change in position relative to time or velocity (Loth & Wadsworth, 1998). The motion of bodies in space may be concerned with a single point in space (i.e., center of gravity), the position of several segments (i.e., the upper extremity), or position of a single joint or motion (Hamil & Knutzen, 1995). It may represent linear or angular movements. Kinematics is not concerned with the causes of motion but rather with the results of the causes.

Osteokinematics describes movement of bones, while *arthrokinematics* describes the movement of articulating surfaces in relation to the direction of movement of the extremities.

Osteokinematics

The movements of bones have been classified using planes and axes as determinants of motion (Figure 2-1). Planes and axes provide a three-dimensional system of recording the descriptions of movements in space of specific points on the body.

The location of movement occurs in three planes that are at right angles to each other:
1. The first plane is the *sagittal plane*, which corresponds to the sagittal suture in the skull. This is a vertical plane that divides the body into right and left halves. Other names for this plane are the anterior-posterior plane or the YZ plane.
2. The second plane is the *frontal/coronal plane*, which corresponds to the coronal suture in the skull. This, too, is a vertical plane that divides the body into front and back portions. Alternative names for this plane are lateral plane or XY plane.
3. The *transverse plane* is a horizontal plane that separates the body into upper and lower (cranial-caudal) portions. The transverse plane is also referred to as the XZ or horizontal plane.

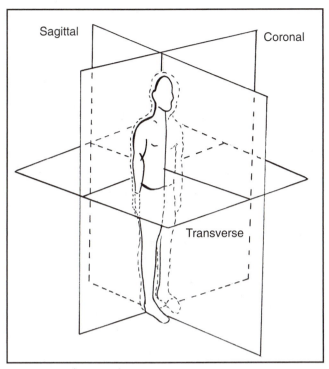

Figure 2-1. Planes and axes.

Table 2-2.
MOTIONS IN EACH PLANE AND AXIS

Motions in a Frontal/Coronal Plane Around a Anterioposterior/Sagittal Axis
Shoulder: abduction and adduction
Wrist: radial and ulnar deviation
Thumb: extension
Hip: abduction and adduction
Foot: eversion and inversion

Motions in a Sagittal Plane Around a Frontal/Coronal Axis
Shoulder: flexion and extension
Hip: flexion and extension
Knee: flexion and extension
Ankle: dorsi and plantar flexion
Thumb: abduction

Motions in a Horizontal Plane Around a Longitudinal/Vertical Axis
Shoulder: internal and external rotation
Forearm: supination and pronation
Hip: internal and external rotation

Planes and Axes

The direction of movement is determined by the axis, which can be thought of as the line around which movement takes place. Axes are related to planes and are perpendicular to them. Three axes divide the three planes into four quadrants.

1. The *anterioposterior* or *sagittal axis* extends horizontally from front to back. The sagittal axis determines the direction of movement in the frontal plane (Table 2-2, Figure 2-2).
2. The *frontal/coronal axis* extends horizontally from side to side. With the sagittal plane, the frontal axis determines the direction of flexion and extension, as well as thumb abduction (see Table 2-2).
3. A vertical line in a cranial-caudal direction is the *longitudinal/vertical axis*, which intersects the *transverse/horizontal plane*. Movements that occur in this transverse plane/longitudinal axis are rotational (see Table 2-2).

Most joint axes are offset from the anatomic planes. For example, the interphalangeal joint of the thumb is in a straight line during extension but pronates and adducts to meet the index finger when flexed. The offset action also influences the action of tendons. For example, flexor pollicis longus flexes and internally rotates the thumb and extensor digitorum extends and externally rotates. Both cross the joint axis of the interphalangeal joint, but extensor digitorum is not perpendicular to the proximal phalange. Only two muscles are required for delicate and precise control, and powerful contractions (Brand & Hollister, 1999).

The importance of understanding planes and axes is in the ability of this three-dimensional system to describe movements clearly and consistently so the movement can be understood explicitly. Anatomic concepts are based on this system and this is the basis for describing these movements.

Movements of Bony Segments

The movement of bony levers is called *swing* (Kisner & Colby, 1990). The amount of swing is measured in degrees of motion using a goniometer. These movements are flexion, extension, abduction, adduction, and rotation.

Angular Movement

Flexion, extension, abduction, adduction, and rotation are all considered *angular* or *rotary* movements. In angular movements, movement occurs around an axis or a pivot point (Smith et al., 1996). Different segments of the same body or object do not move through the same distance (Hamil & Knutzen, 1995) because different segments are at varying distances from the axis. All parts of the object, however, move through the same angle in the same direction at the same time (Watkins, 1999). Everyday examples of angular motion can be seen in a swinging door or a turning doorknob.

In the human body, many motions of the joints are angular. Flexion and extension of the elbow without movement at the shoulder are examples of angular movement. In upward rotation of the scapula, the shoulder girdle as a whole moves with rotary motion. While the inferior angle of the scapula may have moved further than the medial angle of the scapula, and not all parts move an equal distance, the resulting movement is that of angular or rotary movement because all parts of the scapula moved through the same angle in the same direction at the same time.

A child swinging on a swing set demonstrates angular movements about an axis of rotation external to the body, whereas an ice skater in a spin demonstrates rotation of an axis within the body (McGinnis, 1999). McGinnis clarifies this type of motion by imagining any two points on the object. As the object moves, if the paths that each of these points travel is circular with the same center, and if an imaginary line connecting these two points continues to change orientation as the object moves and changes direction, then this would be an angular or rotary movement.

Because of the orientation of the joint axes in the hand, definitions of movements of the thumb are not always as easily visualized as movements at other joints. Figure 2-3 A-E illustrates movements of the thumb.

Translatory Movement

Another type of movement that occurs is *linear* or *translatory movement*. In translatory movement, all parts of an object or person move the same distance in the same direction at the same time (Gench et al., 1995). A person traveling in a car is moving with translatory motion because all parts of that person are moving in the same direction at the same velocity. A figure skater gliding across the ice in a static position or a bicyclist coasting on a flat section of road are examples of linear movement. Protraction and retraction of the scapula are examples of linear motion (McGinnis, 1999). Clarification of this movement would be to again imagine a straight line connecting two points. If the line between the two points maintains the same orientation as the object moves, then this would demonstrate linear movement. If both points move in parallel straight lines, this movement is *rectilinear*; if both points move in parallel but not straight lines, the motion is said to be *curvilinear* (McGinnis, 1999).

General Motion

Many of the movements in the human body are a combination of linear and angular movements. *General motion* is most easily understood when one considers walking or running where there is linear motion of the head and trunk and angular motion of the arms and legs. A person bicycling is actually demonstrating linear motion of the head, trunk, and arms, but also angular motion of the legs to cycle and propel the bicycle. Differences between angular and translatory (linear) movements are:

1. In angular motion, there is movement in a circular path around a central point. In translatory motion, movement starts in one place and ends in another.

2. In angular movement, the object changes orientation during the movement. In translatory movement, the object remains in the original orientation.

3. Two points moving in a segment around a circle move at different velocities. In translatory movement, two points in a line move at the same speed (Greene & Roberts, 1999, p. 47).

Table 2-3 provides a summary of terminology related to movements of the joints.

Joint Classifications

Descriptions of movements that occur in joints is one type of joint classification. A *synarthrodial joint* is one that is immovable (such as cranial and facial bones). An *amphiarthrosis joint* is slightly movable, as seen in some intervertebral articulations. Freely movable joints are called *diarthrosis joints*.

Structural classifications have also been developed to define the composition of the tissue of the joint. *Fibrous joints* are made up of fibrous connective tissue, whereas *cartilage joints* are where cartilage connects joints. *Synovial joints* are more complex and include additional structures such as a joint capsule and synovial fluid.

The movement of between-joint surfaces has also been compared to geometric shapes and mechanical devices. Using this classification system, there are three major types of joints:

1. Uniaxial: movement in one axis (one degree of freedom).

2. Biaxial: movement in two axes (two degrees of freedom, usually flexion/extension and abduction/adduction).

3. Triaxial/multiaxial joints: movement in all axes, including all movements possible.

Uniaxial joints include joints that work like a hinge and are aptly called *hinge joints* or *ginglymus joints* (Figure 2-5). These joints permit flexion and extension, which are angular motions. Examples of

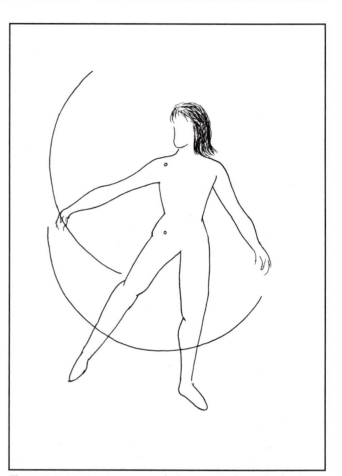

Figure 2-2. Motion in a coronal plane around a sagittal axis.

hinge joints are the humeroradial and humeroulnar joints (also known as the elbow joint). The interphalangeal joints of the fingers are also ginglymus joints.

Another type of uniaxial joint is a *trochoid* or *pivot joint* (Figure 2-6). This is where an arch-shaped process fits around a peg-like process. The axis of movement is longitudinal so the movement is rotary. The proximal radioulnar and the distal radioulnar joint, which are responsible for pronation and supination of the forearm, are trochoid joints.

There are two types of *biaxial joints*. In the first, a *condyloid* or *ellipsoid joint* (Figure 2-7), one oval condyle fits into an elliptical socket. There is flexion and extension in one plane and abduction and adduction in the other. The wrist joint (radiocarpal joint) and the metacarpalphalangeal joints of the hand are examples.

Saddle joints are the second type of biaxial joints (Figure 2-8). In a saddle joint, each joint is convex in one plane and concave in the other and these surfaces fit together. A saddle-shaped bone fits into a socket that is concave-convex-concave in shape. There is movement in two planes as with condyloid joints, which are flexion/extension in one plane and abduction/adduction in the other. The carpometacarpal joint of the thumb is the most universally accepted saddle joint using this classification, although the sternoclavicular joint of the shoulder complex is also considered a saddle joint according to some resources (Konin, 1999).

The shoulder (glenohumeral joint) and the hip are considered ball and socket joints, a type of multiaxial or triaxial joint (Figure 2-9). All movements are possible, including flexion/extension, abduction/adduction, rotation, and combined movements such as circumduction. These joints have three axes perpendicular to each

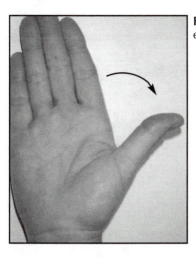

Figure 2-3A. Thumb MP extension.

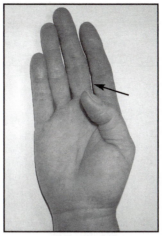

Figure 2-3B. Thumb MP flexion.

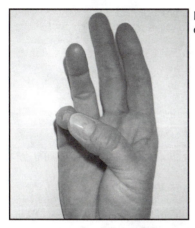

Figure 2-3C. Thumb opposition.

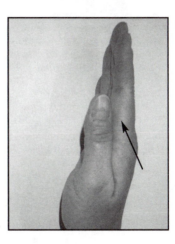

Figure 2-3D. Thumb MP adduction.

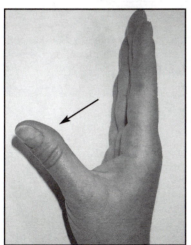

Figure 2-3E. Thumb MP abduction.

other. Independent movement is possible about each of these axes. These types of joints require many muscles for control and stabilization and muscles are placed in the proximal portions of the limbs to be closer to the center of gravity, thereby limiting the amount of movement required (Brand & Hollister, 1999, p. 43).

In addition to ball and socket joints, there are joints that are capable of a gliding motion that can occur in all planes to some slight degree. These are gliding or plane joints, which are also considered multiaxial joints. While discussed here as multiaxial or tri-axial, some sources refer to gliding joints as nonaxial joints. Slight gliding motion occurs in the vertebrocostal, sternocostal, and acromioclavicular joints, for example.

Arthrokinematics is the description of the movement of articulating surfaces in relation to the direction of movement of the extremities. Some authors contend that joints are not flat, cylindrical, conical, or spherical (Kisner & Colby, 1990; Roberts & Falkenburg, 1992). Instead, joints can be classified as ovoid/oval or sellar joints.

Table 2-3.

TERMINOLOGY RELATED TO JOINT MOVEMENTS

Description of Motion	Special Considerations or Alternative Terms
Flexion: the bending of a part (like the elbow) so that surfaces (usually anterior) come closer together. In flexion, the angle of the joint decreases as the joint is moved. Example: when you use your shoulder to reach overhead to retrieve an object from a high shelf.	*Flexion of the thumb:* the thumb moves across the palm of the hand. *Flexion of the knee:* posterior surfaces of the body parts come closer. *Lateral flexion of neck and trunk*: bending movements that occur in a lateral direction either to the right or to the left *Flexion of the foot or dorsiflexion:* when the sole of the foot and toes are pulled up. Example: when you are performing the downward stroke on a bicycle.
Extension: when the angle at the joint increases as the joint is moved. Example: when the elbow is inserted into the armhole of a shirt. Movement of the shoulder when the arm goes behind the body in the coronal plane has been termed both *extension* and *hyperextension,* depending upon the source. For simplicity, this text will assert that shoulder extension occurs from directly overhead to placement at the side of the body.	*Hyperextension*: the movement from hand placement at the side of the body to directly posterior in the coronal plane. *Plantarflexion* of the foot occurs when the sole of the foot and toes are pointed away from the leg. Example: when toes are pointed when one dons a pair of socks.
Abduction: movement away from a defined line, such as the center of the body. In the hand, midline is the third digit and in the foot, the second digit. Example of abduction of the shoulder: when you raise your arm to comb the back of your hair. A special case of abduction is *shoulder abduction in the plane of the scapula*. This motion has several alternative names including scapular plane elevation, elevation in the scapular plane, and "scaption". This motion is approximately "30-40 degrees anterior to the frontal plane" (Smith et al., 1996). The motion is midway between forward shoulder flexion and abduction of the humerus in the plane of the scapula (Nordin & Frankel, 1989). This is a good position to test the motion of the glenohumeral joint since the capsule is in a loose packed position, so one is less likely to impinge on the coracoacromial structures (Smith et al., 1996).	Special considerations of the movement pattern of abduction follow. *Abduction of scapula*, also called *protraction*: movement of the vertebral border of the scapula away from the vertebral column. *Abduction of the thumb:* when the thumb moves in an anterior direction in a plane perpendicular to the palm of the hand. *Abduction of the wrist* is also known as *radial deviation*. Example: when your raise a hammer to strike a nail, your wrist is in radial deviation. *Eversion of the foot:* when the sole of the foot is turned outward. This is not a pure abduction movement in that eversion is actually abduction and pronation of the forefoot; there is much controversy over how to describe this motion.
Adduction is movement toward a defined line, such as the center of the body. When you are sitting with your arms held at the sides of your body, your shoulders are in adduction.	Special cases of adduction follow. *Adduction of the scapula* or *retraction*: movement of the vertebral border of the scapula toward the vertebral column. *Adduction of the thumb*: when the thumb moves back to anatomical position from a position of abduction. *Adduction of the wrist:* referred to as ulnar deviation. Example: when one tightens a lid on a jar. *Inversion of the foot:* when the sole of the foot is turned inward. It is not a pure adduction movement but rather a combination of adduction and supination. There is much controversy over how to describe this motion.

Table 2-3, continued.	
TERMINOLOGY RELATED TO JOINT MOVEMENTS	
	Horizontal adduction occurs at the shoulder joint. Example: when the shoulder is in 90 degrees of flexion, and the arm is moved in a direction toward the midline or toward the anterior.
Internal (medial) rotation occurs at the shoulder and at the hip. This is when there is a transverse rotation oriented toward the anterior side of the body. Example: when you place the back of your hand on your vertebral column.	*Pronation:* when the palm is directed downward . Pronation can actually be considered internal rotation of the forearm. Example: when you are sanding a board.
External (lateral) rotation: when there is a transverse rotation oriented toward the posterior side of the body. Example: when you brush your hair.	*Supination:* the position of the hand in anatomical position where the palm is facing upward. Again, this movement can actually be considered external rotation of the forearm.
Scapular rotation is described in terms of the direction of movement of either the inferior angle of the scapula or movement of the glenoid fossa of the scapula. *Medial (downward) rotation* of the scapula occurs when the inferior angle of the scapula moves toward the midline and movement of the glenoid fossa moves in a downward or caudal direction.	See Figure 2-4.
Lateral (upward) rotation: when the inferior angle moves away from the midline and movement of the glenoid fossa is in an upward or cranial direction. Additional terms are also used to describe joint positions and movements. anterior palmar/volar posterior dorsal medial ulnar lateral radial	

Ovoid joints are joint surfaces that are egg-shaped and may be nearly planar or nearly spherical in shape. Ovoid joints have a convex and concave surface on the articulating bones. In an ovoid joint, the radius of the curvature varies from point to point (Smith et al., 1996). Some joints have a convex and concave surface on each of the articulating bones and are called *sellar joints*. Examples of sellar joints are the carpometacarpal joint of the thumb, the elbow, the sternoclavicular joint, and the talocurcial joints.

The movements of the articulating surfaces of the bones demonstrate convex-concave relationships; there are two principles relative to this convex-concave relationship that determine the movement between joints:

1. When the bone with the convex surface moves on the bone with concavity, then the convex surface moves in the opposite direction to the bone segment. An example of the concave-convex principles could be when abduction of the shoulder occurs. There is a downward rotation of the humeral head on the glenoid fossa when the humerus moves up.

2. When the bone with concavity moves on the convex surface, the concave articulation moves in the same direction as the bone segment (Figure 2-10).

Joint surfaces match each other perfectly in only one position—the *close packed position*. In a close packed position, there is maximum surface contact between the bones. The attaching ligaments are at a point that is the farthest apart and these structures are under tension. In addition, the capsular structures are taut. Due to these factors, the joint mechanisms are compressed and are difficult to distract (separate). Further movement of the joint is not possible. "This factor is used if the metacarpophalangeal (MCP) and interphalangeal (IP) joints must be immobilized after surgery. Each is splinted in its close packed position, or full MCP flexion and full IP extension. This position maximally stretches structures so that scar tissue assumes the length of the tissue in that position. Once the joint is mobile, movement in the direction of tissue slack and scar tissue does not limit motion" (Greene & Roberts, 1999).

All other positions of the joint are called *open* or *loose packed*, where the joint surfaces do not fit perfectly. Loose packed positions permit additional or accessory motions that are necessary for pain-free movement. Accessory motions cannot be performed voluntarily by the client. Component movements accompany active movement, such as when there is upward rotation of the scapula and clavicle during humeral flexion. This movement of the scapula and clavicle occurs without conscious control and full humeral flexion would not be possible without this component, or accessory motion. Joint play, another type of accessory movement, is the distensibility of the joint capsule or the "give" that occurs when joints are passively moved. Joint play movements include distraction (separation), rolling, spinning, sliding, and compression (Kisner & Colby, 1990).

Figure 2-4. Scapular movements.

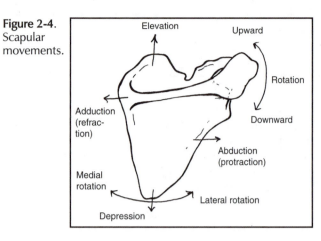

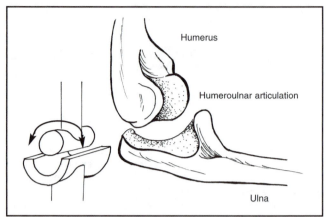

Figure 2-5. Hinge or ginglymus joint.

Figure 2-6. Pivot or trochoid joint.

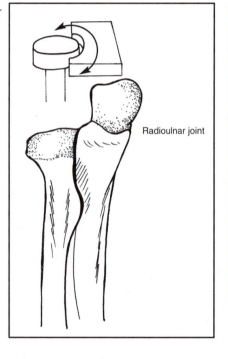

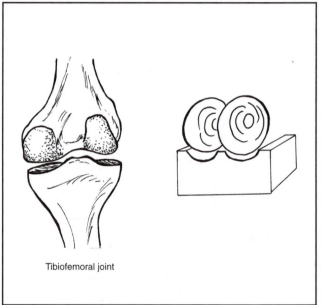

Figure 2-7. Condyloid or ellipsoid joint.

Figure 2-8. Saddle joint.

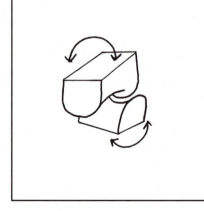

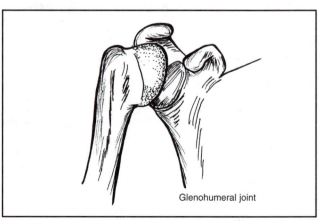

Figure 2-9. Ball and socket joint.

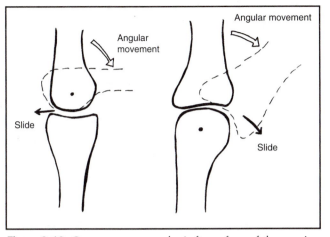

Figure 2-10. Concave-convex rule. Left: surface of the moving bone is convex, so sliding occurs in the opposite direction of the angular movement. Right: surface of the moving bone is concave, so slide and angular motion are in the same direction.

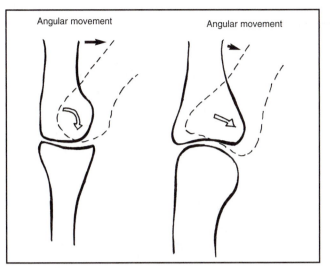

Figure 2-11. Whether surfaces are convex or concave, rolling is in the same direction as angular movement.

Accessory Motion of Bone Surfaces

Motions of bone surfaces within the joint are a combination of rolling, sliding, or spinning. *Rolling* is analogous to a ball rolling on a table where each point on one surface contacts a new point on the other surface (Figure 2-11). Characteristics of one bone rolling on another are:

1. The surfaces are incongruent.
2. New points on one surface meet new points on the opposing surface.
3. Rolling results in angular motion of the bone.
4. Rolling is always in the same direction as the angulating bone motion whether the bone is convex or concave.
5. If it occurs alone, rolling causes compression of the surfaces on the side to which the bone is angulating and separation on the other side. Passive stretching done using bone angulation alone may cause stressful compressive forces to portions of the joint surface, potentially leading to joint damage.
6. In normally functioning joints, pure rolling does not occur alone but in combination with joint sliding and spinning. Some muscles may function to cause the slide with normal active motion (Kisner & Colby, 1990; Nicholas & Hershman, 1990).

Slide is another type of motion of the bone surfaces within the joint. Characteristics of slide are:

1. For pure slide, the surfaces must be congruent, either flat or curved.
2. The same point on one surface comes into contact with new points of the opposing surface.
3. Pure sliding does not occur in joints because the surfaces are not completely congruent.
4. The direction in which sliding occurs depends on whether the moving surface is convex or concave. Sliding is in the opposite direction of the angular movement of the bone if the moving joint surface is convex. Sliding is in the same direction as the angular movement of the bone if the moving surface is concave. This is the basis for determining the

direction of the mobilizing force when joint mobilization gliding techniques are used (Kisner & Colby, 1990).

Combined roll-sliding occurs in joints. The more congruent the surfaces are, the more sliding of one bony segment on another. The more incongruent the surfaces between two bones, the more rolling occurs. The sliding component is used in joint mobilization to restore joint play and reverse joint hypomobility, whereas rolling is not used because it causes joint compression (Kisner & Colby, 1990).

If there is rotation of a segment about a stationary axis, this is called *spin*. The same point on the moving surface creates an arc of a circle as the bone spins. Spinning rarely occurs in joints but in combination with rolling and sliding. Flexion and extension of the hip and shoulder are examples of where spin occurs in the body (Kisner & Colby, 1990) (Figure 2-12A-C).

These accessory motions of rolling, spinning, and sliding provide large amounts of motion at the joints using small articulating surfaces (Smith et al., 1996) and these motions contribute additional motion between joint surfaces. Joint mobilization techniques are used to restore or maintain joint play motions within a joint as well as in treatment of stiffness, hypermobility, and pain. In accessory movements, the joint axis moves, usually in a curved pattern, as the joint motion occurs. It is this changing of the joint axis during movement that creates problems for proper fitting of orthotic devices such as splints and in reliable measure of joint angles as in goniometry.

Accessory movements are essential for pain-free joint movement. For example, if distal movement of the head of the humerus on the glenoid fossa did not occur, then the greater tuberosity would hit the acromium process leading to injury, pain, and loss of ROM (known as "frozen shoulder"). If there is a loss of joint play accompanied by pain, there will be joint dysfunction (Smith et al., 1996). If this occurs, then the joint is not free to move nor are muscles free to move and this can lead to deterioration in the joints (Smith et al., 1996).

Kinematic Chains

Kinematic chains are several joints that unite successive segments. The distal segments have higher degrees of freedom, which enables the body to transform stereotyped angular motion of joints

Figure 2-12A. Examples of spin movements. Glenohumeral joint.

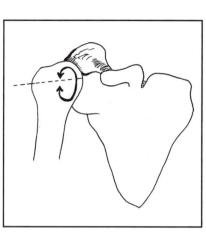

Figure 2-12B. Hip joint.

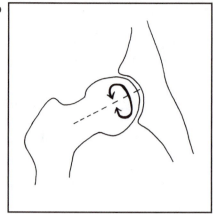

Figure 2-12C. Humeroradial joint.

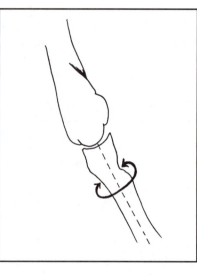

into efficient curvilinear motion (Smith et al., 1996). Smith et al. indicate that the large number of degrees of freedom in kinematic chains is an advantage to maintaining function because one can compensate for loss of motion but at the expense of requiring more energy (1996).

KINETICS

Forces acting in and on the body that produce stability or mobility are the focus of study in kinetics. This study includes consideration of internal forces, such as body mass and muscular forces applied to move body mass, and external forces, such as gravity and forces impacting on the body. An occupational therapist uses this knowledge of forces to plan intervention to minimize deforming positions and detrimental stresses on joints to prevent further disability. Remediation of neuromusculoskeletal system limitations to elongate tissues and to strengthen muscles is based on an understanding of how forces affect these soft tissues. Remediation of these impairments is done to increase performance in meaningful occupations.

External Forces

Gravity

External forces are those that originate outside of the body and may include wind, water, other people, objects, and gravity. *Gravity*

is a constant force that we accommodate without conscious thought. Gravity can and frequently does provide forces for movement and this force is directed vertically downward at a rate of 32 feet/second (9.8 meters/second). Gravity affects the stability of the body as well as movements of the extremities, neck, and head. We adjust to the weight of our arm as we use it in different positions just as we adjust easily, and without a loss of stability, when we use tools or pick up heavy objects.

Balance and Stability

The stability of one's body is dependent upon the relationship of the center of gravity with the base of support. The *center of gravity* is a point of the body at which the entire weight of the body is concentrated. This is the balance point at which the vertical and horizontal planes meet (Greene & Roberts, 1999). In an upright position, the center of gravity position in humans is generally accepted to be at sacral level 1 or 2 (S_1 or S_2), although the precise center of gravity for each person depends on the proportions of that individual. Specific centers of gravity for each body segment have been determined as well.

The position of the body affects the center of gravity so that changes in movement produce changes in the center of gravity. Stability is maintained as long as a line of gravity is maintained within the base of support. Try this exercise: put an object on the floor in front of you a few feet away from a wall; put your heels up against the wall and then try to pick up the object while your feet remain against the wall. What happens? You lose your balance. Why? Not because the weight of the object changes, not because the force of gravity has changed, and not because your mass has changed. What has changed is the base of support relative to your center of gravity. Your center of gravity was no longer within your base of support, and being unable to make postural adjustments, balance and stability were lost.

Postural control enables the body to remain in equilibrium or in balance. Balance is maintained by automatic postural adjustments (equilibrium reactions) that serve to keep the center of gravity over the base of support, to provide a wide base and lower center of gravity (protective extension reactions), and to move the base to keep it under a moving center of gravity.

The larger the base of support, the greater the stability. Consider a toddler who is learning to walk and the wide base of support that the toddler uses to maintain balance. This concept is further elucidated when considering the use of proper body mechanics in transfer and mobility activities with clients. Widening your base of support so that your vertical gravity line falls within a wider base of support and maintaining your center of gravity close to the client's center of gravity provide greater stability and safety in transfer.

Crutches, canes, and walkers are excellent means of increasing mobility because these devices provide a broadened base of support. Clients need to learn to shift their center of gravity so that it lies within the newly broadened base of support when using these devices. In addition to having a wider base of support, if the line of gravity falls at the center of the base of support, this, too, provides greater stability.

Individual client variables also affect balance and stability. Greater mass increases stability. If one considers a football player crouched at the beginning of a play, this position affords much in terms of stability. Not only is there a great deal of mass, but the crouched position also permits a lower center of base of support, which helps to stabilize the player. Changes in posture will cause the center of gravity to move.

Another individual variable is that while we have automatic adjustments to postural displacement, we also can train ourselves to have better balance. Gymnasts, for example, have a high level of learned balance and are skilled in maintaining equilibrium and in the use of spatial judgements. Age is also an individual variable and both static and dynamic balance are most efficient in young adults and middle aged people. The elderly are especially at risk for falls due to problems with balance and mobility secondary to medical condition, fear of falling, and environmental hazards (Thompson & Floyd, 1994).

Maintaining balance depends on:

- Adequate functioning central nervous system (CNS)
- Musculoskeletal system
- Adequate vision
- Vestibular function
- Proprioceptive efficiency
- Tactile input, especially hands and feet
- Integration of CNS with sensory stimuli
- Visuo-spatial perception
- Effective muscle tone that adapts to changes
- Muscle strength and endurance
- Joint flexibility (Galley & Forster, 1987)

The importance of the triad of visual, vestibular, and proprioceptive sensory system input is essential in the maintenance of balance. The vestibular system is vital in detecting motion and the position of the head in space in relation to gravity. This system influences muscle tone, especially in the antigravity extensor muscles, and helps to maintain stable visual perception when the person or environment moves. Proprioception is important in informing the body where the head is in relation to body. The muscle spindles, golgi tendon organs, and proprioceptors are instrumental in informing the body about the current position of joints, whether the joint is static or moving, the range and duration of movement, the velocity and acceleration of body segments, the pressure and tension in joint structures, and the relative lengths of muscles. Vision tells us the relation of the head to the object. The role of vision cannot be overemphasized because vision is the most far-reaching sensory system and strongly dominates our perception of the environment and our adaptation to it.

Other factors that influence balance are adequate hearing, psychological factors (fear of falling increases muscle tension, anxiety, inattention, and mental confusion), environmental factors (good illumination, nonslip even surfaces, suitable clothing and footwear), and undue noise or excessive movement (Galley & Forster, 1987; Thompson & Floyd, 1994).

When posture is disturbed, rescue maneuvers may be done by the person to prevent a fall. The person may sway to correct the imbalance, stagger or perform sweeping motions to prevent the fall.

Vertigo may be associated with damaged vestibular mechanisms, so it is important to determine when loss of balance occurs and in which positions. A person may also experience dizziness or giddiness and other symptoms such as vomiting, nausea, pallor, sweating prostration, or hypotension (Galley & Forster, 1987). Postural hypotension occurs when a person moves from lying to sitting or standing and experiences a drop in systemic systolic blood pressure of 20 mmHg from what was measured when lying down (Galley & Forster, 1987).

Friction

Friction can provide a stabilizing force that can retard movement or contribute to instability. Friction is a resistance force to smooth movement (Lafferty, 1992). Skipping a stone on ice goes far because there is little friction. A house of cards stays up because there is friction between the cards and they stay in place as long as there is a steep angle. Hovercraft use a cushion of air that holds the boat away from the water so friction is reduced, enabling the boat to travel at high speeds (Lafferty, 1992). How much friction limits a movement depends on how firmly the two surfaces are pressed together, as well as the nature of the materials that are in contact and their effects on each other (Galley & Forster, 1987). To change the degree of friction between two surfaces, it is necessary to change the forces that hold the surfaces together or to change the nature of surfaces in contact (Galley & Forster, 1987). This idea is used in ball bearing feeding orthoses (mobile arm supports) where friction is reduced by rolling balls, which enable movement by weak clients. Oil and lubricants also reduce friction, as illustrated in automobiles. Synovial joints in the human body have synovial fluid, which reduces friction during joint movements. The least amount of friction in synovial joints occurs when the joints are moving because the synovial fluid lubricates and smoothes the movement of the articulating surfaces. The loss of smooth, friction-reduced movement is a problem encountered in rheumatoid arthritis, where there is decreased gliding due to injury to synovial tissues.

Magnitude of External Force

While Newton's First Law discusses how forces act in pairs and how externally applied forces bring about changes in inertia, the magnitude of externally applied forces affect motion according to Newton's Second Law, the law of acceleration: "Acceleration of a body is proportional to the magnitude of the resultant forces on it and inversely proportional to the mass of the body." This means that the change in momentum is proportional to the force exerted and the direction of the applied force. If you push a wheelchair with a great force, there is more acceleration. If you push a wheelchair in which a large person is sitting, you will get less acceleration than if the person in the wheelchair has less mass, with force application remaining constant in both cases. A large push on a small object provides rapid acceleration. A small push on a large object provides slow acceleration. A greater force is required to move or stop a large mass than a smaller one. *Acceleration* is defined as the rate of change in velocity, so changes in motion include increased rate, decreased rate, and stopping. Mass and acceleration are the key factors in Newton's Second Law.

An example of Newton's Second Law can be seen in a rocket: the force provided by the rocket both lifts and accelerates the rocket. The rate of acceleration is dependent upon the mass of the rocket so that as the rocket fuel is burned up, there is less mass and greater acceleration (Lafferty, 1992).

This second law of acceleration can be applied to the human body as well. When a muscle contracts, it shortens. The same force is applied on the proximal and distal attachments so that either or both segments may move. One way to reduce weight clinically is by using gravity-eliminated positioning, which will decrease the force of gravity to enable greater and easier movement in weakened muscles.

Newton's Third Law, the Law of Action and Reaction, states: "For every action, there is an equal and opposite reaction." This means that whenever two bodies touch, they exert an equal and opposite force on each other. When you are walking, your feet exert a force on the ground while at the same time, the ground is exerting the same force to your foot. When you jump from a rowboat, you jump in one direction, while the rowboat is pushed in the opposite direction. When you row a rowboat, the oar on the water pushes back but the boat moves forward. Rockets can be used as another example of Newton's Third Law in that the thrust of gases and fuel goes in one direction while the rocket goes in the other.

Forces acting in pairs occur often in the body in order to produce movements of great variety and strength. Often more than one force is acting on the body at a time. For example, flexor digitorum profundus (FDP) and extensor digiti (ED) cross the distal interphalangeal (DIP) joint of the middle finger and attach at the DIP. If FDP contracts, there is flexion of the DIP joint. If ED contracts, there is extension of the DIP. If each muscle exerts a force, there is movement in the direction of the pull of the fibers. Since these muscles effectively cancel the action of the other and co-contraction occurs, there is no movement. Often this type of muscle action is helpful in stabilization of body parts, as in posture. Other times, two or more muscles must act together to produce movements that are not possible by the single action of either muscle alone, such as the synergistic actions that produce wrist ulnar and radial deviation.

Internal Forces

Internal forces are those that act on the body but arise from sources within the body. These forces serve to counteract forces (both internal and external) as well as produce movement. Forces produced internally are the result of movement of muscles, ligaments, and bones. Internal forces provide movement and stability. Stability of the joints depends upon bony architecture (as in the elbow), ligamental support (as in the wrist), and tendon and muscle tension (as in the shoulder) (Flowers, 1998).

As an example, the shoulder complex is capable of a great variety and range of movements and is very mobile. This joint is not very stable. The shoulder serves in a mobilizing function for the arm rather than as a stabilizer. The stability of the shoulder is accomplished by the muscles in and around the joints of the shoulder. In contrast, the elbow is a more stable joint due to the congruence of the bones that make up this joint, but it lacks the variety of the movements possible (Flowers, 1998).

When external forces are applied, this causes stress inside of the object. Stress is the force per unit area and is an internal reaction force within the material. Stress is not visible. These applied forces or loads lead to changes in the size and shape of the object or material and this is called *deformation*. The amount of deformation depends upon the load and the ability of the material or object to resist the load. Deformation is measured by *strain*.

Forces acting upon the body are often a focus of intervention. A frequent goal of health care professionals working with clients who are either bedridden or have decreased sensation is the prevention of decubiti ulcers. Pressure is the total force applied per area of force application, or P = F/A (Galley & Forster, 1987). Compression of tissues causes stress inside of the tissues by occluding blood vessels and decreasing circulation to the area. The compression results in deformation of the skin and is measured by the strain caused by the external load. To minimize the compression forces on skin surfaces, one needs to either decrease the force or increase the area of skin contact to decrease the pressure. This is accomplished by changing the material with which the person is in contact or distributing the body weight over a larger area.

Deformations may be temporary or permanent based on the characteristics of the material and the magnitude of the force. This is an important intervention consideration when techniques are designed to increase the extensibility of tissues by means of stretch. Knowledge about the characteristics of muscles, tendons, ligaments, and the skin will enable the therapist to develop interventions that will provide permanent gains in the amount of ROM for the client. The effects of prolonged immobilization (due to splinting, casts, and orthotic devices) and inactivity are also conditions that pertain to changes in tissues and are often the focus of remedial intervention.

Force Systems

Forces may be grouped to form different types of force systems. *Linear force* systems occur along the same action line. These forces produce tension or compression. Any system of forces acting on the same plane are called coplanar and are *parallel force* systems. The forces are parallel to each other but do not share the same action line. These forces cause rotary movements about an axis. A lever or seesaw is a common example of a parallel force system. A special case of parallel force system is called a *force couple*. The parallel forces are equal in magnitude but opposite in direction. This can be visualized by imagining a steering wheel on a car where both hands on the steering wheel (one pushing up, the other pulling down) combine to turn the steering wheel in one direction (Galley & Forster, 1987). This force couple system is also evident in the wheel and axle mechanics demonstrated by the movements of the scapula.

Esch compares the rotary movements of the scapula to the turning of a wheel (Figure 2-13). If one pulls on vector A, the wheel will turn to the left. Likewise, if one pulls on vector B, the wheel will turn to the right. The next drawing (Figure 2-14) shows a few of the muscles of the scapular region. Contraction of the upper trapezius muscle will produce an upward motion of the scapula. Contraction of the levator scapula will cause the scapula to downwardly rotate. Combined actions occur with many of the scapular and shoulder muscles producing different movements. If the upper trapezius and levator scapula contract, the scapula will elevate, whereas if the lower trapezius and levator scapula contract, retraction of the scapula will occur (Esch, 1989).

The idea of the effect of wheel and axle mechanics continues with the idea that if a wheel is turned by a small force at its rim, a larger force can be generated at the axle. This is the idea behind waterwheels, round door handles, and water faucets (Lafferty, 1992). In the human body, small muscular forces can produce movements of long bony segments.

Concurrent force systems occur when all of the forces meet in one point. The forces do not act along the same line but do act on the same point (McGinnis, 1999). The sternal and clavicular heads of pectoralis major muscle is an anatomical example of a concurrent force system. A *general force* system occurs when all of the forces are in the same plane but are not covered in the above categories.

Forces have both magnitude and direction, which can be represented either graphically or mathematically. In the human body, the number of active muscle fibers determine the magnitude (Roberts & Falkenburg, 1992), while the direction is the resultant force based on the action lines and the point of application of the muscle fibers. Graphic representations are used throughout this book to illustrate the application and results of forces acting on particular muscles at certain joints to produce specific motions.

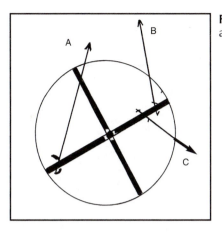

Figure 2-13. Wheel and axle mechanics.

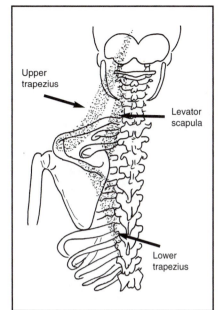

Figure 2-14. Scapular wheel and axle mechanics.

Graphic representation is done via vectors that take into consideration the qualities of magnitude and direction. Analysis of forces can be done by showing the combined effect of one or more forces in the same plane (coplanar) and on the same point (concurrent), which is called *composition of forces*. Or it may be necessary to replace a single force by two or more equivalent forces, which is called the *resolution of forces* (LeVeau, 1992).

Composition of Forces

It is generally accepted that the simplest system to analyze is a linear force system. The parallel forces are coplanar (same plane), concurrent (same object), and are also colinear, or acting along the same line (Figure 2-15A and B). In the figure, force #1 is acting on the same object in the same direction as force #2 along the same line, so the forces may be added together to obtain the resultant force. In the second part of the illustration, the two forces are acting along the same line but in opposite directions. The resultant force is actually the difference in the two forces (LeVeau, 1992).

Concurrent force systems are used when two or more forces act on the same point. Instead of using a linear graphic representation, polygons and parallelograms represent the composition of forces.

Resolution of Forces

Resolution of forces is the opposite process to the description of the composition of forces that was used in determining the combined effect of force. "Any pair of concurrent forces has a resultant. Conversely, any single force can be considered to be the resultant of a pair of concurrent forces" (LeVeau, 1992, p. 74). In other words, a single force can be broken down into its horizontal and vertical components. A muscle force can be seen to act along the length of the muscle with its orientation parallel to the direction of the muscle fibers. However, due to the action line (or line of pull of the muscle) of the muscle being fixed by anatomic attachments, the muscle often pulls in a line other than in the direction of movement and some of the efficiency of the muscle is reduced (LeVeau, 1992) (Figure 2-16).

Diagonal muscle pull has two components: one along the bone and toward the joint to press the articulating surfaces together, which is the stabilizing/dislocating (or sometimes called nonrotary) component; and secondly, vectors at right angles causing the bone to rotate about a joint axis, which is the angular or rotary component (Figure 2-17). Conclusions about the effectiveness of the muscle in terms of stabilization or mobilization can be made based on comparisons of the lengths of horizontal and vertical vectors as well as the angle of muscle pull. The resolved force vector is depicted as a diagonal line located between, and at right angles to, the

two component forces. The tips of the three lines can be connected to form a rectangle. If the stabilizing line is longer than the rotary or angular line, then this muscle is more effective in stabilization in this position than it is in causing rotation or movement. The angle of pull, defined as the angle between the action line of the muscle and the mechanical axis of the bone or segment involved (Galley & Forster, 1987), is important in considering the effectiveness of a muscle as a stabilizer or as a mobilizer. Gench et al. (1995) state that "the farther from the perpendicular the angle of insertion becomes, the weaker the muscle will be as a joint mover" (p. 35) and "The smaller the angle between forces, the greater the resultant." In the example of the levator scapula muscle, the line of pull of the muscle is longer for the vertical component than it is for the horizontal component. Because of this, the levator scapulae muscle functions more effectively as an elevator of the scapula than it does as an adductor. By breaking down the components of a muscle, one can determine the angle of the pull of the muscle, function of the muscle, and the relative strength of that muscle in any position of the muscle fibers. This information is relevant to intervention with the intention of increasing muscle strength by suggesting optimal positioning of the muscle during activities.

Parallel Force Systems

Parallel force systems occur when two or more parallel forces act upon the same object but at some distance from each other. In parallel force systems, parallel forces do not coincide (they are parallel), and these forces do not have the same line of action (LeVeau, 1992).

This application of force at a distance from the pivot point is a *moment* or *torque*. This twisting or turning force can be seen when you open a door. If you push or pull the door at the center of the door, you will not be able to move the door as effectively as if you push the door from as far from the hinges as possible. The hinge acts as an axis and when you push far from the hinges, you increase the force arm (Hamil & Knutzen, 1995). In canoeing, torque is applied by the person using the oar to cause it to rotate. In golf or tennis, torque is applied to the club or racquet to swing these implements (McGinnis, 1999). This same idea applies to manual muscle testing. When testing elbow flexion, resistance is applied at

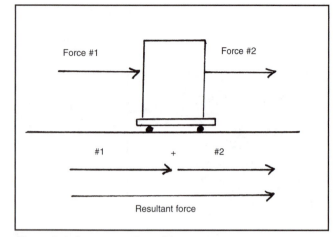

Figure 2-15A. Composition of forces.

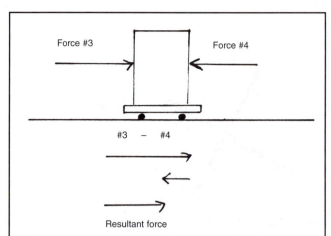

Figure 2-15B. Composition of forces.

Figure 2-16. Resolution of forces.

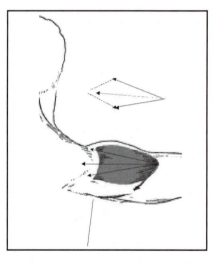

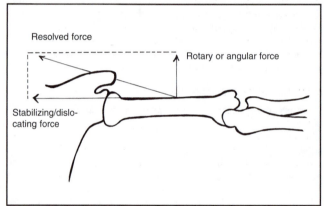

Figure 2-17. Resolution of diagonal muscle pull.

the wrist rather than the middle of the forearm. The torque produced by the patient is the same but the force applied by the therapist is about ½ less at the wrist due to a longer resistance arm (Smith et al., 1996). If force is applied distally, forces might be small but there would be relatively large torques that the muscles must match (Smith et al., 1996). Clinically, external resistance encountered by the body includes forces produced by casts, braces, plates of food, dumbbells, crutches, or exercise equipment, and these are often applied distally. The muscle force required to overcome these forces must be taken into account with the understanding that the maximum resistance torque of the weight occurs when the segment or extremity is horizontal because the action line of the force to the axis is the longest (Smith et al., 1996). The effectiveness of the torque depends upon not only the magnitude of the force but also on the location of force application.

Levers are an example of a parallel force system and levers are found frequently in the human body. A lever is a rigid bar which can turn around a fixed axis or point (Lafferty, 1992). In a lever, there are three parts:

1. A = axis or fulcrum (F); in the human body, this usually is the axis of the joint.

2. R = resistance or weight of a part; this might be a bony segment or an externally applied resistance; this can be a force that is opposing the motion.

3. F = force or effort (E) that is moving or holding; in the body, this is usually the muscle contraction that is the force causing or attempting to cause the motion. The point of force application is often the muscle insertion.

There are three types of levers. A *first class lever* occurs when forces are exerted on opposite sides of each other with the axis or fulcrum in the center (Figure 2-18). One can gain either force or speed depending upon distance from the axis to the resistance and the distance from the axis to the effort force. Greater force can be achieved if the axis is closer to the resistance force, whereas greater speed is accomplished with the axis closer to the effort force (Figure 2-19). In a seesaw, the heavier child sits closer to the axis so that the greater mass can be overcome by a smaller force. Common examples of first class levers are a doorknob, seesaw, scissors (actually a double first class lever), and a steering wheel. Examples in the body include the atlantoccipial joint in which the head is balanced by the neck extensors; the intervertebral joints in

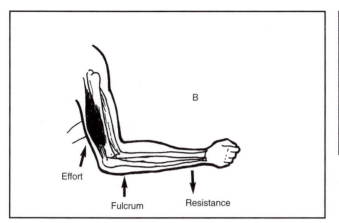

Figure 2-18. First class lever.

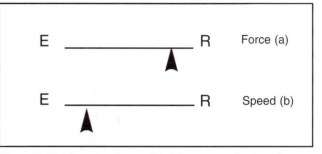

Figure 2-19. First class lever with fulcrum or axis placed nearer to the resistance (a) and nearer to the effort (b).

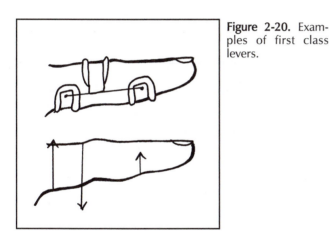

Figure 2-20. Examples of first class levers.

sitting or standing where the trunk is balanced by the erector spinae acting on the vertebral axis; and the triceps muscle acting on the ulna. A clinical example of a first class lever would be when developing seating adaptations. The three-point system of contact is actually a first class lever. Other clinical examples are splints (Figure 2-20) and the balanced forearm orthosis (or mobile arm support).

First class levers can also act to change the direction of the movement as seen commonly around bony prominences by means of pulley systems. An example of this is seen in the angle of pull of the quadriceps muscles as it is altered by the action of the patella on the condylar groove of the femur (Hamil & Knutzen, 1995) in the action of knee extension. Other examples of pulleys are the peroneus longus muscle action around the ankle and the long finger flexors. Pulleys act by applying a force in one direction to move a weight in the other direction (Smith et al., 1996). While pulleys change the direction of the force, the magnitude of the force is not changed (Figure 2-21).

A *second class lever* occurs when a large amount of weight is supported or moved by a smaller force and a second class lever is considered a force magnifier (Lafferty, 1992) (Figure 2-22). Common examples are a wheelbarrow, a nutcracker, or a faucet. In a second class lever, the weight or resistance is in the middle with the effort force and axis on either side. There are few examples of second class levers in the body and those that are identified are seen as controversial. Standing on one's toes is an example in the body where the big toe is seen as the axis, the muscles inserting into the heel are the effort forces, and the weight of the body acting

through the ankle is the resistance force. Other examples are the splenus muscle action in extending the head at the atlantoccipial joint (Lafferty, 1992). The forearm and brachialis are also identified as second class levers because the center of gravity of the forearm is between the elbow and the insertion of the brachialis muscle (Gench et al., 1995) (Figure 2-23).

Third class levers are the most common in the body (Figure 2-24). In third class levers, the effort force is central with the resistance force and the axis on either side. Third class levers permit speed or movement of a small weight for a long distance and are considered force reducers (Lafferty, 1992) since the effort force is greater than the resistance or load. A broom, fishing pole, tweezers, chop sticks, and a crab's pincer are examples of third class levers. The deltoid muscle, extensor carpi radialis muscle, and iliopsoas muscles are examples of third class lever systems in the body.

Mechanical Advantage

Levers differ in their capacity to balance and overcome resistance. This is known as *mechanical advantage*. In looking at lever force configurations, the distance between the axis and the effort force is known as FA (force arm) and the distance between the axis and the resistance force is RA (resistance arm). If the FA is greater than RA, then the joint has mechanical advantage.

Mechanical advantage is FA divided by RA:

$$MA = \frac{FA}{RA}$$

In second class levers, the FA is always greater than the RA, so second class levers have mechanical advantage. Conversely, in third class levers, the FA is less than the RA. In third class levers, there is no mechanical advantage and third class levers have the least capacity to overcome resistance. First class levers can vary in the amount of mechanical advantage, depending on the location of the axis in relation to the resistance force and effort forces.

Gench et al. (1995) point out that it may seem paradoxical that the levers least found in the body are the levers that are capable of the greatest mechanical advantage. They add that this would be true if we used our bodies to move great amounts of weight slowly. However, our bodies are more often used in activities requiring movement of smaller weights or moving quickly and this is consistent with an abundance of third class lever systems.

While it may seem that the predominance of third class levers would make the human body perform inefficiently and ineffectively, there are distinct benefits to this arrangement. In a third class lever, while the magnitude of the force needed to move the joint is great and therefore inefficient, the movement produced distally is through a much greater arc than that produced proximally. "In fact,

Figure 2-21. Example of a pulley mechanism.

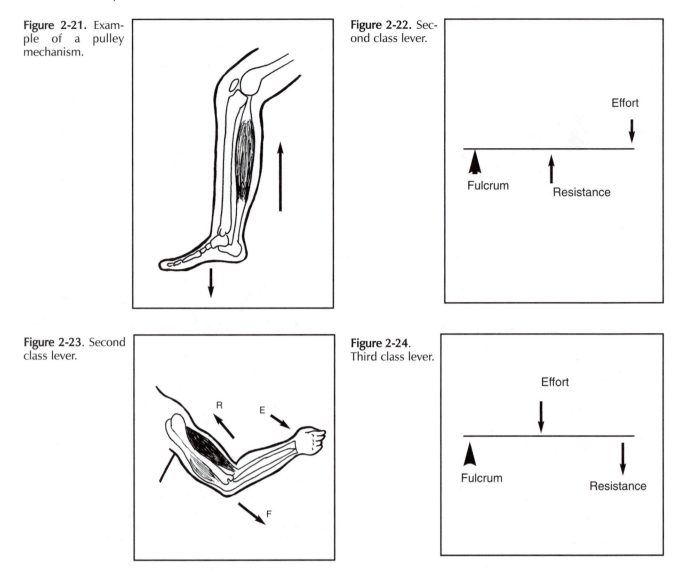

Figure 2-22. Second class lever.

Figure 2-23. Second class lever.

Figure 2-24. Third class lever.

the shorter the lever arm of the effort force (the closer the effort force is applied to the axis), the greater is the movement of the distal end of the lever" (Norkin & Levangie, 1992). This greater movement and speed is not true in a second class lever where there is mechanical advantage and efficiency in terms of force output but relatively little gain in movement distally (Norkin & Levangie, 1992).

Norkin and Levangie summarize these concepts:

- When a muscle is the effort force and the FA is smaller than the RA, the magnitude of the effort force must be large, but the expenditure of muscle force is offset by gains in speed and distance of the distal portions of the segment. This is true for all third class levers and for first class levers in which RA > FA.

- When the external force is the effort force and the FA is larger than the RA, the magnitude of the effort can be small as compared to the resistance, but relatively little is gained in speed and distance. This is true for all second class levers and for first class levers in which FA > RA (p. 40).

These concepts are inherent in the logic behind the joint protection technique to use the strongest joints possible for activities and for body mechanics principles that advocate keeping objects closer to the body, not only for greater stability but also so that less force is needed to lift the objects, as in transfers.

The principle of the leverage factor states that "the greater the perpendicular distance between the action line of the muscle (F) and the joint center (A), the greater the torque" (Smith et al., 1996, p. 61). Joint effectiveness is a function of the tendon's distance from the axis of movement according to the leverage factor. An example of this is the flexor pollicis longus muscle, where there is greater torque at the more proximal joint because the tendon is farthest from the axis of rotation. This is also seen in the biceps muscle, where the greatest torque is produced with the elbow at 90 degrees of elbow flexion and with the least effective force produced during full extension.

A clinical example of the leverage principle can be seen in the contraindication of performing passive stretching after fractures, surgery, or joint pathology when force is applied to the distal end of the bone. The force on the lever arm has greater mechanical advantage over the injured part and the force can be amplified 10 to 20 times (Smith et al., 1996). However, mobilization or passive movement of joint surfaces following normal accessory motion are indicated in pathological conditions to relieve pain and restore movement, but one must consider the following:

- Direction and force must follow normal arthrokinematics of the joint.
- Magnitude of the force must be controlled and gentle.
- Motions of the joint surfaces are small; use very short lever arms with force applied at the base (head) of the bone forming the joints.

SUMMARY

- Movement is complex and involves all aspects of the body.
- Different parts of science study different aspects of movement. Anatomy looks at the production of movement by the muscles of the body. Biomechanics looks at forces relative to the body.
- Dynamics is concerned with movement and is subdivided into kinematics and kinetics. Kinematics describes motion and looks at the result of movement, whereas kinetics studies the forces and causes of motion.
- Newton's Laws of Physics (inertia, acceleration, and action/reaction) apply to the body as well as to other physical objects.
- Movements of the joints are based on the direction of movement in planes around an axis. There are three cardinal planes and three axes used as references when describing motion.
- Movement is angular, linear, or general motion, which is a combination of angular and linear.
- Joints are classified in terms of the motion that is produced, the structure of the joint, or the shape of the bones. Joints are often described as being hinge, pivot, condyloid, saddle, ball and socket, or gliding.
- Accessory motion also occurs at joint surfaces, resulting in rolling, sliding, or spinning motions of bones, which provide additional motion at joints.
- Gravity is a constant force acting on the body. Other external forces include friction, wind, water, other people, or objects. These are forces outside of the body.
- Internal forces are those from within the body that produce movement or counteract other forces. Internal forces are due to muscles, ligaments, and bones.
- Forces acting on the body produce deformation of structures, which is measured by strain.
- Forces can be combined to determine the overall effect of all forces on an object. Composition of forces can be linear or can be represented by polygons and parallelograms.
- Forces can also be resolved into component parts. This is helpful in determining the line of pull of a muscle. By looking at how the muscle pulls on the bone during a muscle action, conclusions about the effectiveness of the muscle in terms of stabilization or mobilization can be made.
- In linear force systems, forces act on the body as first, second, or third class levers. While third class levers are the most common in the body, they are not the type of lever that provides the greatest mechanical advantage. While this seems contradictory, the predominance of third class levers allows for greater speed and mobility than would levers with greater mechanical advantage.

REFERENCES

Brand, P. W., & Hollister, A. M. (1999). *Clinical mechanics of the hand* (3rd ed.). St. Louis, MO: Mosby.

Durward, B. R., Baer, G. D., & Rowe, P. J. (1999). *Functional human movement: Measurement and analysis.* Oxford: Butterworth Heineman.

Esch, D. L. (1989). *Analysis of human motion.* Minneapolis, MN: University of Minnesota Press.

Flowers, K. (1998). Shoulder anatomy and biomechanics. Paper presented at the Ohio Occupational Therapy Association. Columbus, OH.

Galley, P. M., & Forster, A. L. (1987). *Human movement: An introductory text for physiotherapy students* (2nd ed.). New York: Churchill-Livingstone.

Gench, B. E., Hinson, M. M., & Harvey, P. T. (1995). *Anatomical kinesiology.* Dubuque, IA: Eddie Bowers Publishing,Inc.

Greene, D. P., & Roberts, S. L. (1999). *Kinesiology: Movement in the context of activity.* St. Louis, MO: Mosby.

Hamil, J., & Knutzen, K. M. (1995). *Biomechanical Basis of Human Movement.* Baltimore: Williams & Wilkins.

Kisner, C., & Colby, L. A. (1990). *Therapeutic exercise: Foundations and techniques* (2nd ed.). Philadelphia: F.A. Davis.

Konin, J. G. (1999). *Practical kinesiology for the physical therapist assistant.* Thorofare, NJ: SLACK Incorporated.

Lafferty, P. (1992). *Force and motion.* New York: Darling Kindersley Inc.

LeVeau, B. F. (1992). *Williams and Lissner's biomechanics of human motion* (3rd ed.). Philadelphia: W. B. Saunders Co.

Loth, T., & Wadsworth, C. T. (1998). *Orthopedic review for physical therapists.* St. Louis, MO: C.V. Mosby Co.

McGinnis, P. M. (1999). *Biomechanics of sport and exercise.* Champaign, IL: Human Kinetics.

Nicholas, J. A., & Hershman, E. B. (1990). *The upper extremity in sports medicine.* St. Louis, MO: C.V. Mosby Co.

Nordin, M., & Frankel, V. H. (1989). *Basic biomechanics of the musculoskeletal system* (2nd ed.). Philadelphia: Lea and Febiger.

Norkin, C. C., & Levangie, P. K. (1992). *Joint structure and function: A comprehensive analysis* (2nd ed.). Philadelphia: F. A. Davis Co.

Roberts, S., & Falkenburg, S. A. (1992). *Biomechanics: Problem solving for functional activity.* St. Louis: C. V. Mosby Co.

Smith, L. K, Weiss, E. L., & Lehmkuhl, L. D. (1996). *Brunnstrom's clinical kinesiology* (5th ed.). Philadelphia: F. A. Davis Co.

Thompson, C. W., & Floyd, R. T. (1994). *Manual of structural kinesiology* (12th ed.). St. Louis, MO: C.V. Mosby Co.

Trombly, C. A. (Ed). (1995). *Occupational therapy for physical dysfunction* (4th ed.). Baltimore: Williams & Wilkins.

Watkins, J. (1999). *Structure and function of the musculoskeletal system.* New York: Human Kinetics.

BIBLIOGRAPHY

Basmajian, J. V., & DeLuca, C. J. (1985). *Muscles alive* (5th ed.). Baltimore: Williams & Wilkins.

Burstein, A. H., & Wright, T. M. (1994). *Fundamentals of orthopaedic biomechanics.* Baltimore: Williams & Wilkins.

Esch, D. L. (1989) *Musculoskeletal function: An anatomy and kinesiology laboratory manual.* Minneapolis: University of Minnesota.

Frankel, V. H., & Burstein, A. (1970). *Orthopaedic biomechanics: The application of engineering to musculoskeletal system.* Philadelphia: Lea and Febiger.

Jenkins, D. B. (1998). *Hollingshead's functional anatomy of the limbs and back* (7th ed.). Philadelphia: W. B. Saunders Co.

Kendall, F. P., & McCreary, E. K. (1983). *Muscles: Testing and function* (3rd ed.). Baltimore: Williams & Wilkins.

Lehrman, R. L. (1998). *Physics the easy way* (3rd ed.). Hauppauge, NY: Barron's Educational Series, Inc.

MacKenna, B. R., & Callender, R. (1990). *Illustrated physiology* (5th ed.). New York: Churchill Livingstone.

Magee, D. J. (1992). *Orthopedic physical assessment.* Philadelphia: W. B. Saunders Co.

Marieb, E. N. (1998). *Human anatomy and physiology.* Glenview, IL: Addison Wesley Longman Publishers.

Perr, A. (1998). Elements of seating and wheeled mobility intervention. *OT Practice*, 16-24.

Rasch, P. J., & Burke, R. K. (1978). *Kinesiology and applied anatomy: The science of human movement.* Philadelphia: Lea and Febiger.

Shankar, K. (1999). *Exercise prescription.* Philadelphia: Hanley & Belfus, Inc.

Snell, M. A. (1999). Guidelines for safely transporting wheelchair users. *OT Practice*, 35-38.

Spaulding, S. J. Biomechanics of prehension. *Amer J Occup Ther, 43*(5), 302-306.

Zelenka, J. P., Floren, A. E.., & Jordan, J. J. (1966). Minimal forces to move patients. *Amer J Occup Ther, 50*(5),354-361.

Factors Influencing Range of Motion

Chapter 3

Range of motion (ROM) is the amount of movement that occurs at a joint and can be defined as "the measurement of motion available, or the arc of motion available at a joint or through which the joint passes, resulting from the joint structure and surrounding soft tissue" (Norkin & White, 1985; Pedretti, 1996; Trombly, 1995). This motion depends on many variables, which may include the restraining effects of ligaments and muscles crossing the joint as well as overlying skin and other soft tissues, the bulk of tissue in adjacent segments, age, gender, and methodological factors (Table 3-1).

SUBJECT FACTORS

Individual subject factors can vary due to genetic predispositions for greater motion (hypermobility), as is sometimes seen in hyperextension at the elbow. There may be less motion (hypomobility), as when soft tissue tightness or contractures limit full motion. Different activities put different stresses on joints, which may change the amount of motion that occurs. Gymnasts and cheerleaders, for example, may have greater wrist extension due to repeated handstands or placing body weight on extended wrists. This individual variability needs to be considered in assessment when the range of motion (ROM) is different from expected normative values. Questions asked about activities done currently and in the past may help explain variances in flexibility.

Decreased motion occurs for many reasons. The overall health of the client is important in determining the amount of motion that occurs. Joint disease or injury, edema, pain, skin tightness or scarring, muscle or tendon shortening due to immobilization, muscle weakness or muscle hypertrophy, muscle tone abnormalities, and excess adipose tissue are all possible reasons for decreased ROM.

The consequences of decreased motion are many. Supporting structures may become loose, creating joints that are unstable and painful. The joint structures may be insufficient to hold the joint in stable and functional positions during activities. Ligaments and muscles may be stretched and, combined with the effects of gravity, can lead to subluxation of the joint. This is often seen in the shoulders of clients with hemiplegia where the shoulder and scapular muscles are inactive or diminished and the weight of the arm plus gravity pull the humeral head out of the glenoid fossa. Inactivity of the muscles can lead to contractures due to muscle imbalance and the inability to perform normal activities. Muscles and tendons can lose their tensile strength. Scar tissue adhesions, which occur secondarily to chronic inflammation with fibrotic changes, can tear when the muscle is stretched. As muscles lose their normal flexibility, changes occur in the length-tension relationships. The muscles are no longer capable of producing peak tension, which can lead to pain and decreased strength.

Age and gender are subject factors that also influence the amount of motion that occurs at joints. Decreased ROM of joints occurs with increased age as a normal part of the aging process that can be offset somewhat by the types and level of activities in which one engages throughout life. Age-related changes occur symmetrically unless accompanied by other impairments, with the greatest changes occurring in the spine.

Females generally have more flexible joints with greater ROM than do males and this is true throughout life. Few studies have been done that indicate trends in regards to culture, race, or ethnicity (Van Deusen & Brunt, 1997), although positioning in childhood and customary postures may be attributed to variability of lower extremity joint motion (Demeter, Andersson & Smith, 1996) and related to culture.

Another subject-related factor that may influence the amount of ROM a client demonstrates can be observed in the level of effort and cooperation during testing. If limited, this would diminish active motion results. Limited effort also may be due to the effects of pain.

PSYCHOLOGICAL AND PSYCHOSOCIAL FACTORS

Psychological and psychosocial factors also influence ROM. The motivation of the client is a vital component to active movement and is related to the person's emotional state at the time the movement is requested. Fear of injury or reinjury will prevent a client from engaging in activities that are perceived to be potentially painful. By not moving, the part is immobilized and soft tissue changes will result. Anxiety and stress can cause muscle contractions, tightness in tissues, or inactivity. These emotions may be observed in the level of cooperation demonstrated by the client, in the client's discussions about expectations for recovery, and in dialogues about continuation in functional activities.

In providing instructions for movement or engagement in activities, cognition is a variable as well. If the client cannot understand what movement or activity you are requesting, whether due to anxiety, depression, or inability to cognitively attend to the task, efforts at evaluation will be invalid.

ENVIRONMENTAL FACTORS

The physical environment is important in the assessment of ROM, as in many musculoskeletal assessments. The temperature, level of noise, and number of people in the room affect not only the comfort of the client, but the client's ability to attend to the task and the physiological readiness of muscles to respond. The time of day has a bearing on the amount of motion possible, as can be seen in clients with rheumatoid arthritis who are stiff in the mornings and able to move more comfortably later in the day. Less motion may be possible later in the day for some clients (possibly multiple sclerosis patients) due to fatigue.

Skeletal Factors

The amount of movement that occurs in a joint is based on the types of tissue that make up the joint. There are four major types of tissue in the body: epithelial, connective, muscle, and nervous. Of these, connective tissue is the "passive" element of the musculoskeletal system and muscle is considered an "active" element.

Connective tissue includes fibrous tissues, cartilage, and bone. Fibrous tissues are comprised of tendons, aponeuroses, and ligaments characterized by dense collagen fibers arranged in parallel bundles and generally supplied sparingly with blood vessels. These are inelastic structures that can withstand great tension forces but only small compression forces (Goss, 1976). Unorganized dense fibrous tissues, seen in fascial membranes, dermis of the skin, periosteum, or capsule of the organs, can resist tensile stress in many directions, while tendons can only withstand unidirectional tension forces. Fibrous unions of bones create synarthrodial joints of which there are three types: sutures (as in sutures in the skull), syndesmosis joints (inferior tibiofibular articulation), and gomphosis (teeth's insertion into mandible and maxilla). These joints are essentially joints of no movement. Freely movable joints are diarthrosis or synovial joints, the most numerous in the body. The six synovial joint types (hinge, condyloid, saddle, ball and socket, pivot, and gliding joints) are capable of producing the angular and rotational movements of the extremities, trunk, and neck. The shapes of the articulating surfaces also contribute to the movements of the joints by permitting accessory joint movements by having bony surfaces roll, spin, and glide across each other.

Cartilage is a nonvascular structure without a nutrient supply. Hyaline cartilage is the clear covering that protects the ends of bones, and fibrocartilage contains some elastic components to allow for accommodation of pressure, friction, and shear forces (Kisner & Colby, 1990). Fibrocartilage is also called menisci. Cartilage is strong, flexible, and acts as a shock absorber for the joint. Cartilaginous articulations, called amphiarthrosis joints, are classified either as a synchondrosis joint (which is an immovable joint) or as a symphysis, where slight movement is possible, as seen in the articulation of the two pelvic bones. The function of articular cartilage in diarthrosis joints is to "increase load distribution and provide a smooth wear-resistant bearing surface" (Nordin & Frankel, 1989, p. 54).

Bones are the hardest of the connective tissue. Unlike dense connective tissue, bones are highly vascular and can self repair. Bones can alter their properties and configuration based on stresses applied to the body. Adaptive remodeling occurs as a result. The purpose of the skeletal system is to protect internal organs, to provide a rigid lever system and muscle attachment sites, and to facilitate muscle action and body movement.

Fibers of connective tissue are made of either collagenous or elastic types. Collagen, the most abundant protein in the body, offers tensile stiffness and strength. Tendons, which connect skeletal muscle to other structures (usually bone), are made up of 80% collagen fibers. This makes tendons strong enough to sustain tensile forces from muscle contractions but also flexible enough to change the direction of muscle pull (Nordin & Frankel, 1989). Collagen fibers offer little resistance to compression because they tend to buckle under compressive loads. Ligaments, also containing many collagen fibers, allow for little stretch except in one

---

Table 3-1.

FACTORS INFLUENCING RANGE OF MOTION OF JOINTS

Subject Factors
- Health/pathology
- Gender
- Age
- Activity levels
- Cardiovascular fitness

Psychological/Psychosocial Factors
- Motivation
- Expectations
- Fear of injury
- Cognition
- Cooperation
- Anxiety/stress
- Psychological state

Environment
- Temperature
- Noise
- Number of people in room
- Time of day
- Activities done

Skeletal Factors
- Characteristics of bones
- Structure of joints
- Types of joints
- Stability of joints
- Mechanisms of joint movement
- Normal limiting factors

Methodological and Measurement Factors
- Instrument used
- Experience of tester
- Stabilization
- Axis
- Goniometer placement
- Posture
- Instructions

---

direction and shortening with movements in the opposite direction (Irion, 2000).

Due to the predominance of collagen fibers in these dense connective tissues, the function of tendons and muscles varies. Tendons transmit tensile loads from muscle to bone, which produces joint motion. Ligaments and joint capsules, which connect bone to bone, augment stabilization of the joint, guide joint movement, and serve as a protective mechanism in prevention of excessive movements. The more ligaments that cross a joint, the greater the stability. However, since a ligament can only stretch 6% of its length before rupture (called a sprain), in joints where ligaments are the major means of bracing a joint, the joint is not very stable

Table 3-2.

PHYSIOLOGIC (NORMAL) END FEEL

End Feel	Structure	Example
Soft	Soft tissue	Knee flexion
		Elbow flexion
		CMC thumb flexion
Firm	Muscular stretch	Scapular elevation
	Capsular stretch	Depression
	Ligamentous stretch	Abduction
		Adduction
		Rotation
		Shoulder extension, IR, ER, horizontal adduction/abduction
		Forearm: supination
		Wrist: flexion, extension, radial and ulnar deviation
		Fingers: MCP and CMC extension of thumb, PIP extension, DIP flexion and extension, IP flexion and extension of thumb
		Hip flexion
Hard	Bone against bone	Elbow extension
		Forearm pronation
		PIP flexion
		MCP flexion of thumb

Adapted from Norkin, C. & White, D. (1985). *Measurement of joint motion: A guide to goniometry.* Philadelphia: FA Davis Co.

(Konin, 1999). Tendons are a factor in joint stability as well because tendons become taut when muscles are contracted.

Movement is important for cartilage and bone nutrition and growth, for bone density and strength, and for adequate functioning of ligaments and tendons. By assessing both active and passive aspects of movement, intervention not only can be directed toward increased function in work, play, and self-care, but also as prevention of further disability in underlying structures.

Normal limiting factors of joint movement can be felt when passively moving a part to the extreme ends of ROM. Structures that limit the amount of motion that occurs at a joint have a characteristic feel to them that is felt as resistance to further movement and is known as *end feel* (Norkin & White, 1985). While there are some variations in the terminology used to describe an end feel, generally it is accepted that there are six types of end feel; three are descriptions of normal limiting factors and three are pathological impediments to movement.

An end feel that is soft limits further motion due to tissue compression in soft tissue. This is a normal limiting factor and is seen in knee flexion when the soft tissue of the posterior leg comes into contact with the posterior thigh (Norkin & White, 1985).

Firm end feel occurs when there is a tension in the way the joint feels but also a slight give in the structures comparable to pulling a rubber band or a strip of leather, depending upon the structure limiting the motion. Normal firm end feel can occur due to muscles, capsules or ligaments. A firm muscular end feel occurs with hip flexion with the knee straight because there is passive elastic tension in the hamstring muscles. Extension of the metacarpophalangeal joints of the fingers creates tension in the anterior capsule and is an example of firm capsular end feel. Firm ligamental end feel is demonstrated in forearm supination with tension occurring in the palmar radioulnar ligament of the inferior radioulnar joint, interosseous membrane, and oblique cord.

The third type of normal end feel is *hard*, in which there is an abrupt hard sensation at the extreme end of ROM. This is when a bone contacts another bone and can be felt in elbow extension (Table 3-2).

Soft, firm, and hard end feels can also occur in pathological conditions if these sensations are felt in joints not normally attributed to that end feel or if the end feel is felt sooner or later in the total ROM than is expected. Table 3-3 provides examples of conditions that can cause pathological end feels. Other abnormal end feels include the following:

- *Springy block* is when a joint rebounds at the end of range due to internal articular derangement that may be indicative of intra-articular blocks, such as torn meniscus or articular cartilage.
- *Spasm* is felt as a vibrant twang (Marieb, 1998, p. 8) and is the result of a prolonged muscle contraction in response to circulatory and metabolic changes (Kisner & Colby, 1990).
- *Muscle guarding* is an involuntary muscle contraction in response to acute pain (Kisner & Colby, 1990).
- *Muscle spasticity* is increased tone in response to central nervous system (CNS) influences.

METHODOLOGICAL FACTORS

Methodological variables affect the precision of measurement, the accuracy and stability of results, and the worth of the test to functional activities. These variables include how the testing is done, the method of testing, the instruments used, and the knowledge and experience of the testers. Methodology is concerned with the particular assessment chosen, the domain of concern, and the person conducting the assessment.

The purpose of an assessment in general is:

1. To support effective clinical reasoning.
2. To define the nature and scope of clinical problems.
3. To provide baselines against which to monitor progress.
4. To summarize changes that occur as a result of therapy and define areas of treatment requiring revision based on changes in the client.
5. To allow peers and managers to critically evaluate the effectiveness of interventions and develop directions for quality improvements.
6. To aid in the decision-making process regarding allocation of health care resources.
7. To aid in the classification of different kinds of client groups and in justification for the need for ongoing service provision.
8. To aid in the determination of a functional outcome, determination of discharge plans, potentials for work, play, and self-care within the person's own context.
9. To provide an opportunity to establish rapport with the client and as an aid in communication with other professionals.

Table 3-3.

PATHOLOGICAL END FEEL

End Feel	Description	Example
Soft	Occurs sooner or later in range of motion Occurs in a joint normally firm or hard Feels boggy	Synovitis Edema
Firm	Occurs sooner or later In joints normally soft or hard	Increased tone Capsular, muscular or ligamentous shortening
Hard	Sooner or later Joint normally soft or firm Bony grating or block felt	Osteoarthritis Chondromalacia Loose bodies in a joint Myositis Ossificans Fractures
Empty	ROM never reached due to pain No resistance	Acute joint inflammation Bursitis Abscesses Fractures Psychogenic

Adapted from Norkin, C. & White, D. (1985). *Measurement of joint motion: A guide to goniometry.* Philadelphia: FA Davis Co.

Table 3-4.

CONSIDERATIONS IN SELECTING AN IMPAIRMENT METHODOLOGY

Principle	Considerations
Objectivity	Validity, intratester reliability, accuracy. Relevance preferred.
Consistency	Intertester reliability. Small range of normal human variability preferred.
Fairness	Relationship between numerical impairment rating and true alteration of health status and physical function.
Accuracy	Precision, signal-to-noise ratio, specificity, sensitivity; potential to discriminate, intraindividual and interindividual alterations in health status.
Relevance	Correlation between assessment technique and alteration of health status from "normal". Requires comparison to normal functioning.
Convenience	Test must be easy to perform, preferably with techniques known to all potential evaluators. Limited educational requirements. Limited time required for assessment.
Cost	Minimum desirable by parties requesting assessment but not at the price of significantly increased variability. Shortest possible time commitment of expert evaluators. Minimize variability to minimize disputes generally considered worth paying for.

Reprinted with permission from Demeter, S., Andersson, G., Smith, B. J. & Smith G. M. (1996). *Disability evaluation.* St. Louis, MO: C. V. Mosby.

10. To provide a means of tracking improvements, which is often motivational for the client (Asher, 1996; Hinojosa & Kramer, 1998).

There are ethical considerations in choosing and using assessment tools. Therapists are consumers of tests and measurement instruments, and as such are accountable to clients for the choices made. It is the therapist's responsibility to elicit the client's best performance on any assessment by being familiar with the test in advance, by maintaining an impartial and scientific attitude during testing, by establishing a therapeutic and positive rapport with the client, and by providing an optimal environment in which the test is given (Demeter, Andersson, & Smith, 1996) (Table 3-4). Accurate measurements are essential to the development of intervention plans based on the goals and needs of the client, the limitations in performance, and the expected outcome. Accurate measurements are also used to document effective remediation that will ensure reimbursement of therapy services and become part of the legal record of these services. Accurate measurements also are vital in providing research data for treatment efficacy.

It is important that the evaluations used yield results that truly represent the client's function (validity) (Table 3-5) and that yield similar results through time and between testers (reliability) (Table 3-6). Multiple studies have been done to determine the reliability

and validity of ROM assessments but results vary based on the part being measured, measurement error due to mass of body segments, inconsistent operational definitions, variety in instruments used and placement of tools, and variability in identification of body landmarks.

ROM evaluations have what's known as logical validity, in which the performance is clearly defined and the therapist directly observes the behavior. In ROM assessment, the movement itself is being tested, not the ability to move, which would entail aspects of the CNS as well as muscle strength and ROM. ROM assessments have content validity in that testing is based on knowledge of anatomy for proper placement of the goniometer, identification of bony landmarks, and the axis of rotation. Difficulties arise in using explicit definitions of ROM and how the motions are defined. While normative data is available for the motion at each joint, the

Table 3-5.

METHODS FOR DETERMINING VALIDITY IN TESTS

Face Validity

From appearance, and without statistical proof, the test items appear to address the purpose of the test and the variables to be measured; subjective, logical judgment by the author or experts on the topic.

Content Validity

The items on a test represent sufficient, representative samples of the domain or construct being examined; requires selection of a specific aspect of the behavioral domain evaluated; designed to measure the level of mastery of a particular content domain.

Criterion-Related Validity

The ability to determine performance on one test based on the performance on another test; the degree of agreement between two tests; determines the accuracy of prediction that is obtained by squaring the validity coefficient (r'), which tells us how much variance the predictor variable is able to explain.

Concurrent or Congruent Validity

The extent of agreement between two simultaneous measures of the same behaviors or traits.

Predictive Validity

The extent of agreement between the current test results and a future assessment; used to make predictions about future behavior.

Construct Validity

Based on the theoretical framework to test the "goodness-of-fit" between the theorized construct and resulting data from a test; a gauge of the ability of a test to measure a trait or hypothesis that is not observable.

Convergent Validity

The test results should correlate highly with another measure of the same variable or construct; infer degree of agreement measuring the same trait with two different tests of the same trait or construct.

Discriminant Validity

The test results should not correlate with another measure of the same variable or construct; infer degree of disagreement measuring the same trait with two different tests of the same trait or construct.

Factorial Validity

The identification of interrelated behaviors, abilities, or functions in an individual that contribute to collective abilities or functions; correlation of the test with other group to define the common traits it measures.

Reprinted with permission from Hinojosa, J. & Kramer, P. (1998). *Occupational therapy evaluation: Obtaining and interpreting data.* Bethesda, MD: American Occupational Therapy Association.

Table 3-6.

METHODS FOR DETERMINING RELIABILITY IN TESTS

Test-Retest

A measure of test score stability on the same version of the test repeated over two occasions; based on a correlation of the scores obtained during each of two administrations; useful for tools monitoring change over time.

Intrarater Reliability

Consistency in measurement and scoring by the evaluator when two test results from two similar situations are correlated.

Interrater or Interobserver Reliability

The degree of agreement between the scores from two raters following observation and rating of the same subject; correlations of .85 or higher are expected to compare the objective competency between two raters of the same testing condition.

Alternate or Parallel Forms

Useful when multiple, equivalent forms of the same test are needed; particularly useful when one's response to the earlier test items can easily be recalled and influence the responses on the second test after a lapse of time (alternate); while the forms contain different questions, similar items on each test are expected to have item equality, making the tests equal at a given point in time (parallel); correlation should be >.80.

Internal Consistency

Reflects the degree of homogeneity between test items; items measure the same construct; correlation should be >.80.

Split Half

The results from performance on the first half of the test are correlated with the second half or the scores on all even-numbered items are compared to odd-numbered ones.

Covariance Procedures

The average of all split-half tests; expressed as KR20 or KR21; the consistency of response between all items on a test; referred to as interitem consistency.

Reprinted with permission from Hinojosa, J. & Kramer, P. (1998). *Occupational therapy evaluation: Obtaining and interpreting data.* Bethesda, MD: American Occupational Therapy Association.

norms are not sensitive enough to reflect differences based on age, gender, occupation, or sociocultural considerations. However, in a study comparing radiographs (x-rays) with goniometric measurements, there was found to be a high correlation between these two types of measurements, which indicates that this assessment has concurrent or congruent validity, which is a criterion referenced measure. The goniometer is "considered to be the gold standard by which other tools of joint measurement are compared" (Palmer & Epler, 1998). Validity can be improved by controlling for outside variables, for maturation, for sensitivity to the test, and consideration of environmental variables.

Consistent results are also important. When a test is given to a client one time and the same test is given to the same client again by a different tester, this is known as *interrater reliability*. When the same tester assesses the same client at different times, this is called *intrarater reliability*. Comparison of studies of reliability indicate that intrarater reliability is higher than interrater reliability. While some studies suggest that if reliability has been established among testers, there can be a high degree of accuracy, other authors recommend that examiners with little experience may want to take several measurements and record the mean of the values (p. 12) to increase reliability. Error estimates for ROM vary according to the particular joints tested and reliability can be improved by using consistent and well-defined testing positions and anatomic landmarks to align the goniometer.

The type of goniometer or instrument used in the measurement of joint motion must also be considered when comparing results of studies. Universal goniometers have "good to excellent" reliability (Palmer & Epler, 1998). These are simple, uniplanar protractors used commonly in practice. The goniometer has either 360 degree or 180 degree scales (or both), with two arms used to measure the motion. One arm follows the movement and the other aligns with a stationary part of the body. These can be full circle goniometers or half-moon (in the shape of half of a circle).

Gravity dependent goniometers use gravity's effect on pointers and fluid levels. The device is strapped onto a distal leg segment with the proximal limb positioned vertically or horizontally. The pointer or bubble is read at the end of ROM. This type of goniometer does not need to be aligned with skeletal landmarks and makes the measurement of passive ROM easier. Disadvantages are that the gravity dependent goniometer is bulkier, more expensive, not as readily available, and more difficult to use on small joints and for rotational movements than the universal goniometer.

An inclinometer is a pendulum-based device that has a 360 degree scale protractor with a counter-weighted pointer. Electronic versions are available and this type of goniometer is especially good for measurements of spinal ROM.

A fluid goniometer (bubble goniometer or hydrogoniometer) also has a 360 degree scale with fluid in a tube with small air bubbles.

An electrogoniometer is a potentiometer in which movement causes changes in resistance and voltage that can be calibrated to represent ROM. This tool is expensive and often used in research (Tan, 1998). Other methods of measuring joint motion include use of tape measures, photometric (video-based) motion analysis systems, radiographs, photocopies, free hand drawings or tracings, infrared light sources, light emitting diode (or reflectors), or laser lights, which have good validity and reliability but are expensive (Tan, 1998). The type of goniometer chosen reflects the level of accuracy required, resources available, and convenience.

ASSESSMENT OF RANGE OF MOTION

Goniometry is a commonly used measurement of joint motion. The word *goniometer* comes from two Greek words: "gonia" which means angle, and "metron" which means measure (Norkin & White, 1985). A goniometer is a tool that is used to determine the amount of motion available at a specific joint.

ROM can be measured actively and passively with different information gleaned from each procedure. For clarification, the following abbreviations and terminology are defined:
- PROM: arc of motion through which a joint passes when moved by an outside force.
- AROM: arc of motion through which a joint passes when moved by muscles acting on a joint.
- AAROM: arc of motion through which a joint passes when moved initially by muscles then completed by an outside force.

- "Functional ROM": amount of motion necessary to perform essential activities of daily living (ADL) tasks without adaptations or equipment.

Joint ROM can be assessed by means of a goniometer or by screening techniques (Table 3-7). Screening tools are used as a rapid method of assessing multiple joint movements or combined movements to determine if more in-depth and standardized assessments are needed. While visual estimation is often used clinically, this method is unreliable and deemed "not acceptable" (Demeter, Andersson, & Smith, 1996) for a complete joint assessment, but is often used as a screening mechanism. Functional motion tests or motion inventories often use observation to determine decreased motion or use of compensatory motions when achieving combined motions, such as when one is asked to "touch the top of the head", "make a fist", or "touch the top of the shoulder". Generally, a screening tool uses active motion and gives information about patterns of movement and about the client's willingness to move. A disadvantage of functional motion screening tools is the variability of movements that can occur that satisfy the request for movement. For example, if asked to touch the top of the head, the humerus can be abducted or flexed with the elbow and wrist flexed to reach the hand to the head, or the elbow can be flexed with neck and trunk flexed to reach the head to the hand. More detailed descriptions may minimize this problem but may also be more difficult for the client to understand. Scoring of functional motion tests often involves use of nominal scales such as:

n = completes normally
s = completes with substitution
I = initiates movement but cannot complete
u = unable to perform
NT = not tested

Percentages are also used to indicate what part of range is limited, such as:
0 limitation = full ROM
minimal limitation = 1 to 33%
moderate = 33 to 66% full ROM
maximal = 66 to 100% (Tan, 1998).

If deficits have been noted or a more detailed measurement of joint motion is desired, goniometric measurements are made. For each description of the measurement of a joint motion, the following is provided:
1. Testing position or the way patient is to be positioned.
2. Goniometer placement

   a) fulcrum: the rivet of the goniometer, also referred to as the axis because it is aligned to the axis of movement of the joint. A specific bony landmark is often used to represent the joint axis, although the exact axial point may seem to shift during movement. This is especially noticeable with the measurements of shoulder flexion and abduction when the joint axis point does move due to combined, synchronous movements of both the glenohumeral joint and the scapula.

   b) goniometer arms: sometimes referred to as "stationary" and the other as "moveable". The stationary arm usually will lie parallel to the longitudinal axis of a fixed proximal joint segment and/or will point toward a distal bony prominence. The other (moveable) arm lies parallel to a longitudinal axis of the moving distal joint segment and/or points toward a distal bony prominence. To make sense of this, just remember you are measuring a part of the body that moves. One part of the goniometer has to be a reference (stationary arm) and the other part has to follow the movement (moveable arm).

Table 3-7.

RANGE OF MOTION SCREENING TEST

Position of Patient	Motion Being Tested	Instructions to Patient
Sitting	1. Shoulder abduction and lateral rotation	1. Reach behind head and touch opposite scapula, or place hands behind neck and push elbows posteriorly.
	2. Shoulder adduction and medial rotation	2. Reach to opposite shoulder or touch the inferior angle or opposite scapula, or place both hands behind back as high as possible.
	3. Shoulder flexion and extension	3. Raise arms in front of body overhead and reverse to behind back.
	4. Elbow flexion and extension	4. Bend and straighten elbows.
	5. Radioulnar supination and pronation	5. With elbows flexed 90 degrees, supinate and pronate.
	6. Wrist flexion and extension	6. Flex and extend wrists.
	7. Radial and ulnar deviation	7. Move wrist laterally and medially.
	8. Finger abduction and adduction	8. Spread fingers apart and bring them together.
	9. Finger flexion and extension	9. Make a tight fist and open fingers wide.
	10. Thumb flexion and extension	10. Bend thumb across the palm and out to the side.
	11. Neck flexion and extension	11. Place chin on chest, tilt head back.
	12. Neck rotation	12. Turn head to the right and left.
	13. Hip flexion and adduction	13. Sitting, cross one thigh over the other.
	14. Hip flexion, abduction, and lateral rotation	14. Uncross thighs and place the lateral side of foot on opposite knee.
	15. Ankle inversion	15. Turn foot in.
	16. Ankle eversion	16. Turn foot out.
Supine	17. Hip abduction and adduction	17. Spread legs apart and bring them together.
Supine or sitting	18. Hip extension	18. Flex hips and knees; lift buttocks as in bridging. Rise to standing from sitting position.
	19. Knee flexion and extension	19. Pull knees to chest, heels toward buttocks, and return.
Standing	20. Trunk flexion	20. Bend forward and reach for toes with knees straight.
	21. Trunk extension	21. Bend backward while I stand beside you.
	22. Trunk lateral bending	22. Lean to the left, then right while I stabilize your pelvis.
	23. Trunk rotation	23. Turn to the right and to the left while I stabilize your pelvis.
	24. Ankle plantarflexion and toe extension	24. Stand on tiptoes.
	25. Ankle dorsiflexion	25. Stand on heels.

Reprinted with permission from Palmer, M. L. & Epler, M. (1998) *Fundamentals of musculoskeletal assessment.* 2nd ed. Philadelphia: Lippincott Williams & Wilkins.

To fully assess ROM, not only is the arc of motion measured, but a general assessment of the joint itself is a part of the assessment. With visual observation, one is looking for symmetry between limbs, the use of compensatory motions, overall body posture, muscle contour and proportion, and the color and condition of the skin. Palpation, or examination of body surfaces by touch, will help to determine bony and soft tissue contours, soft tissue consistency, skin temperature and texture. Palpation is necessary to identify bony skeletal landmarks used as reference points when measuring the arc of motion (Table 3-8).

RECORDING OF RANGE OF MOTION RESULTS

While the method of performing a ROM assessment is consistent, there are different methods of recording ROM results. There are two systems used in clinical practice: the 360 degree system and the 180 degree system. The 180 degree system is more commonly used (i.e., Academy of Orthopedic Surgeons) and accepted in clinical practice. In this system, the neutral zero or starting position is with the body in anatomical position with the zero position toward the feet. The body is in the plane in which the motion is to occur, with the axis of the joint acting as the arc of motion (Pedretti, 1996).

In the 360 degree system, the zero starting position is overhead with the arc of motion related to a full circle. In both systems, some motions do not readily lend themselves to movements around a semicircle or a full circle. These are generally rotational movements such as pronation, supination and internal and external rotation, radial and ulnar deviation, and thumb carpometacarpal flexion and extension.

The arc of motion for shoulder flexion is generally accepted to be 180 degrees which would be recorded as 0 to 180 degrees in the 180 degree system. A separate movement of shoulder hyperextension (movement from the arm held at the side then moved in a posterior direction) would be recorded as 0 to 60 degrees. In the 360 degree system, this same arc of motion would include the additional movement of hyperextension and the total movement would be recorded as 0 to 240 degrees. It is clear that identification of the system of recording is vital to clear communication and documentation of ROM results.

Another method of recording is the SFTR system. In this system, the measurement of ROM is completed as in either the 180 or 360 degree systems. The recording of the results is related directly to the cardinal planes, with "S" indicating the sagittal plane, "F" the frontal, "T" the transverse plane, and "R" indicative of rotational movements. Neutral zero is the anatomical position with three numbers used to record the motion rather than a ROM. The first number indicates movements away from the body such as abduction, flexion, or external rotation; the second number indicates the starting position (usually zero); and the third number represents movements toward the body such as extension, adduction, and internal rotation. An SFTR recording of the shoulder movement of full flexion and hyperextension would be: 180 degree-0-60 degree to indicate full flexion, starting position, and hyperextension.

Usually in clinical practice, the recording of shoulder flexion and extension uses the 180 degree system. The ROM result for shoulder flexion would be 0 to 180 degrees because the "0" signifies the starting position of full extension and the "180" is indicative of the motion overhead. This one ROM describes both flexion and extension. Other motions where one set of ROM values describes two motions are: shoulder abduction and adduction, elbow and knee flexion and extension, finger flexion and extension (PIP, DIP, MCP). Separate measurements are required for shoulder internal rotation, shoulder external rotation, pronation, supination, wrist flexion, wrist extension, ulnar deviation, radial deviation, hip adduction, hip abduction, hip flexion, hip extension, hip internal rotation, hip external rotation, dorsiflexion, plantarflexion, inversion, and eversion.

In the recording of results, it is important to record both numbers, as these signify the starting and the end positions. Limitations will be readily apparent in the designation of these values. If normal shoulder ROM is 0 to 180 degrees, a value of 15 to 180 degrees would indicate a deficit in the ability to assume the zero starting position, or an inability to assume full extension. Similarly, 0 to 165 degrees would indicate a 15 degree deficit in shoulder flexion. Familiarity with normative values is helpful in determining deficits in ROM.

However, lack of achievement of the norms for a given motion does not necessarily signify this as a intervention goal because consideration of client goals and limitations in functional activities are the determinants of treatment planning.

The use of negative recordings leads to reporting of unclear data (Trombly, 1995). For example, if the client lacked 20 degrees of shoulder flexion, a negative recording would be -20 degrees. This lack of 20 degrees does not indicate the total ROM that occurred and can be easily misunderstood. Fused joints have the same starting and end points and results should state: "fused at x _".

Table 3-8.

GENERAL PROCEDURE FOR RANGE OF MOTION EVALUATION

1. Make sure the patient is comfortable and relaxed.
2. Tell the patient what you will be doing; why and how. Demonstrate the motion, ask the patient if he/she has any fused joints or any previous fractures.
3. Uncover the joint (remove clothes) if it interferes with full motion. Access to the joint is needed for palpation of bony landmarks and for alignment of goniometer.
4. Position the body part in the test position (usually 0° in anatomical position except for rotary movements).
5. Proper test position is important since desired joint movement is in one plane with one joint.
6. Stabilize the joint proximal to the joint being measured. A stable position will ↓ substitution movements, ↑ accuracy, ↓ patient fatigue.
7. Try to keep changes in position to a minimum to ↓ fatigue, and ↑ therapist efficiency.
8. Have the patient perform the movement or you move the part passively. Indicate if patient moved actively or if you moved the joint passively.
9. Observe and/or palpate for joint axis.
10. Position the goniometer. Record the number of degrees of motion at the starting position.
11. Hold part securely but gently—do not force joints to move. Be aware of pain or discomfort, and if any is noted, indicate this on the recording form.
12. Record number of degrees of motion at final position.

INTERPRETATION OF RANGE OF MOTION RESULTS

The values recorded give an indication of how the joint motion of the client compares with normative values. In interpreting the results, it is important to recognize that these norms are not specific in regards to age or gender, and that there is variability in what is considered "normal" based on environmental, methodological, individual, and skeletal factors (Table 3-9).

The amount of range achieved is determined, too, by the type of motion performed. Normally PROM is greater than AROM due to accessory motions and joint play in the joints. These motions are not under voluntary control of the client and serve to protect joint structures. PROM gives the examiner information about the integrity of the articular surfaces, the extensibility of the joint capsule, ligaments, and muscles. Joint play is the "give" or distensibility of the joint capsule and soft tissues that can only be obtained passively. It is usually a motion less than 4 mm that must be tested in the loose packed (resting) position, for this is the position in which the joint is under the least amount of stress. The joint capsule works at its greatest capacity in this position and there is minimal congruency between articular surfaces and the joint capsule. The ligaments are in a position of greatest laxity, which allows joint distraction via rolling, spinning, and sliding. The close-packed position should be avoided because in this position, the two joint surfaces fit together perfectly, ligaments and tendons are maximally tight, and the joint is under maximal tension.

Table 3-9.

COMPARISON OF RANGE OF MOTION NORMATIVE VALUES

	Wiechec and Krusen	Dorinson and Wagner	JAMA	Daniels and Worthingham	Esch and Lepley	Gerhardt and Russe	Boone and Azen	AAOS	CMA	Clarke
Shoulder										
Flexion	180	180	150	90	170	170	167	180	170	130
Extension	45	45	40	50	60	50	62	60	30	80
Abduction	180	180	150	90	170	170	184	180	170	180
Internal rotation	90	90	40	90	80	80	69	70	60	90
External rotation	90	90	90	90	90	90	104	90	80	40
Horizontal abduction						30	45			
Horizontal adduction						135	140	135		
Elbow										
Flexion	135	145	150	160	150	150	143	150	135	150
Pronation	90	80	80	90	90	80	76	80	75	50
Supination	90	70	80	90	90	90	82	80	85	90
Wrist										
Flexion	60	80	70	90	90	60	76	80	70	80
Extension	55	55	60	90	70	50	75	70	65	70
Radial deviation	35	20	20	25	20	20	22	20	20	15
Ulnar deviation	75	40	30	65	30	30	36	30	40	30
Hip										
Flexion	120	125	100	125	130	125	122	120	110	120
Extension	45	50	30	15	45	15	10	30	30	20
Abduction	45	45	40	45	45	45	46	45	50	55
Adduction		20	20	0	15	15	27	30	30	45
Internal rotation		30	40	45	33	45	47	45	35	20
External rotation		50	50	45	36	45	47	45	50	45

continued

Table 3-9, continued.

COMPARISON OF RANGE OF MOTION NORMATIVE VALUES

	Wiechec and Krusen	Dorinson and Wagner	JAMA	Daniels and Worthingham	Esch and Lepley	Gerhardt and Russe	Boone and Azen	AAOS	CMA	Clarke
Knee										
Flexion	135	140	120	130	135	130	143	135	135	145
Ankle										
Plantarflexion	55	45	40	45	65	45	56	50	50	50
Dorsiflexion	30	20	20		10	20	13	20	15	15
Inversion		50	30		30	40	37	35	35	
Eversion		20	20		15	20	26	15	20	

Reprinted with permission from Baxter, R. (1998). *Pocket guide to musculoskeletal assessment.* Philadelphia: WB Saunders.

Table 3-10.

CONTRAINDICATIONS FOR ASSESSING RANGE OF MOTION

1. Dislocation or unhealed fracture.
2. Immediately following surgery to tendons, ligaments, muscle joint capsule or skin.
3. In presence of myositis ossificans.

Table 3-11.

PRECAUTIONS FOR ASSESSING RANGE OF MOTION

Use extra care:
1. In presence of infectious or inflamed joint.
2. Client is on pain or muscle relaxants; he or she may not feel pain from ROM that is too vigorous.
3. In regions of marked osteoporosis.
4. In assessment of hypermobile or subluxed joints.
5. In painful conditions where ROM may increase the suffering.
6. In people with hemophilia.
7. In regions of hematomas, especially elbow, hip or knee.
8. In assessing joints if bony ankylosis is suspected.
9. Immediately after injury with soft tissue damage.

Joint integrity tests are passive tests to rule out or confirm joint or capsule lesions. These would include:

- Traction, where there is separation of joint surfaces. Note if pain increases/decreases and how easily they move apart.
- Approximation of joint surfaces, which occurs with compression. Again, it is important to note if pain increases/decreases under the compressive forces. If pain increases, it is likely due to some structures within the joint and not a muscle.
- In gliding, note the quality and quantity of joint play and whether these accessory motions cause pain (Irion, 2000).

PROM may be considered more objective because the motion is controlled by the examiner and is free of control by the subject (Demeter, Andersson, & Smith, 1996),

Measurement of ROM is not always indicated or safe for clients (Tables 3-10 and 3-11). Measurement of AROM may be a safer method for the client for assessment of joint assessment since there is voluntary cooperation. Active motion assesses the physiologic movement of the joint. Additional information that can be gathered during active motion may include the degree of coordination, the level of consciousness, the length of the attention span, indications about pain, the ability to follow directions, and the skill in performance of functional activities. An unintended effect of AROM is that of self-limitation of end ranges. While PROM provides information about the amount of motion permitted by joint structures, AROM indicates a person's ability to produce motion at a joint (Norkin & White, 1985). If there are tissue changes, PROM may be diminished. If AROM is less than PROM, decreased strength or muscle weakness is suspected.

SUMMARY

- Range of motion is the arch of motion that occurs at a joint and is often measured with a tool called a goniometer.
- Individual factors such as genetic disposition, types of preferred activities, overall health of the person, age, and gender influence the amount of ROM at a joint. Anxiety and stress also influence joint mobility.
- The amount of movement that occurs in a joint is based on the types of tissue that make up the joint. Not only is the joint structure important for movement, but movement is also important to the joint structure for cartilage and bone nutrition and growth, and adequate functioning of ligaments and tendons.
- Structures limit the amount of motion at a joint and these structures have a characteristic resistance called end feel. End feel can be firm, soft, or hard in normal joints and these end feels also occur in joints with pathology. Other pathological end feels are springy blocks, spasms, muscle guarding, and muscle spasticity.

- Variations in the measurement of ROM occur due to different methods, devices, means of recording, and other variables that influence the reliability and validity of goniometric measurement. Goniometry measurements generally are seen to have better intrarater reliability than interrater and measurement of the upper extremity is a more reliable measurement than lower extremity. Using consistent test procedures with the same client under the same environmental conditions enhances reliability and validity.

REFERENCES

Asher, I. E. (1996). *Occupational therapy assessment tools: An annotated index* (2nd ed.). Bethesda, Md: American Occupational Therapy Association.

Demeter, S. L., Andersson, G. B. J., & Smith, G. M. (1996). *Disability evaluation.* St. Louis, MO: C.V. Mosby Co.

Goss, C. M., Ed. (1976). *Gray's anatomy of the human body* (29th ed.). Philadelphia: Lea and Febiger.

Hinojosa, J., & Kramer, P. (1998). *Evaluation: Obtaining and interpreting data.* Bethesda, MD: American Occupational Therapy Association.

Irion, G. (2000). *Physiology: The basis of clinical practice.* Thorofare, NJ: SLACK Incorporated.

Kisner, C., & Colby, L. A. (1990). *Therapeutic exercise: Foundations and techniques* (2nd ed.). Philadelphia: F. A. Davis.

Konin, J. G. (1999). *Practical kinesiology for the physical therapist assistant.* Thorofare, NJ: SLACK Incorporated.

Marieb, E. N. (1998). *Human anatomy and physiology.* Glenview, IL: Addison Wesley Longman Publishers.

Nordin, M., & Frankel, V. H. (1989). *Basic biomechanics of the musculoskeletal system* (2nd ed.). Philadelphia: Lea and Febiger.

Norkin, C. C., & White, D. J. (1985). *Measurement of joint motion: A guide to goniometry.* Philadelphia: F. A. Davis Co.

Palmer, M. L., & Epler, M. E. (1998). *Fundamentals of musculoskeletal assessment techniques* (2nd ed.). Philadelphia: J. B. Lippincott.

Pedretti, L. W. (1996). *Occupational therapy : Practice skills for physical dysfunction* (4th ed.). St. Louis, MO: C. V. Mosby.

Tan, J. C. (1998). *Practical manual of physical medicine and rehabilitation*. St. Louis, MO: C. V. Mosby.

Trombly, C. A., Ed. (1995). *Occupational therapy for physical dysfunction* (4th ed.). Baltimore: Williams & Wilkins.

Van Deusen, J., & Brunt, D. (1997). *Assessment in occupational therapy and physical therapy*. Philadelphia: W. B. Saunders Co.

BIBLIOGRAPHY

Baxter, R. (1998). *Pocket guide to musculoskeletal assessment*. Philadelphia: W. B. Saunders Co.

Christiansen, C., & Baum, C. (1997). *Occupational therapy: Enabling function and well being* (2nd ed.). Thorofare, NJ: SLACK Incorporated.

Durward, B. R., Baer, G. D., & Rowe, P. J. (1999). *Functional human movement: Measurement and analysis*. Oxford: Butterworth Heineman.

Dutton, R. (1995). *Clinical reasoning in physical disabilities*. Baltimore: Williams & Wilkins.

Esch, D. L. (1989). *Analysis of human motion*. Minneapolis: University of Minnesota.

Galley, P. M., & Forster, A. L. (1987). *Human movement: An introductory text for physiotherapy students* (2nd ed.). New York: Churchill-Livingstone.

Gench, B. E., Hinson, M. M., & Harvey, P. T. (1995). *Anatomical kinesiology*. Dubuque, IA: Eddie Bowers Publishing, Inc.

Greene, D. P., & Roberts, S. L. (1999). *Kinesiology: Movement in the context of activity*. St. Louis, MO: C. V. Mosby.

Hayes, C. (Ed.). (1980). *Sample forms for occupational therapy*. Rockville, MD: American Occupational Therapy Association.

Magee, D. J. (1992). *Orthopedic physical assessment*. Philadelphia: W. B. Saunders Co.

Melvin, J. L. (1982). *Rheumatic disease: Occupational therapy and rehabilitation* (2nd ed.). Philadelphia: F. A. Davis Co.

Norkin, C. C., & Levangie, P. K. (1992). *Joint structure and function: A comprehensive analysis* (2nd ed.). Philadelphia: F.A. Davis Co.

Shankar, K. (1999). *Exercise prescription*. Philadelphia: Hanley & Belfus, Inc.

Van Ost, L. (2000). *Goniometry: An interactive tutorial*. Thorofare, NJ: SLACK Incorporated.

Zimmerman, M. E. (1969). The functional motion test as an evaluation tool for patients. *Am J Occup Ther, 23*(1), 49-56.

Factors Influencing Strength

Chapter 4

Strength can be defined simply as a *muscular force or power*, which is a vague, unscientific definition. A more elaborate definition might be a force or torque produced by a muscle during maximal voluntary contraction. The differentiation of strength, power, and endurance is necessary at this point. Strength and power are not the same. Strength is a force that is directly related to the amount of tension a muscle can produce. Power is the product of force and velocity (Hamil & Knutzen, 1995) or the amount of work per unit of time. Endurance is the ability to maintain a force over time or for a set number of contractions or repetitions. Whether muscles contract for strength, power, or for endurance, the development of active force comes from the muscles and many factors contribute to this development of force in the muscles (Table 4-1).

Muscular Factors

The major function of the muscular system is to stabilize and support the body and to allow movement. Muscle actions generate tension that is then transferred to bone. Muscles contribute significantly to joint stabilization when the muscle tension is generated and applied across joints via tendons. This is especially true in the shoulder and knee joints (Hamil & Knutzen, 1995). The tension developed by muscles applies a compression force to the joints, enhancing stability. Muscles could also pull segments apart and create instability, depending upon the line of pull of the muscle and the direction of movement. Muscles support and protect visceral organs and internal tissues, develop tension in muscle tissue that alters and contributes to pressure inside body cavities, and contribute to maintenance of body temperature.

There are three kinds of muscles in the body. *Voluntary/striated/skeletal* muscles appear striped, attach primarily to the skeleton, and have contractions that are usually rapid and intermittent. *Involuntary/unstriated/smooth* muscles are found in areas where movement occurs without conscious thought such as in the stomach, intestines, and blood vessels. Smooth muscles contract slowly and rhythmically as is seen in peristalsis. *Cardiac* muscle is the specialized heart muscle that has characteristics of both smooth and skeletal muscles.

Skeletal muscles are different from smooth and cardiac muscles in that each skeletal muscle receives a branch from a nerve cell called an *alpha motor neuron*, which is part of the somatic nervous system. These alpha motor neurons signal the muscle fibers to contract. Contraction of muscle fibers and not the muscle as a whole enable fine gradations of force to be produced by these muscles. Cardiac and smooth muscles are innervated by the autonomic nervous system and muscle contraction is not determined directly by a single message from the nerve (Irion, 2000).

Irion (2000) states that "muscles act as a transducer to convert chemical energy into mechanical energy producing the force necessary to provide movement, support, and other mechanical functions" (p. 206). This being true, it is reasonable that skeletal muscles are the main energy consuming tissues in the body. However, of the energy produced during a muscle contraction, only 20% of that energy is used to produce movement; the rest is lost as heat (Hamil & Knutzen, 1995).

Muscles are also the most abundant tissue in the body making up 40 to 45% of the total body weight. While it is obvious that muscles contribute to joint movement and strength, muscles also add protection to the skeleton by distributing loads and acting as shock absorbers.

Skeletal muscles have four general characteristics. *Contractility* is the ability to produce tension between the ends of two bones to exert a pull, as when a muscle contracts. *Irritability* is the ability of the muscle to respond to stimuli and transmit impulses. A muscle is *distensible* because it can be lengthened or stretched by a force outside the muscle itself, which is used therapeutically to increase range of motion (ROM). *Elasticity* describes the ability of a muscle to recoil from a distended stretch. Not all parts of the muscle have each of these characteristics; some parts of the muscle contain the contractile elements and other parts the elastic components (one of two major parts of connective tissue with the other part being collagen).

The structural unit of skeletal muscle is the muscle fiber. Fibers range in thickness and length. Fibers are organized into various sized bundles called *fascicles*; there may be as many as 200 muscle fibers in one fascicle. Fascicles are encased in dense connective tissue (perimysium), which creates pathways for nerves and blood vessels. While each muscle is covered externally by epimysium, each muscle fiber is encased in a membrane (endomysium), which carries capillaries and nerves that innervate and nourish each muscle fiber. The connective tissue in the perimysium and epimysium gives the muscle the ability to be stretched. Perimysium is the focus of flexibility training because it can be stretched, which enables muscle elongation (Hamil & Knutzen, 1995). The function of the epimysium is to transfer muscular tension to tendons and then to bone.

Each muscle fiber is composed of a large number of delicate strands called *myofibrils*. Each muscle fiber is filled with 80% myofibrils and the remaining 20% is made up of mitochondria, sarcoplasm, reticulum, and T tubules (Hamil & Knutzen, 1995). Myofibrils are made up of *filaments*. One unit consists of thin, light bands of myofilaments and thick, dark bands and is called a *sarcomere*, which is the basic contractile unit of the muscle. The dark, thick bands are made up of myosin (tropomyosin) proteins and the light, thin bands are actin proteins (Figure 4-1). The bands of light and dark myofilaments are what give skeletal muscles the charac-

Table 4-1.

FACTORS INFLUENCING STRENGTH

Subject Factors

General health status

Pathology/comorbidity

Gender

Age

Usual activity level

Psychological/Psychosocial Factors

Motivation

Cognitive status/learning

Perceived effort

Expectation

Depression

Distress and anxiety

Level of skill

Self-efficacy

Fear of injury

Methodological Factors

Manual

Instrument

Device

Device settings

Individual vs. group muscles

Stabilization

Position of subject

Joint position of test

Position in range

Warm-up

Prestretch

Rest periods

Muscle Factors

Innervation ratio

Fiber type

Fiber arrangement/architecture

Muscle length

Cross-sectional area

Angle of pull

Type of contraction

Location of muscle

Number of joints crossed

Vascularity

Velocity of contraction

Training effect

Fatigue

Measurement Factors

Operational definitions

Reliability

Interrater

Intrarater

Test-retest

Validity

Face

Construct

Discriminative

Predictive

Adapted from Van Deusen, J., & Brunt, D. (1997). *Assessment in occupational therapy and physical therapy*. Philadelphia: W. B. Saunders Co.

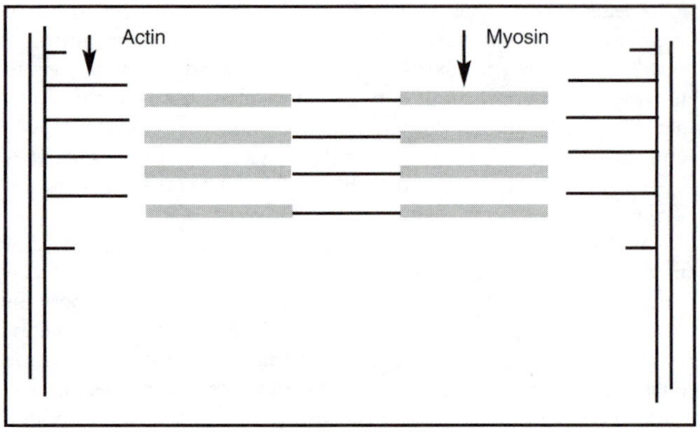

Figure 4-1. Myofilament movement of actin and myosin. Adapted with permission from Brand, P. W., & Hollister, A. M. (1999). *Clinical mechanics of the hand* (3rd ed.). St. Louis, MO: C. V Mosby.

teristically striped (or striated) appearance. These two proteins, actin and myosin, create muscle fiber contraction due to the creeping action of actin protein along the thicker myosin protein.

The *sliding filament theory* of muscle fiber contraction describes this creeping action of the thick and thin filaments as they increase or decrease their degree of overlap. Once a muscle is stimulated to contract via neurochemical stimulation, calcium is released, which causes the sliding of actin to the center of the sarcomere, which is likened to "pulling on a rope hand over hand" (McPhee, 1987). This stimulation of single muscle cells occurs in an "all-or-none" manner where the cells either respond completely or they don't respond at all. If the stimulus is adequate, the myosin protein moves along the actin forming cross-bridges between the head of the myosin and the actin filaments. Each cross-bridge acts independently and it is the simultaneous sliding of many filaments that creates a change in length and force in the muscle, which is proportional to the number of cross bridges formed. The action of the myofibril cross-bridging of actin and myosin is the active, contractile element of the muscle.

There are two elastic or passive components of the muscle that serve to absorb, transmit, and store energy (Hamil & Knutzen, 1995). *Series elastic components* are found primarily in tendons (85%) with the remaining found in actin-myosin cross-bridges. When the active contractile components shorten, this stretches the series elastic components, which act like a spring to maintain the tendon-muscle length and slows down the forces generated (Hamil & Knutzen, 1995). The second passive element, parallel elastic component, is found in the sarcolemma, epimysium, perimysium, and endomysium. These parallel components are important when a passive muscle is being elongated (when the contractile elements are active, the parallel elastic components do not function) (Kisner & Colby, 1990). As the passive muscle is lengthened, the parallel component offers an opposing force and prevents the contractile elements from being torn apart by external forces. When a muscle is stretched prior to testing, it will have greater tension because elastic energy is stored in the noncontractile elements and is converted to kinetic energy when stretched (Kisner & Colby, 1990).

Nordin and Frankel (1989) cite several ways in which the elastic components are valuable to the muscle:

- "They tend to keep the muscle in readiness for contraction and assure that muscle tension is produced and transmitted smoothly during contraction.
- They assure that the contractile elements return to their original (resting) length when contraction is terminated.
- They may help the passive overstretch of the contractile elements when these elements are relaxed, lessening the danger of muscle injury" (p. 96).

Skeletal muscles as a whole are capable of responding with great variances of force, time, and speed rather than the all-or-none responses of muscle cells. This is due to the nerve-muscle functional unit called the *motor unit*, which is a single motor neuron and all muscle fibers innervated by it. The number of muscle fibers in a motor unit relates to the degree of control required of that muscle. Small muscles that perform fine movements may have less than a dozen muscle fibers, whereas large muscles performing grosser movements may have several thousand fibers in one motor unit. This innervation ratio has a direct bearing on the skill level achieved by the muscle. The fibers of each motor unit are dispersed throughout the muscle with fibers of other units. This means that if a single motor unit is stimulated, a large portion of the muscle

appears to contract, when in fact only a single motor neuron is contracting. Motor units affect the functioning of a muscle in:

- The number of muscle fibers, which affects the magnitude of the response.
- The diameter of the axon, which determines the conduction velocity.
- The number of motor units firing at any one time, which affects the total response of the muscle.
- The frequency of the motor unit firing (Nordin & Frankel, 1989).

When a single, brief threshold stimulus is applied to a muscle, a muscle twitch occurs. Once stimulated, there is a latent period before the muscle contracts, followed by a period of contraction and then a period of relaxation. Twitch contractions are sometimes rapid and brief, while others are slow and more long-lasting due to differences in the metabolic properties of the myofibrils and enzymes in the muscles (Konin, 1999). Muscle twitches are often studied in laboratories in vitro and muscle twitches are rarely expressed in normal movement patterns.

A muscle as a whole contracts as larger numbers of motor units are added to contraction, which is called the *graded strength principle*. Graded muscle responses occur in two ways: increasing the rapidity of stimulation, which produces a wave summation, and by recruiting more motor units to produce a multiple motor unit summation.

Wave summation or *temporal summation* occurs when more than one stimulus is received and the second contraction is induced before the muscle fully relaxes after the first contraction. Since the muscle was already partially contracted, the tension produced by the second contraction causes more shortening than the first by actually "summing" the contractions (Konin, 1999). If the stimulus is applied at a constant rate, the muscle is stimulated at faster rates and relaxation time decreases. The summation becomes greater until a smooth, sustained contraction occurs called *tetanus*. Since continuous, prolonged contraction cannot continue indefinitely, prolonged tetanus leads to muscle fatigue.

Fiber Type

Multiple motor unit summation serves to control the force of muscle contractions more precisely by neural activation of increasingly larger numbers of motor units (Konin, 1999). If weak and precise movements are required, few motor units are activated. When many motor units are stimulated, the muscle contracts more forcefully. The smallest motor units (with the fewest muscle fibers) are controlled by the most excitable motor neurons and are activated first. Larger motor units, activated by less excitable neurons, are activated only when stronger contractions are needed. This illustrates the *size principle of recruitment*, where small motor units are activated initially and as the force of contraction increases, gradually larger motor neurons and larger numbers of motor units are required. Small motor neurons generally innervate the types of muscle fibers (type I/slow-twitch) that are required for sustained muscle actions and that fatigue slowly. This insures weak but sustained postural contraction. By recruiting motor units controlling larger numbers of fibers, more cross-bridges are formed so more tension is produced. Smooth skeletal movements occur because different motor units fire asynchronously, so that while one motor unit is firing, another is relaxing, ensuring that even weak contractions are smooth.

There are three types of fibers based on varied physiologic features.

1. *Type I/tonic (antigravity-postural)/red/slow twitch oxidative (SO)* are muscle fibers with a small diameter that are slow to fatigue because there is a good capillary supply and less build-up of lactate. Type I fibers are recruited early but respond with weak contractions due to a small number of fibers activated. Type I fibers are generally involved in maintaining posture against gravity, and are generally more deeply located and more medial. Examples of muscles with a predominance of Type I fibers are the massiter, gluteus maximus, quadriceps, and soleus muscles.

2. *Type IIB fibers/phasic/white/fast twitch glycolic (FG)* are basically anaerobic because the capillary supply is not as abundant as Type I fibers. Type IIB fibers have large diameters and are recruited later to produce more powerful contractions of the muscle. Type IIB fibers are usually more numerous, producing sharp bursts of energy that enable quick postural changes or skilled movements. While Type IIB fibers contract more readily than Type I, these fibers also fatigue more readily. Generally, Type IIB muscles are more superficial and laterally located, are often longer muscles, and cross more than one joint. Examples of fast twitch muscles are tibialis anterior and gastrocnemius muscles.

3. *Type IIA fast twitch oxidative glycolic (FOG)* tends to be intermediate in physiological characteristics as compared to Type I and Type IIB fibers. FOG fibers have fast conduction rates and are able to engage in both aerobic and anaerobic muscle activities. In terms of tension development, Type IIB muscles are capable of the greatest tension, followed by Type IIA and finally by Type I fibers. The differentiation of muscles by fiber type is an important consideration when developing intervention that focuses on strengthening muscles because consideration of intensity and duration of muscle contraction will be variables directly linked to fiber type (Table 4-2).

Fiber Architecture

Muscle fibers are arranged either in a parallel or an oblique manner within the muscle. *Parallel* or *series fibers* are longer muscles that are capable of producing greater ROM. Parallel fibers can be subdivided further. *Strap* fibers are long and thin, running the entire length of the muscle, as is seen in the sartorius muscle. *Fusiform* fibers are spindle-shaped or wider at the middle, tapering off at each end (brachialis). *Rhomboid* fibers are arranged in a flat, rectangular, or square shape (rhomboid, pronator quadratus), whereas *triangular* fibers are flat and fan-shaped, with fibers coming from narrow attachment at one end and broad attachment at the other (pectoralis major).

The muscle fibers are arranged parallel to the line of pull in a longitudinal manner. The fiber length is greater than the tendon length so these muscles have the potential for shortening through greater distances. Contraction occurs through the maximal distance allowed by the length of the muscle fibers so one can achieve maximum ROM but with limited power.

Oblique fibers can be seen in the tibialis posterior, flexor pollices longus, and semimembranosus muscles as a series of short fibers attaching diagonally along the length of a central tendon. These are *unipennate* fibers, which look like a one-sided feather. *Bipennate* oblique fibers obliquely attach to both sides of a central tendon (the rectus femoris muscle). Many tendons with oblique fibers (the deltoid or subscapularis muscles) are multipennate fibers (Kisner & Colby, 1990) (Figure 4-2).

Table 4-2.

FIBER TYPES

	Fast twitch glycolic (FG) (light work) White type II	Fast twitch oxidative glycolic (FOG) intermediate fast twitch red Type II A	Slow twitch oxidative (SO) (heavy work muscles) Slow twitch red Type I
Other Names			
Diameter	Large	Intermediate	Small
Color	White	Red	Red
Capillary supply	Sparse	Dense	Dense
Speed of contraction	Fast	Fast	Slow
Rate of fatigue	Fast	Intermediate	Slow
Motor unit size	Large	Intermediate to Large	Small
Axon conduction velocity	Fast	Fast	Slow

Adapted from Norkin, C. C., & Levangie, P. K. (1992). *Joint structure and function: A comprehensive analysis.* (2nd ed.). Philadelphia: F. A. Davis Co.

The oblique arrangement of the fibers makes a diagonal force to line of pull and the muscle cannot shorten to the degree that parallel muscles can. However, due to the greater number of muscle fibers in the same area, oblique fibers are capable of greater power. Therefore, the arrangement of the fibers influences whether the muscle is primarily functioning for greater movement and mobility or whether it is more functional for strength and stability.

Angle of Pull

When a muscle contracts, it creates a force that causes the body segment in which it inserts to rotate around an axis of the joint. This turning effect, or torque, is the product of the muscle force and the perpendicular distance between the axis of rotation and the muscle force (Gench, Hinson, & Harvey, 1995). The optimal angle of muscle pull occurs when the muscle is pulling at a 90 degree angle or perpendicular to the bony segment. It is at this point that all of the muscle force is acting to rotate the segment and no force is wasted acting as a distracting or stabilizing force on the limb (Gench et al., 1995). If the muscle is pulling at an optimal length or is perpendicular to the bony segment, then this will produce a stronger contraction.

The angle of pull and length-tension relationships interact to produce this force. Generally there is a decrease in force production in the extreme outer and inner ranges, with greater force pro-

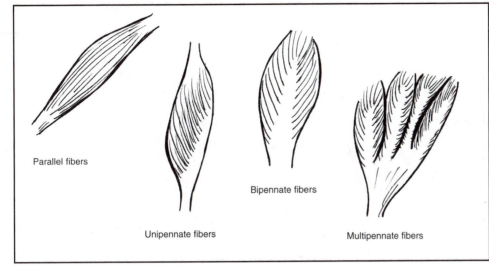

Figure 4-2. Fiber architecture.

Parallel fibers

Unipennate fibers

Bipennate fibers

Multipennate fibers

duced in the middle ROM. As a muscle begins contracting through its full range of shortening, it begins in a weakened condition, gradually becomes stronger, and then it approaches its shortest length and becomes weakened again. The force resolution of the biceps muscle demonstrates that mechanically the biceps muscle reaches peak strength at 90 degrees of elbow flexion or in the middle of full ROM. If the elbow is in full extension, the angle of the biceps insertion is small and there is a long stabilizing component that makes the biceps muscle less effective or forceful in this position. In elbow flexion greater than 90 degrees, the resolution of forces yields an angular and a dislocating force that runs along the bone and away from the joint. These forces decrease the effectiveness of the biceps muscles as an elbow flexor because the forces are now directed toward dislocating the joint, not in force production (Gench et al., 1995).

Length of Muscle

The tension developed within a muscle depends upon the initial length of the muscle. A muscle is capable of generating maximal force at or near resting length because a maximal number of cross-bridges of actin and myosin can be formed. Moderate tension is produced when the muscle is lengthened and minimal tension is possible in a shortened or contracted muscle. In a shortened state, the maximum number of possible cross-bridges have already been formed and no additional tension can be produced.

In the shortened state, tension in muscle is equal to the tension in the series elastic components. As tension-developing characteristics of active components diminish with muscle elongation, tension in the total muscle increases due to the passive elements in muscle. As the series elastic component is stretched and tension develops in the tendon and cross-bridges, significant tension in the parallel component occurs as the connective tissue offers resistance to stretch. When the muscle is lengthened, passive tension is generated. At extreme lengths, tension is almost exclusively elastic or passive tension (Hamil & Knutzen, 1995). This factor has ramifications not only for strengthening programs but also for stretching of muscles and soft tissues.

Types of Muscle Contraction

When muscle fibers change in length, different forces are generated. In isotonic muscle contractions, internal forces result in movement of the joint, which may include lengthening (eccentric) or shortening (concentric) (Figure 4-3).

Many texts refer to concentric and eccentric contractions as isotonic contractions, although some texts define muscle contractions not only in terms of tension/energy/length but also in terms of the leverage effects at the joint (Richards, Olson & Palmiter-Thomas, 1996). By strict definition, isotonic means "equal tension," and since the muscle force changes through ROM, muscle tension must also change. Norkin and Levangie (1992) add that "the tension generated in a muscle cannot be controlled or kept constant" and that the concept of equal or constant tension in a muscle is "unphysiologic" (p. 107). So in the strictest sense, isotonic contractions do not exist in the production of the joint motion. In general use, the term "isotonic" refers to a description of muscle length and not tension, and isotonic contractions may be one of two types: concentric or eccentric.

Concentric contractions occur when the internal force produced by a muscle is greater than the external force or resistance that produces a shortening of the muscle. An example of this is when one is walking up stairs. The quadriceps is demonstrating concentric contractions in the extending knee.

Eccentric contractions produce a lengthening of the muscle as a whole because the internal force produced by the muscle is less than the external force or resistance. Eccentric contractions help to regulate movements caused by external forces such as gravity and can be seen when one lowers an object onto a table or one eases into a chair. Eccentric contractions act as a brake to decelerate motion of the joint as seen in the quadriceps muscles when one descends stairs. Muscle tension is less than gravity pulling the body down but sufficient to allow controlled movement. Eccentric contractions occur in every movement in the direction of gravity. In eccentric contractions, active muscles are those which are antagonists of the same movement when it is made against gravity. For example, when lowering a load, there is an eccentric contraction of the shoulder flexors as they are lengthening and decelerating the movement.

Figure 4-3. Types of muscle contractions.

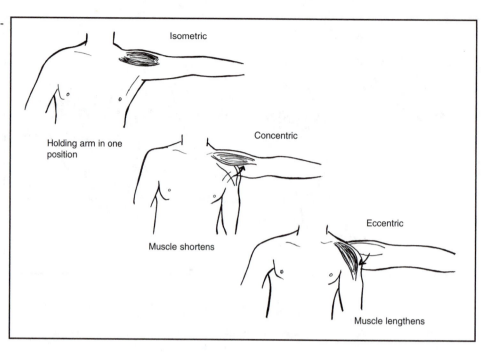

Isometric

Holding arm in one position

Concentric

Muscle shortens

Eccentric

Muscle lengthens

Isometric contractions of muscles happen when the internal force generated by the contractile elements of the muscle does not exceed the external force of resistance. The tension produced against resistance is in equilibrium and there will be no change in the external muscle length, no motion, and no mechanical work. This is an example of static work where physiologic work is done (energy is expended), but no joint (mechanical) work is done. It is important to point out that all dynamic work involves an initial static (isometric) phase as the tension develops. Isometric contractions enable muscles to act in a restraining or holding action. Muscles acting as stabilizers and some synergists produce tension equal to the resistance that it needs to overcome. An example of an isometric contraction is a contraction in which a constant external load is lifted at the extreme ends of motion. When you grasp the handle of a coffee cup, there is muscle tension but no movement. The sustained contraction helps to hold the cup.

Of the muscle contraction types, the most force can be generated by eccentric (lengthening) contractions because the muscle is able to create more cross-bridges. The next greatest force generator is a muscle contracting isometrically followed by concentric (shortening) contractions.

An additional type of muscle activity is called *isokinetic* movement at a joint, which is characterized by constant angular velocity and speed in the ROM so that shortening and lengthening of the muscle is controlled via machines such as computerized dynamometers and Cybex or Biodex. While not a naturally occurring contraction, when used in exercise, the advantage of isokinetic resistance is that the device provides resistance that is proportional to the resistance produced by the muscle throughout all points in the ROM (Nordin & Frankel, 1989). *Isoinertial* contractions are another "made up" (Nordin & Frankel, 1989) variable where a muscle acts against a constant load or resistance. If the resistance to the muscle is equal to that of the machine, an isometric contraction occurs; if the resistance is greater than that produced by the muscle, the muscle will lengthen. Similarly, if the muscle strength is greater than the resistance, the muscle will shorten. Isoinertial exercise is seen as superior to isokinetic in that isoinertial more closely simulates daily life activities.

Location of Muscle and Axis

Muscles that move a part usually do not lie over that part but are often proximal to the part moved. The distance of the origin and the insertion of the muscle to the joint axis has an influence on type of movement produced. If the distance from the insertion to the joint axis is greater than the distance from the origin, this is considered to be a *shunt muscle*. Shunt muscles tend to have the line of pull along a bone, so the muscle tends to pull bones together creating a more translatory effect and the muscle acts as a stabilizer. Examples of shunt muscles are the sternocleidomastoid muscle and the brachioradialis muscle where the origin is near the axis and the insertion is far.

A *spurt muscle* is one where the origin is farther from the joint axis and the insertion nearer. Spurt muscles have their line of pull across bones so that there is a larger rotary component to the movement produced. While shunt muscles act to stabilize joints, spurt muscles help to overcome inertia and produce rapid movements throughout a wide ROM. Two joint muscles may possess spurt characteristics at one joint and shunt at the other joint. Spurt and shunt classifications are based on 19th century engineering terms, with spurt defined as a force "which provides energy to impel a body into motion or keep it in motion", which basically is a restatement of Newton's Second Law (Gench et al., 1995).

The muscle's location or line of action in regards to the location of the joint axis determines what motion the muscle will perform. Muscles crossing anterior to joint axis in the upper extremity, trunk, and hip are flexors, while muscles located posterior to the axis are extensors. Muscles located laterally and medially are abductors and adductors (Nordin & Frankel, 1989; Gench et al., 1995). By applying knowledge about anatomy and muscle fiber arrangement, one can determine optimal angles of pull and locations of muscles to use muscles most advantageously in everyday occupations.

Cross Section of the Muscle

Larger muscles with larger cross sectional areas are capable of producing greater strength. By exercising, muscle cells hypertrophy, causing an increase in size and therefore an increase in

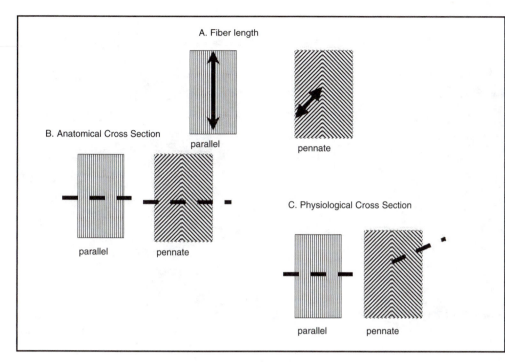

A. Fiber length

parallel

pennate

B. Anatomical Cross Section

parallel

pennate

C. Physiological Cross Section

parallel

pennate

Figure 4-4. Cross section differences. A. Longer fiber length in parallel fibers. B. Anatomical cross sections are similar. C. Pennate fibers have a greater sum of fibers in the muscle in area perpendicular to the muscle pull. Pennate muscles are usually stronger.

strength. Because pennate muscles generally have more muscle fibers and shorter fibers that run diagonally into the tendon, pennate muscles have a much larger physiologic cross section than parallel muscles, which enables greater force generation.

Physiologic cross section is defined as "the sum total of all of the cross sections of fibers in the muscle, measuring the area perpendicular to the direction of the fibers" (Hamil & Knutzen, 1995). *Anatomic cross section* is the cross section made at right angles to the longitudinal axis of the muscle (Hamil & Knutzen, 1995). In parallel fibers, the anatomic and physiologic cross sections are the same, whereas in pennate fibers, the physiologic cross section is greater than the anatomic cross section. Because of the greater number of fibers in a pennate muscle, even if a pennate muscle and a parallel muscle had the same anatomic cross section, the pennate would still be capable of producing greater force due to the larger physiologic cross section. The physiological cross sectional area will give an indication of maximum tensile force capable of producing (Marieb, 1998)(Figure 4-4).

Velocity of Contraction

Not only is muscle length an important variable in the development of maximum tensile force, but the velocity of the shortening of the muscle is also to be considered. Greater force is achieved at lower speeds due to greater opportunities for recruitment. As the speed of shortening (concentric) increases, tension decreases. In concentric contractions, velocity is increased at the expense of a decrease in force. The maximum force is at zero velocity because a large number of cross-bridges are attached and maximum velocity is achieved at the lightest load. As the velocity of the muscle shortening (concentric) increases, fewer cross-bridges are formed so force production is negligible (Hamil & Knutzen, 1995). Conversely, as the speed of lengthening (eccentric) increases, tension increases.

If a concentric muscle action (shortening) is preceded by an eccentric (lengthening) action, the resulting concentric action is capable of generating greater force. This prestretch changes a muscle's characteristics by increasing the tension through storage of potential elastic energy in series elastic component. When a muscle is stretched, small changes occur in the muscle and tendon length and in the maximum accumulation of stored energy. When concentric action follows, there is an enhanced recoil effect adding to the force output. Stored elastic energy in parallel components in connective tissue also contributes to high force output at initial portions of concentric action as the tissue returns to a resting length. The parallel elastic contribution drops off as the muscle continues to shorten. If the stretch is held too long before shortening occurs, stored elastic energy is converted to heat and lost (Hamil & Knutzen, 1995; Irion, 2000).

Number of Joints Crossed by the Muscle

Norkin and Levangie (1992) call muscles that cross more than one joint "economic" since they are able to produce motion at more than one joint (p. 116). However, one-joint muscles are recruited first for single joint motions because additional muscle fibers or motor units may be required to prevent unwanted motions of a two-joint muscle.

Two-joint or multi-joint muscles are able to be stretched over a greater ROM. A multi-joint muscle is most effective when shortened at one end and lengthened at the other, so that the muscle works most effectively at one joint while being disadvantaged at the other. ROM and manual muscle tests are designed to put one end of multi-joint muscles "on slack". Weak positions are avoided in normal activities with favorable length-tension relationships maintained. When the muscle attachments are close together, only weak muscle contractions can be achieved. This is known as *active insufficiency*. An example of this is when the two-joint muscle rectus femoris crosses the hip and the knee and is both a hip flexor and knee extensor. Rectus femoris is more effective as a hip flexor if the knee flexes simultaneously because the muscle can contract within a favorable range. Likewise, the hamstrings are more effective in generating force as a hip extensor when the knee also extends (Smith, Weiss, & Lehmkuhl, 1996).

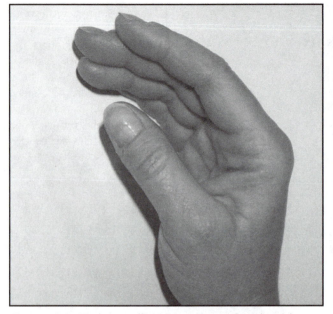

Figure 4-5A. Passive insufficiency with wrist flexed and fingers extended.

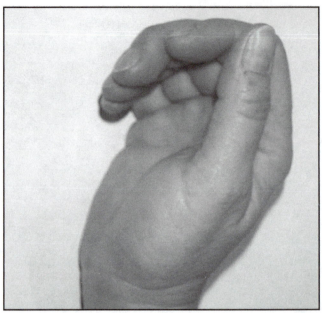

Figure 4-5B. Passive insufficiency with wrist extended and fingers flexed.

Figure 4-6. Active and passive insufficiency. Note passive tension in extensor muscles, active tension in flexor muscles.

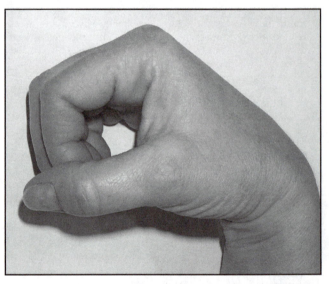

Passive insufficiency occurs when a muscle is of insufficient length over all of the joints the muscle crosses to develop sufficient tension to act at both joints at the same time. Passive tension will develop, which may be significant enough to cause joint movement, as in the tenodesis action of the wrist and fingers. The finger extensors become passively insufficient as they lengthen over the wrist during wrist flexion, causing passive tension to produce finger extension. The opposite occurs when the finger flexors develop passive tension when the wrist is extended. Passive insufficiency is usually felt as an uncomfortable or painful sensation and can be felt when one tries to simultaneously flex the wrist and fingers at the same time (Figure 4-5A, B).

Muscles that become actively insufficient due to excessive shortening are likely to develop passive insufficiency in the opposite or antagonistic muscle group (Nordin & Frankel, 1989) (Figure 4-6). The force generated by the position of the multi-joint muscles can be seen by noting that the greatest isometric grip strength is achieved when the wrist is in slight extension. When the wrist is in full flexion, there is a combination of active insufficiency of the long finger flexors and passive insufficiency of the antagonistic long finger extensors (Smith et al., 1996). Muscles that become actively insufficient due to excessive shortening are likely to develop passive insufficiency in the opposite or antagonistic muscle group (Nordin & Frankel, 1989).

McGinnis (1999) proposes this self-experiment relative to muscle length and insufficiency.

Consider the muscles that flex or extend your fingers. The finger flexor muscles are located in your anterior forearm, whereas the finger extensor muscles are located in your posterior forearm. Their tendons cross the wrist joint, the carpometacarpal joints, the metacarpophalangeal joints and the interphalangeal joints. Flex your fingers and grip a pencil as tightly as you can. Now flex your wrist as far as you can. You may notice that you cannot flex your wrist as far with your fingers flexed as you can without your fingers flexed. You may also notice that your grip on the pencil weakened as you flexed your wrist (try to pull the pencil out in both positions). If you push on your hand and cause it to flex further, the pencil may even fall out of your grip. The finger flexor muscles were unable to produce much tension. The finger extensor tendons were lengthened at each joint they cross and were stretched by the extensor muscles beyond 160% of their resting length. Passive tension created by the stretching of the connective tissue resulted in an extension of the fingers when you pushed your hand further into wrist flexion (p. 272).

SUBJECT AND PSYCHOLOGICAL/PSYCHOSOCIAL FACTORS

In addition to the muscular factors that influence strength, other factors include subject factors, psychological factors, methodological factors and measurement factors. Males with larger bones and larger muscles are stronger than females. Generally, females are 40 to 50% weaker in the upper body and 20 to 30% weaker in the lower body (Tan, 1998). Developmentally, both genders develop the greatest strength capacities from birth through adolescence, with peak strength between 20 to 30 years of age. Large variations occur in each gender due to diet, exercise, and level of activity. Both genders experience a decrease in strength with increasing age due to deterioration of muscle mass, decreased muscle fiber size and number, increases in connective tissue and fat, decreased vascularization, alterations in capacity to generate force, and decreased respiratory capacity of the muscle. Again, while these changes are age related, the amount of decreased strength is a function of training and regular exercise.

Pain is a subject-related variable important in strength assessment. Pain is a multidimensional phenomenon with cognitive and affective components as well as physiologic properties that also have culturally determined values. How one perceives pain and reacts to it is part of a culturally sanctioned role that contributes to a person's ability to function in his or her environment. When assessing strength, indicators of the client's willingness to endure discomfort or pain can be observed. Pain invalidates the assessment of strength if the person is unable to provide a maximal voluntary contraction of the muscle being tested, so observation of discomfort and pain is important in the assessment of strength.

When assessing a client's strength, the ability to follow directions, plan and execute the motor action, and the ability to pay attention are all factors influencing the test that can be observed during the testing. Controlling environmental variables such as noise and number of people may facilitate better performance on tests of strength with clients. Temperature has a direct bearing on muscle activity because a rise in muscle temperature causes an increase in conduction velocity, increasing the frequency of stimulation, thereby increasing muscle force. Further increases in temperature increases enzymatic activity, making muscle contractions more efficient, and increasing the elasticity of the collagen in the passive components. This increases prestretch capabilities of the muscle. Whether the person cannot complete the test motion due to apraxia or due to cognitive impairments can also be determined during assessments. The inability to follow directions may be due to language difficulties as well, whether pathological in nature (as in aphasia) or due to English as a second language. Testing muscle strength can also lead one to make inferences regarding the true

effort of muscle contraction and a desire to do well or an effort to seem more impaired than one actually is for possible secondary gains. Lassitude and depression can present as indifference to the test where true effort will not be given by the client. Cultural, social, and gender issues also are evident, especially when palpation and exposure of body parts are required for assessment purposes.

STRENGTH TESTING

Screening for muscle weakness is appropriate for conditions where muscle weakness is not the primary symptom or the primary limiting factor in performance of daily activities. Screening tools are designed to provide a general estimate of strength and if deficits are indicated, further discrete testing may be done. Functional motion tests vary in what they assess and how the assessment is done. Some tests look at the active movement of a client as an assessment of joint ROM and active, volitional movement patterns. The Zimmerman Functional Motion test screens for strength, ROM, and coordination for the upper extremity (Zimmerman, 1969). In some tests, the part being tested is passively placed and the client is asked to hold the part in that position while resistance is applied. In other tests, active movement into the test position is required. Some tests describe first and second positions designed to take into account the effect of gravity on the part during testing, while others do not.

More discrete testing of muscle strength is actually a measurement of impairment rather than function (Van Deusen & Brunt, 1997). Tan (1998) describes the potential uses of strength testing:

- For physical medicine and rehabilitation
- Prescribing treatment and establishment of a baseline
- Monitoring progress
- Evaluating level of impairment
- Medical-legal
- Test effort consistency
- Determine maximal exertion
- Assess disability
- Industry
- Provide ergonomic and rehabilitation guidelines
- Screen for job placement and return to work
- Compliance with ADA (p. 54)

Other stated purposes for strength testing are to determine how muscle weakness limits performance, to prevent deformities caused by muscle imbalance, to establish the need for assistive or technological devices, and to aid in the selection of appropriate activities. Results are useful in establishing differential diagnoses and prognoses.

Strength testing can be done in various ways. Manual testing would involve the active contraction of the muscle by the client with the application of resistance by the tester. Several muscles can be tested as a group that produces a particular motion. For example, the anterior deltoid, coracobrachialis, pectoralis major, and biceps muscles might be tested as a group of muscles that produce shoulder flexion. Individual muscles can be isolated and tested separately. In addition, inferences about strength can be made when observing a person engage in daily life activities. This type of assessment enables one to assess other factors that may also be interfering with successful performance in tasks such as balance or cognition, as well as the dynamic interaction of muscles.

Manual muscle testing by definition is "the application of resistance by the tester or by the force of gravity to the voluntary maximum contraction of the patient's muscle" (Jenkins, 1998).

Manual muscle testing is appropriate for those clients who are able to voluntarily contract muscles, which excludes those with CNS dysfunction, with tone problems or stereotypic, automatic movements. Manual muscle testing is often not performed with children and is contraindicated for those with dislocations. Extra care and attention in testing should be taken for clients with cardiovascular and chronic respiratory diseases (ie, COPD), as well as those clients just recovering from abdominal surgery. It is possible to tear muscle fibers if excess application of resistance is applied and muscle cramping can occur if resistance is applied for too long a duration. An advantage to manual muscle testing is that no equipment is required.

The definition provided identifies three variables that are used in determining the grade of the muscle (Table 4-3). *Contractility* is the first variable and is determined by palpation of the muscle. If the client is unable to contract a muscle and no muscle tension is felt with palpation, the muscle grade is zero (0). Palpation is best performed by using the middle finger, which is the most sensitive finger to identification of tension. Every muscle tested must be palpated to be sure the correct muscle is being tested and to minimize substitution actions by synergists or other muscles. The muscle that demonstrates the ability to contract by volitional control would be rated a trace or 1/5.

Gravity, the second variable, affects muscle contraction. Muscles that can contract volitionally in a gravity eliminated plane would be considered a poor muscle (or 2/5). If the person can move the extremity in a position against gravity, the muscle grade is fair or 3/5.

The third variable, *resistance*, is used to differentiate the good muscle (4/5) from the normal muscle (5/5). The application of manual resistance is seen as a subjective variable, which may account for the poor reliability and validity of muscle grading above the fair muscle grade. The amount of resistance is dependent upon the muscle being tested (for example, less resistance should be applied to muscles with a predominance of Type II fibers or those of parallel arrangement because they are less likely to be as strong as those that are Type I or pennate) and individual characteristics of the client such as age and gender. Muscle grades can be further defined by adding a "+" or "-" to the muscle grade . Trombly (1995) identifies a muscle of G- or below to be weak, and therefore a possible focus of remediation.

Manual muscle testing follows muscle length-tension relationships and joint mechanics in the positioning of the client for assessment. One-joint muscles often have external force applied at the end of range, whereas two-joint muscles often have the point of maximum resistance at or near midrange.

In manual muscle testing advocated by Lovett and by Daniels and Worthingham, motions using agonists and synergists are the focus of assessment. Group muscle testing is seen as more functional than individual muscle testing and the assessment occurs through the full test ROM. The patient performs a concentric contraction or holds the test position at the end of the available ROM while the muscle is in a shortened position. Not as objective as individualized muscle testing, group strength testing can help to identify where in the range weakness exists (Palmer & Epler, 1998).

Testing at the end of range with the muscle providing the isometric hold is referred to as the *break test or method*. Resistance that is applied throughout the test range in a direction opposite to the muscle's rotary component is known as *make test or method* while the muscle is performing a concentric type of contraction (Palmer & Epler, 1998).

Kendall and McCreary (1983) propose methods for testing specific, individual muscles. This type of manual muscle testing requires a greater knowledge of anatomy and kinesiology. While seen as more accurate, this type of testing is also more time con-

Table 4-3.

FACTORS RELATED TO MUSCLE GRADES

Related to evidence of contraction	Zero = 0: or 0/5	No muscle contraction felt.
	Trace = T: or 1/5	Evidence of contractility on palpation. No joint motion.
Related to gravity	Poor = P: or 2/5	Movement with gravity eliminated but not against gravity or complete ROM with gravity eliminated.
	Fair = F: or 3/5	Can raise part against gravity or complete ROM against gravity.
Related to resistance	Good = G: or 4/5	Can raise part against outside resistance and against gravity or complete ROM against gravity with some resistance.
	Normal = N: or 5/5	Can overcome a greater amount of resistance than a good muscle or complete ROM against gravity with full resistance.

suming to perform. The test is performed while the client contracts isometrically with the segment aligned in the direction of the muscle fibers in a midrange position. The client is then asked to "hold" this position against resistance. Similarly, the Medical Research Council Scale uses resistance as an isometric hold at the end of the test range, and this group advocates using numbers rather than words for muscle grades (for example, a good muscle grade is a 4/5) (Table 4-4).

Those performing manual muscle testing need a thorough knowledge of the location and directional line of pull of muscles and of anatomy. This is especially true when palpating muscles to determine muscle grades of zero and trace. Knowledge of muscles with the same innervation can help in identifying patterns of weakness or those that may be related to specific diagnostic categories. The function of participating muscles (synergist, prime mover, etc.) is important, as is familiarity with patterns of substitution. Experience in positioning and stabilization required in the specific muscle tests enables more accurate test results. Sensitivity to differences in normal muscle contours and joint laxity is invaluable to the assessment of muscles. The effects of fatigue and of sensory loss on the ability to move also cannot be disregarded (Table 4-5).

Manual muscle testing, while used extensively clinically, has not demonstrated good reliability and validity. It is considered inaccurate in testing strength greater than fair muscle grades (or 3/5) and is insensitive to change (Van Deusen & Brunt, 1997). There is a tendency to overestimate the normalcy of muscle strength and manual muscle testing has been seen as inadequate in determining functional capacity (Tan, 1998).

Manual muscle testing has been determined to be reliable within one muscle grade 60 to 75% of the time (Palmer & Epler, 1998) and others have found that results do not vary more than one half of a muscle grade (Palmer & Epler, 1998; Van Deusen & Brunt,

Table 4-4.

COMPARISON OF GRAVITY-RESISTED MUSCLE GRADING CRITERIA

Lovett and Daniels and Worthingham	*Kendall and McCreary*	*Medical Research Council*
N (Normal): Subject completes range of motion against gravity, against maximal resistance.	100%: Subject moves into and holds test position against gravity, against maximal resistance.	5
G+ (Good Plus): Subject completes range of motion against gravity, against nearly maximal resistance.		4+
G (Good): Subject completes range of motion against gravity, against moderate resistance.	80%: Subject moves into and holds test position against gravity, against less than maximal resistance.	4
G- (Good Minus): Subject completes range of motion against gravity, against less than moderate resistance.		4-
F+ (Fair Plus): Subject completes range of motion against gravity, against minimal resistance.		3+
F (Fair): Subject completes range of motion against gravity with no manual resistance.	50%: Subject moves into and holds a test position against gravity.	3
F- (Fair Minus): Subject does not complete range against gravity but does complete more than half the range.		3-
P+ (Poor Plus): Subject initiates range of motion against gravity or completes range with gravity minimized against slight resistance.		2+
P (Poor): Subject completes range of motion with gravity minimized.	20%: Subject moves through small motion with gravity minimized.	2
P- (Poor Minus): Subject does not complete range of motion with gravity minimized.		2-
T (Trace): Subject's muscle can be palpated, but there is no joint motion.	5%: Contraction is palpable with no joint motion.	1
0 (Zero): Subject exhibits no palpable contraction.	0%: No contraction is palpable.	0

Reprinted with permission from Palmer, M. L. & Epler, M. (1998). *Fundamentals of musculoskeletal assessment.* 2nd ed. Philadelphia: Lippincott Williams & Wilkins.

1997). Further, there is approximately 50% complete agreement on muscle grades, including the addition of + and -, 66% agreement within + or -, and 90% agreement within one full grade (Palmer & Epler, 1998).

There is poor interrater reliability in muscle grades below fair (Palmer & Epler, 1998; Tan, 1998), with better discrimination between zero to fair + muscle grades. It is vital to follow procedures, provide clear directions, demonstrate and explain movement, and passively move the client to facilitate understanding. Other factors that need to be considered to improve reliability are:

- Cooperation of the client
- Experience of tester
- Tone of voice of tester
- Ambient temperature
- Temperature of limb
- Distractions to patient and to tester or other environmental conditions
- Posture
- Fatigue
- Operational definitions of muscle grades (Trombly, 1995).

It is generally accepted that manual muscle testing has face and content validity since the testing is based on anatomic and physiologic structures (Palmer & Epler, 1998), but there is little credence placed on the ability to generalize the results to immediate and future behavior of patients (Palmer & Epler, 1998). Validity is improved by palpating each muscle being tested, stabilizing proximal segments during testing, and preventing substitution movements and muscle actions.

Strength testing done with dynamometers is generally regarded as more reliable and valid than with manual resistance. Using a hand-held dynamometer for strength testing yielded a greater than .84 test-retest value when performed by an experienced therapist (Trombly, 1995). Hand-held dynamometers are a portable force measuring device that the examiner holds while the client exerts maximal force. Some hand-held dynamometers that are commercially available include: Lafayette hand dynamometer, Lafayette Pediatric hand dynamometer, Nicholas manual muscle tester

(Lafayette Manual Muscle Test System, Lafayette, IN), Jamar dynamometer, Tech power-track II, and MicroFet dynamometer.

Isometric dynamometers for assessment of limb muscle groups measure peak and average force, reaction time, rate of motor recruitment of motor units, and maximal voluntary exertion and fatigue (Tan, 1998). In this test, the muscle length is held constant, which is a preferred method in conditions where joint motion causes pain. The disadvantage to this type of testing using strain gauges is that the movements are not well correlated with real life dynamic activities (Tan, 1998). The Baltimore Therapeutic Equipment Co. (Hanover, MD) has both isometric and isotonic testing capacities.

Isotonic dynamometers use constant weight or resistance with muscle contractions at an accommodating speed and at an accommodating resistance. An example of a commercially available isotonic dynamometer at an accommodating speed would be the Ariel Computerized Exercise System (Tan, 1998).

With isokinetic dynamometers, strength is measured as the joint moves at a constant preselected speed. Resistance is applied through the ROM. Passive isokinetic instruments include Cybex and Universal Merac, and active isokinetic tools include Biodex and Kin-Com (Tan, 1998).

Grasp and Pinch Assessment

As with body strength, age and gender are factors in the assessment of grasp and pinch. Men are stronger than women and this is true throughout adult life. Men have higher grasp values in all postures and joint angles. While men are stronger, some studies suggest that women are more dextrous (Durward, Baer, & Rowe, 1999; Richards, Olson, & Palmiter-Thomas, 1996). For both genders, strength increases curvilinearly until age 20, peaks between 19 to 50 years of age, then declines. With females, the strength increases until age 13 then remains constant until 20 to 29 years of age. Males demonstrate linear increases before peaking at ages 30 to 39 years, after which decline in strength occurs (Durward et al., 1999). Shiffman found a significant effect of aging on functional performance with statistically significant differences with age on grip strength, prehension, and time to perform tasks (Durward et al., 1999). Desrosiers, Bravo, Hebert, & Dutil (1995) state that "grip strength in persons aged 60 years and older varies negatively and curvilinearly with age and that the loss seems more marked across older subjects" (p. 641). These authors propose that reductions in the number and size of muscle fibers (especially fast twitch fibers), decreased ability to achieve maximum tension levels, as well as normal age-related changes in the nervous system and vascular and circulatory systems, account for decreased grip strength with increased age.

Hand dominance differences in strength are discrepant. Some studies indicate no statistically significant differences in grip strength between right and left hands for left-handed persons (Richards et al., 1996), while Lunde et al. and Desrosiers et al. (1995) found that the dominant hand is 10 to 13% stronger than the nondominant hand (Petersen, Petrick, Connor, & Conklin, 1989; Richards et al., 1996). Many studies resulting in normative values for grip strength reflect the greater grip strength values for the preferred hand.

The measurement of grip strength has been the focus of many studies that consider the position of the shoulder, elbow, forearm, and wrist; type and complexity of directions; position of the body (sitting, standing); instruments used to measure grasp; terminology; and protocols of testing (see Appendix A).

The American Society of Hand Therapists suggests that grip be measured with the client seated in a straight chair with the feet flat on the floor. The upper extremity should be adducted against the body in neutral rotation with the elbow flexed to 90 degrees and

---

Table 4-5.

MANUAL MUSCLE TESTING PROCEDURES

1. Assure that the client is comfortable, warm, rested as possible.
2. Arrange the environment so that the room is quiet, well lit.
3. Explain to the client how the testing will be done, why, and how the results will be used as well as who will see the results.
4. Place the client in the described test position.
5. Provide fixation (stabilization, support, counterpressure) as specified in test procedure.
6. Apply resistance slowly. Tell the patient to "hold" the test position (if using break test).
7. Palpate the contacting muscle.
8. Determine muscle grade.
9. Record results.

---

the forearm in neutral rotation. Several studies support this positioning during grasp and pinch testing (Richards et al., 1996).

Several instruments are used predominantly in clinical practice to evaluate grasp and pinch. The *Jamar hand-held dynamometer* is a sealed hydraulic strain gauge system that measures force exerted on the device in pounds or kilograms. Calibration accuracy is important to validity and Mathiowetz (Richards et al., 1996) determined calibration accuracy of the Jamar dynamometer to be +3 to 5%. This means that if one scored 50 pounds using the Jamar dynamometer, the actual value is somewhere between 47.5 to 52.5 pounds. Grasp values are considered abnormal when associated with functional limitation and/or if value is + 3 standard deviations from normative values. Mathiowetz and Flood-Joy further tested the Jamar dynamometer and found using the second handle position yielded high interrater reliability with a correlation coefficient of 0.97 or above for all tests; test-retest reliability using the mean of three tests was most consistent with a correlation coefficient of 0.80 or better. Lowest correlations occurred when only one trial was done. The Jamar dynamometer is considered the most precise of the instruments used to measure grasp (Desrosiers et al., 1995) (Table 4-6).

Use of the Jamar dynamometer measures strength in pounds with norms based on age and gender. There is generally a 5 to 10% difference between the right and left hands. The procedure for use is:

1. Adjust the handle to fit the patient's hand size and to allow MCP flexion. It was found that with the handle in the second position, the grasp values were the strongest and values obtained in each of the five handle positions would represent a bell-shaped curve (Palmer & Epler, 1998).
2. The client is permitted to rest the forearm on a table if desired but not any part of the dynamometer. The elbow should be flexed to 90 degrees.
3. Three trials with each hand are performed with the mean value recorded. An alternate method is to perform two separate trials where the person exerts maximum pressure (two times with hand) and the higher score is recorded. In each method, both hands are tested alternately with care taken not to fatigue the client.

The *Martin vigorometer* is an air-filled bulb connected to a pressure gauge (Durward et al., 1999) with three different sized bulbs for testing grip and pinch. Measurements are expressed in kiloPascals and unlike the Jamar dynamometer, involves an isotonic contraction due to the movement necessary to compress the

		\multicolumn{12}{c}{Table 4-6.}										

JAMAR GRASP DYNAMOMETER NORMS IN POUNDS (MEAN OF THREE TRIALS)

		\multicolumn{12}{c}{*Norms at Age (years)*}										
		20	25	30	35	40	45	50	55	60	65	70	75+
Male	Right	121	121	122	120	117	110	114	101	90	91	75	66
	SD	21	23	22	24	21	23	18	27	20	21	21	21
	Left	104	110	110	113	113	101	102	83	77	77	65	55
	SD	22	16	22	22	19	23	17	23	20	20	18	17
Female	Right	70	74	79	74	70	62	66	57	55	50	50	43
	SD	14	14	19	11	13	15	12	12	10	10	12	11
	Left	61	63	68	66	62	56	57	47	46	41	41	38
	SD	13	12	18	12	14	13	11	12	10	8	10	9

n=628; age range 20-94 years

Reprinted with permission from Trombly C. *Occupational Therapy for Physical Dysfunction*. 4th ed. Philadelphia: Lippincott Williams & Wilkins; 1995; pg. 150.

bulb (Desrosiers et al., 1995). The vigorometer measures with high test-retest reliability with coefficients of .96 for the mean of three measures on the dominant hand and .98 for the nondominant hand. Norms are available for age and gender.

The third instrument, a *sphygmomanometer* or *modified sphygmomanometer* (blood pressure cuff) is often used for clients with fragile hands. The sphygmomanometer ratings had a strong and linear relationship to Jamar, with r =.83 for right hand and r =.84 for left. The sphygmomanometer measurement is in millimeters of mercury (mmHg). Procedure for use of the use of the sphygmomanometer in measuring hand strength:

1. Roll cuff into cylinder shape and inflate to 100mmHg.
2. Deflate to 30mmHg to establish the baseline.
3. Record as maximum versus baseline average (x mm Hg/30mmHg).

A value of 300mmHg/30mmHg is considered within normal limits and conversion tables have been developed that compare the sphygmomanometer results with Jamar results.

The Baltimore Therapeutic Equipment (BTE) power grip attachment has also been used to assess grasp and pinch. The BTE values had a test-retest value of >.98 on the right dominant hand in clients aged 20 to 45 with a day-to-day variability of 5% for right and 3% for left.

The difficulty in comparing grasp values and determining reliability and validity is that there is such an array of methods and protocols used. Different instruments use different units of measurement, different hand configurations, and different force transmission. For example, the modified sphygmomanometer measures pressure produced within the sphygmomanometer cuff and the Jamar dynamometer measures force exerted on the handle. These tools use different joint and muscle mechanics. Even when the same tools are used, the use of different testing procedures, positions, and lack of standardization in terms of description and testing protocols make comparison of results difficult (Durward et al., 1999).

Assessment of pinch generally involves testing of tip, lateral and palmar pinches, although there is much discrepancy in the description of pinch and in terminology used. The B & L Pinchmeter or the Osco Pinchmeter are often used for testing and the client squeezes the pinchmeter using various pinches. One to three trials are used to test tip, lateral, and palmar pinches and usually three trials are taken with the mean calculated. Pinchmeter values are accurate to within +1%, interrater reliability is >.979, and test-retest reliability is >.81 (Table 4-7). Client results are compared to norms that are based on age and gender. Other ways of assessing pinch and grasp would be observation of hand use during functional activities and by using standardized coordination tests.

SUMMARY

- Muscle strength is the amount of tension that a muscle can produce. Power is the product of force and velocity. Endurance is the ability to maintain a force over time.
- Many factors influence muscle strength. Skeletal muscles have the properties of contractility, elasticity, irritability, and distensibility.
- The sliding filament theory is used to explain the contraction of single muscle cells in an all-or-none fashion where the myosin and actin filaments increase or decrease the amount of overlap.
- Tension in a muscle depends on the initial length of the muscle, the innervation ratio of muscle fibers to motor units, the fiber arrangement and cross section, the type of contraction, the location of the muscle in relation to the joint axis, the type of fiber, the number of joints crossed by the muscle, and the level of fatigue.
- The greatest tension can be produced in fast twitch glycolic fibers, and by shorter muscle fibers that are able to generate higher levels of passive tension and higher peak tension.

Muscles with greater cross sectional areas are able to produce greater tension. Muscles stretched prior to testing are stronger since passive elastic energy in the noncontractile elements are converted to kinetic energy when stretched.

- Tension in muscles can also be increased by increasing the frequency of the firing of motor units and by increasing the number and size of motor units participating.
- Subject related factors (age, gender, activity level) and psychological factors also influence strength and muscle testing.
- Strength testing can be done by manually applying resistance to a part (manual muscle testing) or by using instruments to measure peak strength. Screening for muscle weakness may precede strength testing where muscle weakness is not the primary limiting factor in performance.
- Manual muscle testing has face and content validity but variable reliability. Reliability is enhanced when using dynamometers or instruments.
- Pinch and grasp strength are affected by subject factors, hand dominance, position of the arm and body, devices used for measurement, and variances in testing protocols.

REFERENCES

Desrosiers, J., Bravo, G., Hebert, R., & Dutil, E. (1995). Normative data for grip strength of elderly men and women. *Amer J Occup Ther, 49*(7), 637-643.

Durward, B. R., Baer, G. D., & Rowe, P. J. (1999). *Functional human movement: Measurement and analysis.* Oxford: Butterworth-Heineman.

Gench, B. E., Hinson, M. M., & Harvey, P. T. (1995). *Anatomical kinesiology.* Dubuque, IA: Eddie Bowers Publishing, Inc.

Hamil, J., & Knutzen, K. M. (1995). *Biomechanical basis of human movement.* Baltimore: Williams and Wilkins.

Irion, G. (2000). *Physiology: The basis of clinical practice.* Thorofare, NJ: SLACK Incorporated.

Jenkins, D. B. (1998). *Hollingshead's functional anatomy of the limbs and back.* (7th ed.). Philadelphia: W. B. Saunders Co.

Kendall, F. P., & McCreary, E. K. (1983). *Muscles: testing and function.* (3rd ed.). Baltimore, MD: Williams and Wilkins.

Kisner, C., & Colby, L. A. (1990). *Therapeutic exercise: Foundations and techniques.* (2nd ed.). Philadelphia: F.A. Davis Co.

Konin, J. G. (1999). *Practical kinesiology for the physical therapist assistant.* Thorofare, NJ: SLACK Incorporated.

Marieb, E. N. (1998). *Human anatomy and physiology.* Glenview, IL: Addison Wesley Longman Publishers.

McGinnis, P. M. (1999). *Biomechanics of sport and exercise.* Champaign, IL: Human Kinetics.

McPhee, S. D. (1987). Functional hand evaluations: A review. *Am J Occup Ther, 41*(3), 158-163.

Nordin, M., & Frankel, V. H. (1989). *Basic biomechanics of the musculoskeletal system.* (2nd ed.). Philadelphia: Lea and Febiger.

Norkin, C. C., & Levangie, P. K. (1992). *Joint structure and function: A comprehensive analysis.* (2nd ed.). Philadelphia: F.A. Davis Co.

Palmer, M. L., & Epler, M. E. (1998). *Fundamentals of musculoskeletal assessment techniques.* (2nd ed.). Philadelphia: J. B. Lippincott.

Petersen, P., Petrick, M., Connor, H., & Conklin, D. (1989). Grip strength and hand dominance: Challenging the 10% rule. *Amer J Occup Ther, 43*(7), 444-447.

Table 4-7.

B&L (60) PINCHMETER NORMS IN POUNDS (MEAN OF THREE TRIALS)

		Norms at Age (years)						
		20	30	40	50	60	70	75+
Tip								
Male	Right	18	18	18	18	16	14	14
	Left	17	18	18	18	15	13	14
Female	Right	11	13	11	12	10	10	10
	Left	10	12	11	11	10	10	9
		(average SD: males=4.0; females=2.5)						
Lateral								
Male	Right	26	26	26	27	23	19	20
	Left	25	26	25	26	22	19	19
Female	Right	18	19	17	17	15	14	13
	Left	16	18	16	16	14	14	11
		(average SD: males=4.6; females=3.0)						
Palmar								
Male	Right	27	25	24	24	22	18	19
	Left	26	25	25	24	21	19	18
Female	Right	17	19	17	17	15	14	12
	Left	16	18	17	16	14	14	12
		(average SD: males=5.1; females=3.7)						

n=628; age range=20-94 years.

Reprinted with permission from Trombly C. *Occupational Therapy for Physical Dysfunction.* 4th ed. Philadelphia: Lippincott Williams & Wilkins; 1995.

Richards, L. G., Olson, B., & Palmiter-Thomas, P. (1996). How forearm position affects grip strength. *Amer J Occup Ther, 50*(2), 133-138.

Smith, L. K., Weiss, E. L., & Lehmkuhl, L. D. (1996). *Brunnstrom's clinical kinesiology.* (5th ed.). Philadelphia: F. A. Davis Co.

Tan, J. C. (1998). *Practical manual of physical medicine and rehabilitation.* St. Louis, MO: C. V. Mosby.

Trombly, C. A. (Ed.). (1995). *Occupational therapy for physical dysfunction.* (4th ed.). Baltimore: Williams & Wilkins.

Van Deusen, J., & Brunt, D. (1997). *Assessment in occupational therapy and physical therapy.* Philadelphia: W. B. Saunders Co.

Zimmerman, M. E. (1969). The functional motion test as an evaluation tool for patients. *Am J Occup Ther, 23*(1), 49-56.

BIBLIOGRAPHY

Asher, I. E. (1996). *Occupational therapy assessment tools: An annotated index.* (2nd ed.). Bethesda, Md: American Occupational Therapy Association.

Baxter, R. (1998). *Pocket guide to musculoskeletal assessment.* Philadelphia: W. B. Saunders Co.

Berne, R. M., & Levy, M. N. (1998). *Physiology.* (4th ed.). St. Louis, MO: C. V. Mosby.

Brand, P. W., & Hollister, A. M. (1999). *Clinical mechanics of the hand* (3rd ed.). St. Louis, MO: C. V. Mosby.

Christiansen, C., & Baum, C. (1997). *Occupational therapy: Enabling function and well being*. (2nd ed.). Thorofare NJ: SLACK Incorporated.

Demeter, S. L., Andersson, G., & Smith, G. M. (1996). *Disability evaluation*. St. Louis, MO: C. V. Mosby.

Epler, M. (2000). *Manual muscle testing: An interactive tutorial*. Thorofare, NJ: SLACK Incorporated.

Esch, D. L. (1989). *Musculoskeletal function: An anatomy and kinesiology laboratory manual*. Minneapolis: University of Minnesota.

Galley, P. M., & Forster, A. L. (1987). *Human movement: An introductory text for physiotherapy students*. (2nd ed.). New York: Churchill-Livingstone.

Goss, C. M. (Ed.). (1976). *Gray's anatomy of the human body*. (29th ed.). Philadelphia: Lea and Febiger.

Greene, D. P., & Roberts, S. L. (1999). *Kinesiology: Movement in the context of activity*. St. Louis, MO: C. V. Mosby.

Hinkle, C. Z. (1997). *Fundamentals of anatomy and movement: A workbook and guide*. St. Louis, MO: C. V. Mosby.

Hinojosa, J., & Kramer, P. (1998). *Evaluation: Obtaining and interpreting data*. Bethesda, MD: American Occupational Therapy Association.

Hislop, H., & Montgomery, J. (1995). *Daniels and Worthingham's muscle testing: Techniques of manual examination*. (6th ed.). Philadelphia: W. B. Saunders Co.

Pedretti, L. W. (1996). *Occupational therapy: Practice skills for physical dysfunction*. (4th ed.). St. Louis, MO: C. V. Mosby.

Smith, R. O., & Benge, M. W. (1985). Pinch and grasp strength: Standardization of terminology and protocol. *Amer J Occup Ther*, 39(8), 531-535.

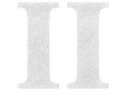

Normal Joint Movement

The Shoulder

Chapter 5

The shoulder is a complex joint made up of many articulations capable of a wide variety of motions. It is widely accepted that the shoulder joint complex consists of three to four major joints and other sources cite at least one and as many as three additional articulations that permit wide variances of movement (Caillet, 1980; Norkin & Levangie, 1992; Smith, Weiss & Lehmkuhl, 1996; Perry, Rohe, & Garcia, 1996). The connections of the thorax with the humerus and scapula enable the positioning of the arm and hand in functional positions (Hartley, 1995).

ANATOMY OF THE SHOULDER JOINT COMPLEX

The shoulder complex is made up of the clavicle, the humerus, the sternum, the scapula, the ribs, and the vertebral column (Figure 5-1A, B).

DESCRIPTION OF STRUCTURES AND PALPATION

Clavicle

The clavicle provides the connection between the sternum and the scapula. The clavicle also increases the mobility of the glenohumeral joint to permit reaching and climbing activities.

Palpation

- Lateral /acromial end: this prominence of the lateral end of the clavicle, which articulates with the acromion process of the scapula and projects above it, is easily palpable (Esch, 1989).
- Medial/sternal end: palpate the rounded projection above the superior aspect of the manubrium sterni. The line of the sternoclavicular joint can be identified (Esch, 1989).
- Shaft: palpate the anterior and superior surfaces from medial to lateral. Note that the anterior surface is convex medially and concave laterally (Esch, 1989).

Scapula

The scapula acts as a platform on which movements of the humerus are based (Gench, Hinson & Harvey, 1995, p. 51).

Palpation

- Inferior angle: palpate the lowest portion of the scapula, i.e., the junction of the medial and lateral borders of the scapula. If your subject consciously relaxes the shoulder girdle musculature, the angle will be more easily palpated (Esch, 1989).
- Medial/vertebral border: this border is easily palpated about 1.5 inches lateral to the vertebrae.
- Acromion process: palpate this flat process at the lateral point of the shoulder where it forms a shelf over the glenohumeral joint.
- Spine of the scapula: palpate from the acromion process to its base on the vertebral border.
- Coracoid process: palpate with deep pressure through the medial border of the anterior deltoid muscle, just inferior to the clavicular concavity. If you have difficulty, ask your subject to protract the shoulder slightly.
- May be palpated approximately 2.5 cm below the junction of the lateral one third and the medial two thirds of the clavicle.
- Sternum: "The sternum is made up of the manubrium, the body and the xiphisternum. The manubrium and body are palpable as is the suprasternal notch, which is located on the superior aspect of the manubrium. The xiphisternum is less easily palpated" (Lumley, 1990).

Humerus

The humerus "represents the first link in the chain of bony levers of the upper limbs; this is the only bone of the upper arm" (Esch, 1989).

Palpation

- Greater tubercle: with the arm in internal rotation, palpate just distal to the anterior portion of the acromion process. As your subject internally rotates the arm, you will feel it move under your fingers (Esch, 1989).
- Lesser tubercle: with the humerus in external rotation, palpate anterior to the greater tubercle.
- Intertubercular groove: palpate between the greater and lesser tubercles.
- Epicondyles (medial and lateral): with the elbow extended, palpate in the upper part of the medial and lateral fossae on the posterior surface of the elbow. Also, the ulnar nerve can be located in the medial fossa between the olecranon process and the medical epicondyle.

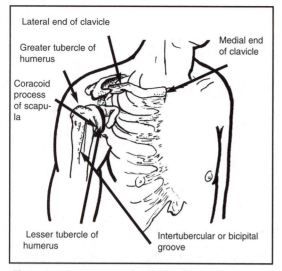

Figure 5-1A. Bones and palpable structures of the shoulder complex.

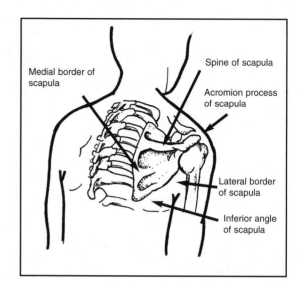

Figure 5-1B. Bones and palpable structures of the shoulder complex.

ARTICULATIONS

Sternocostal and Vertebrocostal Articulations

The ability to achieve full shoulder flexion and abduction is accomplished by the ribs gliding on both the sternum and on the vertebrae. This occurs at the *sternocostal (costosternal)* articulation, where the ribs glide on the sternum, and the *vertebrocostal (costovertebral)* articulation, where the ribs glide on the vertebrae (Flowers, 1998; Gench et al., 1995) (Figure 5-2).

The sternocostal joint is a series of gliding joints with the exception of the first rib, which is fused, making this a synchondrosis joint. The vertebrocostal, also a gliding joint, allows some rotation during depression and elevation and some rotation around its own axis as contributory movements for the total shoulder motion.

The *suprahumeral* or *subacromial* articulation is a functional joint (as opposed to an anatomic joint) serving in a protective capacity. This is the articulation between the acromion and the coracoacromial ligament and arch. The head of the humerus slides beneath the acromion and the tendon of the long head of the biceps muscle slides in the bicipital groove. Tendons of the rotator cuff muscles (supraspinatus, infraspinatus, teres minor, and subscapularis), the long head of the biceps, the joint capsule, capsular ligaments, subdeltoid, and subacromial bursae lie in this area and may be susceptible to impingement or compression syndromes. This articulation prevents trauma from above, prevents upward dislocation of the humerus, and mechanically limits abduction of the humerus.

The *scapulothoracic joint* is also a functional joint where the scapula glides on the thorax to enable greater motion of the scapula. This joint provides a movable base for humerus and permits wide ranges of movement with the scapula and thorax as well as

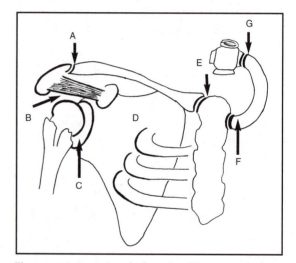

Figure 5-2. Joints of the shoulder complex. A. Acromioclavicular; B. Suprahumeral; C. Glenohumeral; D. Scapulocostal; E. Sternoclavicular; F. Costosternal; G. Costovertebral.

providing stability in the glenohumeral joint for overhead activities. Rather than being a bone-to-bone articulation, this is a bone-muscle-bone articulation between the scapula and thoracic wall where the serratus anterior and the subscapularis muscles glide on each other (Nordin & Frankel, 1989). This functional articulation also acts as shock absorber for forces applied to outstretched hands and permits elevation of the body when crutch walking and during depression transfers.

Glenohumeral Articulation

The glenohumeral joint is the major joint of the shoulder complex. The joint is made up of the glenoid fossa of the scapula articulating with the head of the humerus. Since the glenohumeral joint is a ball and socket joint, there are 3 degrees of movement at this articulation.

The glenohumeral joint is considered an incongruous joint because the articulating surfaces are not in direct contact. In fact, two-thirds of the humeral head is not covered by the glenoid fossa of the scapula, which creates a marked discrepancy between the curvature of the glenoid fossa and the convex surface of the humeral head (Caillet, 1980). The glenoid fossa is deepened somewhat by the glenoid labrum (which consists of the joint capsule, glenohumeral ligaments and the long head of the biceps), but is still shallow, allowing only a small surface area of bone-to-bone contact. The humeral head is particularly incongruent when the shoulder is: 1) adducted, flexed, and internally rotated; 2) abducted and elevated; or 3) adducted at the side with the scapula rotated downward (Saidoff & McDonough, 1997, p. 196).

Unlike the hip joint, another ball and socket joint, the stability of the glenohumeral joint is not accomplished due to the articulation of bony segments but is achieved instead by the muscles and soft tissues of and around the glenohumeral joint. Joint stability is achieved dynamically by the rotator cuff muscles (supraspinatus, infraspinatus, teres minor, subscapularis [SITS]), the biceps tendon and the glenohumeral joint capsule, which attaches around the glenoid rim, arises from the glenoid fossa, and inserts into the anatomical neck of the humerus. When these muscles contract simultaneously, the humeral head is pressed into the glenoid socket. By selective contraction of these muscles to resist displacing forces (as when the lateral deltoid initiates shoulder abduction), the supraspinatus muscle and the long biceps tendon actively resist displacement of the humeral head relative to the fossa. When the pectoralis major and anterior deltoid elevate and flex the shoulder, they tend to push the humeral head posteriorly out the back of the fossa. This displacement is resisted by subscapularis, infraspinatus, and teres minor muscles (Saidoff & McDonough, 1997).

The tendon of the biceps brachii muscle arches over the head of the humerus and under the joint capsule. When there is a strong contraction of the biceps muscle, as in flexion with a load in the hand, there is depression of the head of the humerus, which prevents elevation of the humeral head (Nordin & Frankel, 1989).

Supraspinatus, infraspinatus, and teres minor are the major structures limiting internal rotation during the first half of abduction. Once abduction or flexion occurs, the passive support of the superior joint capsule and supraspinatus muscle is eliminated and stabilization is due to muscles.

Zuckerman and Masten identified five factors that are important for the stability of the glenohumeral joint:
1. Adequate size of the glenoid fossa.
2. Posterior tilt of the glenoid fossa; these authors cite a finding from Saha where anteriorly tilted glenoid fossae were found in 80% of 21 unstable shoulders as compared with 27% of 50 normal shoulders.
3. Humeral head retroversion.
4. Intact capsule and glenoid labrum.
5. Function of muscles that control the anterioposterior position of the humeral head (Nordin & Frankel, 1989, p. 230).

Static stability of the humeral head on the glenoid fossa is accomplished when gravity pulls downward in a direction parallel to the humeral shaft (negative translatory force) creating adduction (counterclockwise torque). Gravity is offset by the superior joint capsule, superior and middle portions of the glenohumeral ligaments and by the coracohumeral ligaments, which are tight when the arm is adducted. This provides stabilization as well as limiting external rotation in the lower ranges of abduction. If the limb has external loads applied in addition to gravity, supraspinatus contracts to aid with stabilization and may be assisted by the posterior deltoid. Supraspinatus and posterior deltoid also help to prevent downward displacement of the humerus (Figure 5-3A, B).

The coracohumeral ligament and the acromion of the scapula form an arch which prevents excessive upward dislocation of the humeral head. In addition, the coracohumeral ligaments blend with the rotator cuff muscles, which provide stability superiorly and joins with the joint capsule. When the humerus is externally rotated, flexed, or extended, the coracohumeral ligament gets taut and this helps to resist inferior subluxation and downward displacement of the humerus. This is considered the most important ligamental structure in maintaining glenohumeral integrity and stabilization (Gench et al., 1995).

The glenohumeral ligament is part of the glenoid labrum and it has three parts: superior, inferior, and middle. The superior and middle portions tighten on external rotation, thereby providing anterior stabilization. The inferior portion is taut when the arm is abducted to 90 degrees or more, providing anterior and posterior stabilization to the joint.

Since this ball and socket joint is a synovial joint with a joint capsule and synovial fluid, friction is decreased. In addition, more movement is available due to the subacromial bursa, which comprise the subacromial and subdeltoid bursae. These bursae allow small motions between the rotator cuff and the acromion and the acromioclavicular joints. The subscapular bursae protect the tendon of the subscapularis muscle and go under the coracoid and the neck of the humerus.

Osteokinematics: Glenohumeral Joint

The glenohumeral joint permits rotation around all three axes, all of which pass through the head of the humerus (Figure 5-4). Glenohumeral flexion and extension move the humerus in a sagittal plane around a coronal axis, glenohumeral abduction and adduction move the humerus in a coronal plane around a sagittal axis, and internal and external rotation of the humerus moves the humerus in a horizontal plane around a vertical axis. The close packed position of the joint in which the bones have the greatest congruency is in maximum abduction and external rotation. Accessory movements of the glenohumeral joint are possible in the loose packed position of 55 degrees of abduction and 30 degrees of horizontal adduction.

Arthrokinematics: Glenohumeral Joint

The glenohumeral joint is a ball and socket, freely movable, synovial joint with 3 degrees of freedom or motion in all planes. The joint surfaces engage in all types of movements to include

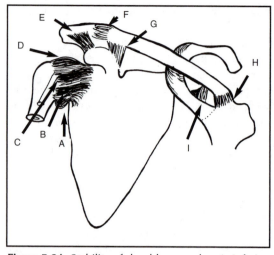

Figure 5-3A. Stability of shoulder complex. A. Inferior glenohumeral ligament; B. Middle glenohumeral ligament; C. Superior glenohumeral ligament; D. Coracohumeral ligaments; E. Coracoacromial ligament; F. Acromioclavicular ligament; G. Coracoclavicular ligament, made up of trapezoid and conoid ligaments; H. Sternoclavicular ligaments; I. Costoclavicular ligaments.

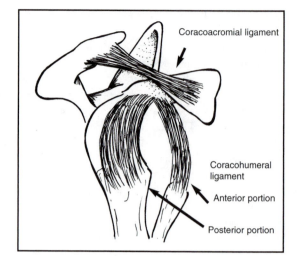

Figure 5-3B. Lateral aspect.

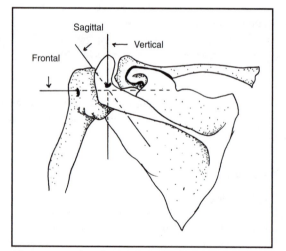

Figure 5-4. Glenohumeral axes of motion.

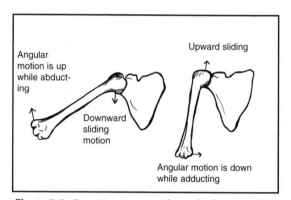

Figure 5-5. Convex-concave rule applied to shoulder motions.

rolling, spinning, and gliding and combinations of these to produce the wide variety of movements seen at this joint. While the movements at the glenohumeral articulation of rolling, spinning, and gliding occur, rotation is the primary movement. Since the convex head of the humerus is not parallel to the concave glenoid fossa, rotation of the joint cannot take place as pure spin but requires that motions of the humerus be accompanied by combined rolling and gliding of the head of the humerus on the glenoid fossa in a direction opposite to the movement of the shaft of the humerus (Norkin & Levangie, 1992). This prevents impaction of the

humeral head on either the acromion or the coracoacromial ligament in the normal glenohumeral joint (Norkin & Levangie, 1992) (Figure 5-5).

With the physiologic motions of the humerus, the convex head of the humerus slides in the opposite direction of the shaft of the humerus. For example, during shoulder abduction, when the humerus moves up, the head of the humerus slides inferiorly. Likewise, during adduction as the arm comes to rest at the side of the body, the humeral head slides upward or superiorly. However, when the humerus is stabilized and the scapula moves, the concave

Table 5-1.

PHYSIOLOGIC MOTION OF THE HUMERUS

Motion of Humerus	*Slide of Humeral Head*
If flex humerus	head of humerus moves posteriorly
If extend humerus	head of humerus moves anteriorly
If IR humerus	head of humerus moves posteriorly
If ER humerus	head of humerus moves anteriorly
If horizontal abduction	head of humerus moves posteriorly
If horizontal adduction	head of humerus moves anteriorly
If abduct humerus	head of humerus moves inferiorly (down)
If adduct humerus	head of humerus moves superiorly

glenoid fossa slides in the same direction as the scapula (Kisner & Colby, 1990). This information is invaluable to the therapist who is trying to provide mobilization to the shoulder by means of passive ROM or soft tissue stretching (Table 5-1).

Acromioclavicular Joint

The acromioclavicular is a small joint formed by the articulation of the acromial (lateral) end of the clavicle with the acromion of the scapula. Articular disks may or may not be present at this articulation. At the acromioclavicular joint, ligaments suspend the scapula from the clavicle. Like the glenohumeral joint, the articular capsule is weak and due to the size and shapes of articulating bones, this joint is considered to be incongruent (Norkin & Levangie, 1992). The joint position of greatest stability is the close packed position, which is 30 to 90 degrees of glenohumeral abduction (Hartley, 1995). The weak joint capsule is reinforced by the *superior and inferior acromioclavicular ligaments*, which restrict anteriorposterior horizontal movements of the joint. The trapezius and deltoid muscles add to the stability of the superior portion of the joint.

The *coracoclavicular ligament* serves as the primary stabilizer of the joint because it connects the coracoid process and the clavicle. The coracoclavicular ligament has two parts:
1. The conoid ligament, located more medially, which aids in producing the motions of protraction/retraction by producing posterior rotation of the clavicle. This ligament also serves to restrict inferior separation of scapula from clavicle.
2. The trapezoid ligament, which is located lateral to the conoid ligament, tends to restrict medial displacement of scapula on the clavicle. Nordin and Frankel (1992) describe the action of this ligament as "a hinge for scapular motion about a transverse (horizontal) axis in the frontal plane" (p. 231).

When the acromioclavicular joint is dislocated, it is often due to a torn coracoclavicular ligament. The ligaments together contribute to the horizontal stability of the joint and are critical to pre-venting superior dislocation of the clavicle on the acromion (Norkin & Levangie, 1992). Both the conoid and trapezoid ligaments limit scapular rotation and these ligaments assist in transmission of compression forces from the scapula to the clavicle (Norkin & Levangie, 1992).

Osteokinematics

The acromioclavicular joint is a gliding joint with 3 degrees of freedom in three axes of motion. Movements of this articulation are seen as two different types: 1) a gliding motion of the clavicle and the acromion, and 2) rotation of the scapula on the clavicle (Goss, 1976). Because the articulating surfaces of this articulation are small and there are wide individual variations, there are inconsistencies in identifying the movements and axes of motion for this joint (Norkin & Levangie, 1992). Rotation of the scapula is the primary motion of the acromioclavicular joint, followed by tipping and winging.

Scapular rotation occurs around an anterioposterior axis and allows the glenoid to tilt upward or downward. Hamill defines this movement as "swinging out and back in the frontal plane" and this motion is accomplished by having the trapezoid ligament act as a hinge for this scapular motion (Nordin & Frankel, 1989) (Figure 5-6A-C).

Winging of the scapula is usually a term applied to a pathological condition whereby the medial border of the scapula moves away from the chest wall (Magee, 1992). While Nordin and Frankel (1989) indicate that there is no consensus regarding a label for this motion, it is defined as "the normal posterior movement of the vertebral border of the scapula (or anterior movement of the glenoid fossa) that must occur to maintain the contact of the scapula with the horizontal curvature of the thorax as the scapula slides around the thorax in abduction and adduction" (p. 215). The motion of abduction (protraction) and adduction (retraction) is accomplished by the conoid ligament, which acts as a longitudinal (vertical) axis for scapular rotation (Nordin & Frankel, 1989).

Tipping is similar to winging of the scapula but is defined as "posterior displacement of the inferior angle of the scapula" (Konin, 1999). According to Norkin and Levangie (1992), both winging and tipping of the scapula function to position the glenoid fossa toward a more anterior or inferior position as well as changing the position of the humeral head.

The small amount of anterior and posterior movement of acromion (abduction/adduction) keeps the glenoid fossa aligned with the humeral head during flexion and abduction, which is permitted and initiated by anterior and posterior acromioclavicular ligaments and coracoclavicular (conoid and trapezoid) ligaments.

Arthrokinematics

Movements at the acromioclavicular joint involve the convex portion on the lateral end of the clavicle and a concave facet on the acromion. The movements of tipping, rotation, and winging of the scapula and the clavicle are in the same direction. For example, if the scapula rotates downward, then the clavicle also rotates in a downward direction.

Figure 5-6A. Acromioclavicular Joint Axes. Frontal Axis.

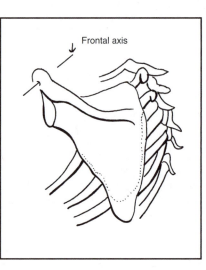

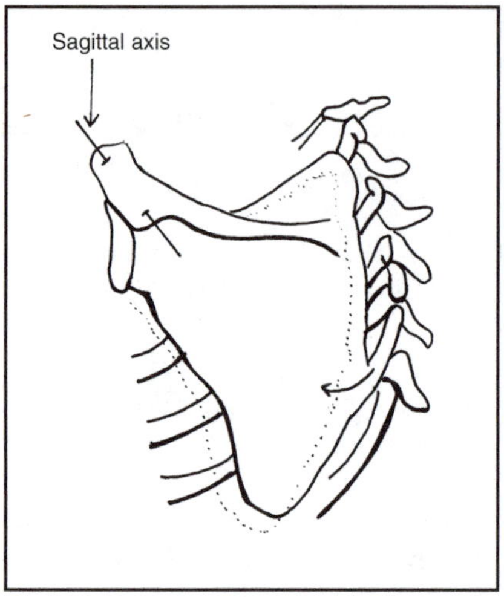

Figure 5-6B. Sagittal axis.

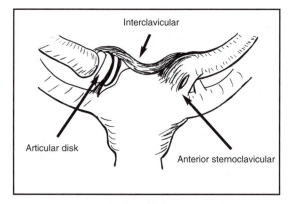

Figure 5-6C. Vertical axis.

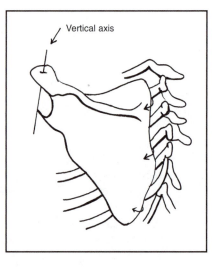

Figure 5-7. Ligaments of the sternoclavicular joint.

Sternoclavicular Joint

The sternoclavicular joint is the articulation of clavicle and manubrium of sternum and first rib cartilage. This is the only true bony articulation of the shoulder girdle with the trunk and is considered the "base of operation" (Nordin & Frankel, 1989).

There are intra-articular discs between manubrium, first costal cartilage, and clavicle. These disks divide the sternoclavicular joint into two functional units for gliding.

The first unit is at the sternal end of the clavicle. This is considered an incongruous joint because not all of the articulating surfaces are in contact. In fact, the superior portion of the medial clavicle serves only as an attachment for the disk and the interclavicular ligament and does not contact the sternum at all (Nordin & Frankel, 1989).

The second unit is formed by the manubrium of the sternum and the first costal cartilage. These two saddle-shaped surfaces permit the movement of the clavicle on the disk and of the disk on the sternum. Since this articulation is considered incongruous, stabilization depends upon ligaments. The ligaments providing stability are the articular capsule, sternoclavicular ligaments, interclav-

icular ligament, costoclavicular ligament and the articular disk (Figure 5-7).

The articular capsule varies in thickness and strength and forms the anterior and posterior sternoclavicular ligaments. The ligaments and capsule are reinforced by attachment of the sternocleidomastoid muscle.

The sternoclavicular joint is supported by *anterior and posterior sternoclavicular ligaments*, which attach the clavicle to sternum and reinforce the joint capsule. The anterior ligament covers the anterior surface of the articulation, while the posterior portion of the joint is covered by the posterior ligament. This ligament tends to limit rotation of sternoclavicular joint during depression of clavicle and the posterior sternoclavicular ligament is the strongest, preventing upward and lateral displacement of clavicle.

The *interclavicular ligament* is a curved ligament that goes from the superior portion of sternal end of one clavicle to that of the other. Due to the attachment to the superior margin of sternum, the interclavicular ligament serves to limit shoulder depression or downward glide along with the articular disk, which helps to protect the brachial plexus and subclavian artery (Norkin & Levangie, 1992).

The *articular disk* or meniscus increases contact between incongruous joint surfaces. The disk also limits shoulder depression as well as serving as a hinge for motion and as a shock absorber for forces transmitted along the clavicle from the lateral end (Nordin & Frankel, 1989; Norkin & Levangie, 1992). Due to the attachments of the disk above, below, and to the sternoclavicular and interclavicular ligaments, the disk also adds strength to the joint and helps to prevent medial displacement of the clavicle.

In elevation and depression, the medial clavicle glides in a superior to inferior direction on the upper attachment of the disk; in protraction and retraction, the clavicle and disk glide anterioposteriorly on the manubrium as a unit, pivoting around the inferior attachment of the disk. It can be considered that the disk functions as part of the manubrium during elevation and depression and acts as a part of the clavicle during protraction and retraction. Because of this changing function of the disk, mobility of the joint is maintained and stability is enhanced (Norkin & Levangie, 1992).

The *costoclavicular ligament* provides an axis for the movements elevation and depression and for protraction and retraction. This ligament serves to limit clavicular elevation and superior glide of clavicle (Norkin & Levangie, 1992) and is considered the "principle stabilizing structure" (Nordin & Frankel, 1989) of the joint. The costoclavicular ligament assists in restricting upward displacement and downward rotation of the medial clavicle by its attachment to the superiormedial part of first rib carriage and to costal tuberosity of inferior surface of clavicle.

Osteokinematics

While the sternoclavicular joint is an incongruent saddle-shaped (sellar) joint, it acts like a double gliding joint, or as some authors suggest, as a modified ball and socket joint (Greene & Roberts, 1999). As such, this joint can move in all axes with 3 degrees of freedom. The movements of elevation and depression, protraction and retraction are described by the movement of the distal segment of the lever, i.e., the movements are visualized as movements of the lateral end of the clavicle (Nordin & Frankel, 1989). In addition, rotation of the clavicle around its own longitudinal axis occurs, but as an accessory motion when the humerus is elevated above 90 degrees and the scapula is upwardly rotated (Kisner & Colby, 1990).

Elevation and depression occur in the sagittal axis. Scapular elevation of 30 to 45 degrees occurs during 30 to 90 degrees of glenohumeral elevation. Further elevation is limited by costoclavicular and interclavicular ligaments and subclavius muscle. The clavicle moves on the disk as a hinge and there is superior-inferior gliding between clavicle and meniscus or disk. The axis is oblique through the sternal end of clavicle and takes a backward and downward course. Due to this orientation, elevation is actually an upward-backward movement and depression a movement in a forward-downward direction. Depression has a range of 5 to 15 degrees and the motion of the clavicle is stopped by the first rib.

Protraction and retraction occur between the articular cartilage, disk, and sternum in a nearly vertical axis, which produces an anterior-posterior gliding as the disk moves with clavicle on the manubrium. The vertical axis lies at the costoclavicular ligament. The ROM for protraction is 0 to 15 degrees, with further movement limited by posterior sternoclavicular ligament and costoclavicular ligament. Retraction also has a range of 0 to 15 degrees, with the anterior sternoclavicular ligament restraining further movement (Smith et al., 1996).

Approximately 30 to 40 degrees of transverse rotation of scapula on the clavicle occurs around the long axis of the clavicle following 90 degrees of shoulder flexion or abduction. This motion occurs in a frontal axis as the disk and clavicle roll on the sternum. This rotational element is essential for full flexion or abduction and should the rotation not occur, only 110 degrees of flexion or abduction would be possible (Smith et al., 1996). Upward rotation occurs due to the tightening of acromioclavicular ligament (trapezoid and conoid). As the conoid ligament tightens, this becomes the axis for upward rotation of the sternoclavicular joint. Given the "s" shape of the clavicle, the acromial end is higher and therefore able to further elevation and upwardly rotate the scapula.

Arthrokinematics

Given that the medial end of the clavicle is convex top to bottom (superiorly to inferiorly) and concave front to back (anterior to posterior), and that the manubrium and first costal cartilages are concave top to bottom and convex front to back, the physiologic motions of the clavicle depend upon the direction of slide of the clavicle on the manubrium.

Since there is a convex superior-inferior clavicular surface and concave surface formed by manubrium and first costal cartilage in a frontal plane around a sagittal, anterior-posterior axis and with inferior-superior motion of the clavicle, arthrokinematically the convex surface of the clavicle must slide on the concave manubrium and first costal cartilage in the direction opposite to movement of the lateral head of the clavicle. For example, elevation of the clavicle results in a downward sliding of the medial clavicular surface on manubrium and first costal cartilage (Kisner & Colby, 1990; Nordin & Frankel, 1989). Conversely, the medial end of anterioposterior clavicle is concave and the manubrial side is convex; arthrokinematically the clavicular surface will now slide on manubrium and first costal cartilage in the same direction as the lateral end of the clavicle. The movement of these surfaces allows protraction/retraction or horizontal forward/backward motion in a horizontal plane around a vertical axis. For example, protraction of the clavicle is accompanied by anterior sliding of the medial clavicle on the manubrium and first costal cartilage (Kisner & Colby, 1990; Nordin & Frankel, 1989).

Rotation of the scapula around its own axis results in a spin motion. This rotation occurs in one direction only from posterior placement to neutral position, which brings the anterior surface of the clavicle facing toward the front or anteriorly (Nordin & Frankel, 1989).

Combined Movements of Sternoclavicular and Acromioclavicular Joints

Motion at the sternoclavicular joint is reciprocal, with the acromioclavicular joint for protraction and retraction and elevation/depression; however, this reciprocity is not true for rotational movement. For example, if the clavicle moves up at the medial end, it moves down at the lateral end.

COMBINED MOTIONS AT THE SHOULDER JOINT

The shoulder girdle is capable of such mobility due to the integrated, coordinated, and synchronous action of all of the joints acting together. The contributions of each joint at any time are dependent upon the plane and axis of motion, the amount of elevation of the humerus, the total load applied to the extremity, and individual anatomical variations (Hamil & Knutzen, 1995; Kisner & Colby, 1990). The contributions of the acromioclavicular and sternoclavicular joints are that movement at these joints permits movement of the scapula, which places the glenoid fossa facing downward, upward, or forward while the costal surfaces remain close to the thorax for stabilization.

Movement at the scapula occurs because when a muscle contracts, whether the origin or insertion moves depends upon which moves easier (Greene & Roberts, 1999). In addition, the acceleration is related to its mass according to Newton's Second Law "since the scapula is less massive than the entire upper extremity when the glenohumeral muscles contract, they move the scapula unless other factors intervene" (Greene & Roberts, 1999, p. 83).

The contributions from these joints allow the synchronous gliding of the scapula, which permits the humerus to move freely in a large arc of motion at the glenohumeral joint.

Scapulohumeral (Scapulothoracic) Rhythm

The scapulothoracic joint, with the acromioclavicular and sternoclavicular joints, contributes to the motions of flexion and abduction of the humerus, which elevates the arm by upwardly rotating the glenoid fossa for a total of 60 degrees from resting position. The glenohumeral joint then moves an additional 120 degrees to give total ROM for flexion and abduction 180 degrees (Nordin & Frankel, 1989). This relationship of glenohumeral contribution to shoulder motion with scapulothoracic, acromioclavicular, and sternoclavicular motions is called *scapulothoracic* or *scapulohumeral rhythm*. Overall, the ratio of glenohumeral contribution to scapulothoracic is a 2 to 1 ratio, i.e., if there is 15 degrees of motion, 10 degrees are due to the glenohumeral joint and 5 degrees are due to the scapulothoracic articulations. This ratio has been disputed, with some authors stating the ratio is 3:2, while others state the ratio is closer to 5:4 (Nordin & Frankel, 1989; Norkin & Levangie, 1992; Smith et al., 1996). Some of the differences are due to the measurement of abduction (measured in the plane of the scapula and in the frontal plane, which yields different values for ROM) and due to the fact that each joint contributes differently to the motion depending upon when in the arc of motion the measurement is taken. Not only do the glenohumeral and scapulothoracic joints contribute differently, so do the sternoclavicular and acromioclavicular joints. Hamil and Knutzen (1995, p. 150) indi-

cate that for flexion and abduction of the humerus, of the 60 degrees contributed by the sternoclavicular and acromioclavicular joints, 65% of the motion was due to the sternoclavicular joint and 35% was due to the acromioclavicular joint, although the amount of contribution of these joints is also disputed (Hamil & Knutzen, 1995; Smith et al., 1996). It is important to realize, too, that these synchronous and coordinated movements occur concomitantly and not sequentially, which produces smooth movements.

Norkin and Levangie (1992) identified three purposes of scapulothoracic rhythm:
1. By distributing motion between two joints, this permits large ROM with less compromise of stability than would occur if the same ROM occurred in one joint.
2. Maintaining the glenoid fossa in optimal position to receive the head of humerus increases joint congruency while decreasing shear forces.
3. Permitting muscles acting on the humerus to maintain good length-tension relationships, which minimizes or prevents active insufficiency of glenohumeral muscles.

The coordinated actions can be visualized by separating humeral flexion and abduction into four phases (Caillet, 1980). In phase 1 of abduction, the arm is held at the side in full adduction. There is no abduction of the humerus, no scapular rotation, no movement at the glenohumeral, sternoclavicular, scapulothoracic, or acromioclavicular joints (Figure 5-8).

In phase 2, considered the "setting phase" (Norkin & Levangie, 1992), the initial portion of movement occurs within the first 30 degrees of humeral abduction or first 45 to 60 degrees of flexion (Hamil & Knutzen, 1995). At this point, the scapula moves toward or away from the vertebral column in order to find a position of stability on the thorax (Hamil & Knutzen, 1995; Norkin & Levangie, 1992). A force couple is formed by the trapezius muscle and the serratus anterior muscle, which produces movement at the sternoclavicular and acromioclavicular joints, ultimately producing 60 degrees of upward rotation (Norkin & Levangie, 1992). The upper and lower trapezius and the upper and lower serratus anterior apply a rotary force on the scapula at the acromioclavicular joint, but movement is prevented by the conoid and trapezoid (coracoclavicular) ligaments. The movements that do occur at the acromioclavicular joint are 10 degrees of winging and tipping of the scapula, which maintains the scapula against the ribs. The spinoclavicular angle (from the spine of the scapula to the clavicle) increases by 10 degrees. The outer end of the clavicle is elevated 12 to 15 degrees, but there is no clavicular rotation (Figure 5-9).

In phase 3, the humerus moves an additional 60 degrees, so total abduction is 90 degrees. Of this 90 degrees of total humeral abduction, 60 degrees are due to movement at the glenohumeral joint and 30 degrees are due to scapulothoracic contributions. The scapula will then move laterally, anteriorly, or superiorly during movements of upward rotation, protraction (abduction), and elevation. The upward rotary force created by serratus anterior and trapezius muscles continues, and this produces movement at the sternoclavicular joint, which forces the clavicle to elevate. Since the clavicle is attached to the scapula, elevation of the clavicle produces elevation of the scapula as it is carried through 30 degrees

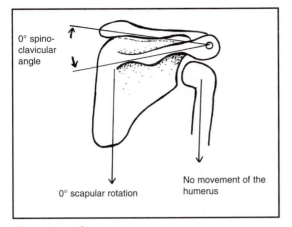

Figure 5-8. Phase 1.

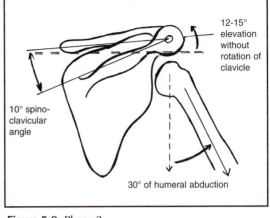

Figure 5-9. Phase 2.

of upward rotation. Further elevation of the clavicle is prevented when the costoclavicular ligament becomes taut (Norkin & Levangie, 1992). There is no change in the movement in the acromioclavicular joint and no increase in the spinoclavicular angle (Figure 5-10).

Maximal ROM for abduction requires external rotation of the humerus in order for the greater tubercle of the humerus to clear coracoacromial arch once the arm is elevated above the horizontal. If there is weakness or inadequate external rotation, there will be impingement of soft tissues in suprahumeral space, causing pain, inflammation, and loss of function (Kisner & Colby, 1990). Once the humerus is externally rotated, an additional 30 degrees of abduction is possible.

Similarly, internal rotation of the humerus is required to achieve full elevation through flexion and this rotation occurs at 50 degrees of passive shoulder. Since most of the shoulder flexor muscles are also medial rotators, as the arm elevates above horizontal in sagittal plane, the anterior capsule and ligaments get taut, causing humerus to medially rotate (Kisner & Colby, 1990).

Phase 4 completes the abduction range to 180 degrees, with the glenohumeral joint providing 120 degrees of the total and the scapulothoracic joints contributing 60 degrees. The coracoid process of scapula is pulled down, tugging on coracoclavicular ligament (Figure 5-11A, B).

Thirty degrees of clavicular rotation occurs around the longitudinal axis, which elevates the lateral end of the clavicle without additional elevation of the sternoclavicular joint. Since the lateral end of the clavicle is elevated, the scapula will be carried through an additional 20 degrees of upward rotation around an anterior-posterior axis through the acromioclavicular joint, where the scapula will reach the maximum of 20 degrees of tip and 40 degrees of winging.

Given that 180 degrees is considered the maximum range of motion for humeral abduction and flexion (some sources say 170 degrees with the additional 10 degrees due to trunk movement), horizontally 60 degrees of glenohumeral and 30 degrees of scapulothoracic motion occurred, with scapular movement due to clav-

icular elevation at the sternoclavicular joint; horizontally to vertically, an additional 60 degrees of glenohumeral motion (plus medial rotation in the sagittal plane for flexion and lateral rotation for abduction in frontal plane), and 30 degrees of scapular movement due to clavicular rotation and acromioclavicular motion (Norkin & Levangie, 1992) (Table 5-2).

A summary of values of ROM for each motion follows:
- Glenohumeral flexion or abduction 120 degrees
- Glenohumeral external or internal rotation 70 to 90 degrees
- Clavicular backward rotation 30 to 50 degrees
- Clavicular elevation 30 to 60 degrees
- Scapular upward rotation 30 to 60 degrees

INTERNAL KINETICS

During hand use, there are large forces that occur in the shoulder because the resistance arm of the lever that is formed can be 2 feet with a tool but the force arms of the muscles are measured in inches (Smith et al., 1996). Calculating the reaction forces of the shoulder is challenging because of the large number of muscles, and the force contribution of each muscle varies with differing loads, planes of shoulder elevation, and degrees of elevation (Nordin & Frankel, 1989). Smith et al. (1996) indicate that the greatest strength of shoulder muscles occurs when muscles contract in an elongated position and torque decreases as the muscles shorten. They add that favorable length-tension relationships over such a large ROM is accomplished by movement of the base of support of the humerus by the scapula and by changes in muscle lever arms. For example, lever arm lengths for the deltoid increased with the motion of abduction; the middle deltoid almost doubled its leverage, and the anterior deltoid increased leverage by eight times (p. 256). Hamil and Knutzen (1995) indicate that the greatest strength output in the shoulder muscles occurs in adduction due to latissimus dorsi, teres major, and pectoralis muscles acting as major contributors. The strength of adduction is twice that of abductor strength even though abduction is used more frequently in activities of daily living or sport (p. 156).

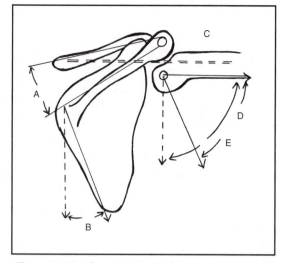

Figure 5-10. Phase 3. A. 10 degree spinoclavicular angle (no change from Phase 2); B. 30 degrees of scapular rotation; C. 30 degrees of clavicular elevation; D. 60 degrees of glenohumeral movement; E. 90 degrees abduction of humerus.

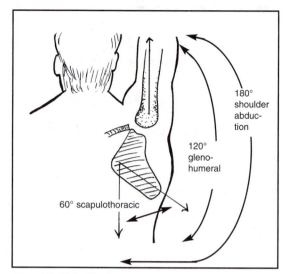

Figure 5-11A. Phase 4.

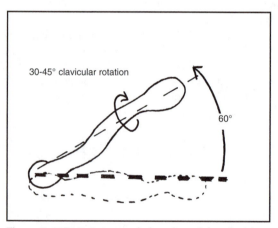

Figure 5-11B. Rotation and elevation of the clavicle.

Extension is the next strongest action because muscles of extension involve the same muscle as adduction. Extension is seen as slightly stronger than flexion. The weakest muscles of the shoulder are the rotators. The muscles of external rotation are weaker than the muscles of internal rotation. The motions of internal and external rotation are most influenced by arm position, with the greatest internal rotation occurring in neutral and the greatest external rotation in 90 degrees of flexion (Hamil & Knutzen, 1995). Rotator cuff muscles as a group can generate forces of 9.6 times the weight of the limb. Since each arm weighs 7% of body weight, the rotator cuff muscles can generate forces in the shoulder joint of approximately 70% of body weight. Forces in the shoulder joint at 90 degrees of abduction have been shown to be close to 90% of body weight, whereas the forces are diminished to half of that if forearm flexes to 90 degrees at elbow (Hamil & Knutzen, 1995).

Nordin and Frankel (1989) indicate that muscle actions at the shoulder have three unusual aspects:

1. Since glenohumeral joint lacks rigid stability, muscles exerting an effect on the humerus must act in concert with other muscles to avoid producing a dislocating force on the joint.
2. The existence of multiple linkages in the shoulder (clavicle, humerus, scapula) gives rise to an interesting situation in which a single muscle may span several joints, exerting an effect on each.
3. The extensive range of shoulder motion causes muscle function to vary depending on the position of the arm in space.

While it is generally true that one can infer the action of a muscle given knowledge of origin and insertion, this is not always the case in shoulder muscles. "For example, when the arm is at the side, contraction of the fibers of the middle portion of the deltoid lifts the humerus along its axis but does not produce the motion of elevation because the line of action of the middle deltoid fibers is essentially parallel to the long axis of the humerus and if 'coupled' with other muscles, elevation can occur" (Nordin & Frankel, 1989, p. 239). A *force couple* is defined as "two forces whose points of application occur on opposite sides of an axis and in opposite directions to produce rotation of the body" (1989). Several examples occur in the shoulder.

The trapezius and serratus anterior muscles form a force couple to produce elevation of the arm due to combining forces to create lateral, superior, and rotational movements of the scapula, producing abduction and upward rotation. The deltoid and supraspinatus muscles contract together to produce abduction or flexion at glenohumeral joint (Smith et al., 1996) "...but their tendency to move the least massive segment rotates the scapula downward; isometric contractions of upward scapular rotators produce scapular stabilization preventing downward rotation while teres minor and deltoid work to depress humeral head and stabilize it" (Greene &

Table 5-2.

SUMMARY OF PHASES OF SHOULDER ABDUCTION

Phase	Humerus	Scapula	Acromioclavicular Joint (Spinoclavicular Angle SCA)	Sternoclavicular Joint	Clavicle	Figure
Phase 1: resting arm	No abduction	0 degree scapular rotation	0 degree spinoclavicular angle	0 degree movement and no elevation of the clavicle	No elevation	Figure 5-8
Phase 2: setting phase	0 to 30 degree abduction	Winging & tipping of scapula	Angle increases 0 to 10 degrees due to rotary force of muscles but movement is minimal due to coracoclavicular ligament	Movement produces elevation	Outer end elevated 12 to 15 degrees No rotation	Figure 5-9
Phase 3	30 to 90 degrees abduction 60 degrees glenohumeral; 30 degrees scapulothoracic External rotation of humerus also occurs for full abduction	0 to 30 degrees scapular rotation	No change in spinoclavicular angle or movement at the acromioclavicular joint	Further movement produces maximal clavicular elevation; further movement prevented by costo-clavicular ligaments	15 to 30 degrees elevation; no rotation	Figure 5-10
Phase 4	90 to 180 degrees abduction 120 degrees glenohumeral 60 degrees scapulo-thoracic (some sources attribute the final 10 degrees of flexion to thoracic spinal movements)	Coracoid depresses	Spinoclavicular angle has increased to 20 degrees due to clavicular rotation; maximal tipping of 20 degrees and wing-ing of 40 degrees	No further elevation due to taut coraco-clavicular and costo-clavicular ligaments	0 to 30 degrees clavicular rotation	Figure 5-11

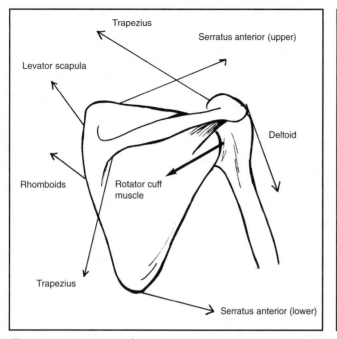

Figure 5-12. Force couples. Trapezius + serratus anterior produce lateral superior and rotational movements of the scapula. Deltoid + supraspinatus produce glenohumeral abduction or flexion. Deltoid + teres minor (rotator cuff) depress humeral head and stabilize it.

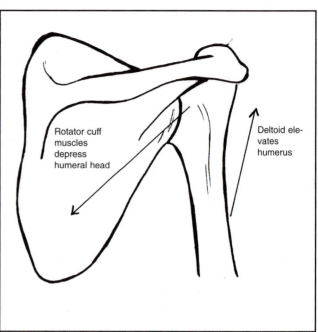

Figure 5-13. Force couple of deltoid and rotator cuff.

Roberts, 1999, p. 83). This tends to illustrate that rotator cuff muscles are unique in that not only do these muscles produce (or contribute) to specific joint motions, but they are also considered dynamic stabilizers of the glenohumeral joint since they combine to stabilize and resist displacement of the humeral head (p. 240). The combinations of movements are achieved by collaboration of many muscles which favorably position the separate joint articulations for greater movement (Figure 5-12). Some muscles act simultaneously and others follow in sequence. In early flexion or abduction, teres minor and deltoid work together to depress the humeral head and stabilize it. Since the muscle force of teres minor is equal and opposite to deltoid, this is a force couple. Subscapularis and infraspinatus muscles join later in flexion or abduction to assist with humeral head stabilization; latissimus dorsi contracts eccentrically to assist with stabilization and this muscle increases in activity as the angle of motion increases; deltoid and rotator cuff work together in flexion and abduction in that the rotator cuff acts to depress the humeral head and the deltoid elevates the arm (Figure 5-13). Serratus anterior and trapezius now form a force couple to create lateral, superior, and rotational movements of scapula after deltoid and teres minor have initiated elevation.

An example of the force couples that operate in the shoulder would be when one places the hand behind the head when combing the hair. There is elbow flexion, sternoclavicular elevation and upward rotation, scapular elevation with upward rotation, and abduction and glenohumeral abduction and external rotation. The biceps muscle is flexing the elbow while the trapezius and serratus anterior are acting as a force couple at the scapula. The deltoid and

supraspinatus are a force couple at the glenohumeral joint, as are infraspinatus and teres minor. When the arm is overhead, there would also be a contraction of the triceps muscle. These muscles all cooperate to enable successful performance in daily activities.

KINETICS

The actions of many muscles working alone or in combination produce movement and stability of the shoulder (Figure 5-14). By knowing the angle of muscle pull, the length and cross section, type of muscle fiber, and location of the muscle in relation to the joint axis, one can tell much about the action and strength of that muscle.

Elevators of the Scapula

Upper Trapezius

Because the upper trapezius attaches on the base of the skull and clavicle, these fibers will pull upward on the clavicle when it contracts. The resolution of the line of pull force on the clavicle is transferred to the scapula via the acromioclavicular joint to elevate the scapula (Gench et al., 1995) (Figure 5-15). The upper trapezius is seen as solely responsible for elevating the lateral angle of the scapula (Jenkins, 1998).

Upper/Lower Trapezius and Serratus Anterior

The upper portions of these muscles form a force couple that moves the scapula in during elevation. These muscles, with levator scapula, support the shoulder girdle against the pull of gravity and act as stabilizing synergists for deltoid action working on the gleno-

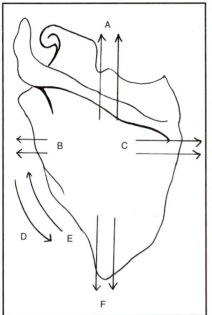

Figure 5-14. Actions of the shoulder muscles. A. Levator scapula, rhomboids trapezius; B. Serratus anterior, pectoralis minor; C. Rhomboids trapezius, levator scapula; D. Levator scapula, rhomboids, pectoralis minor; E. Serratus anterior, trapezius; F. Trapezius, pectoralis major.

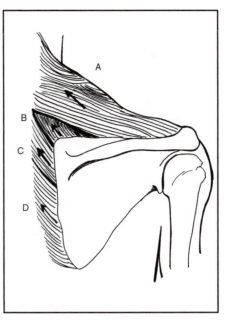

Figure 5-15. Scapular elevators. A. Upper trapezius; B. Levator scapula; C. Rhomboid minor; D. Rhomboid major.

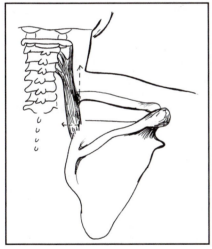

Figure 5-16. Levator scapula force resolution.

this muscle when you palpate in neck region anterior to trapezius but posterior to the sternocleidomastoid (Esch, 1989; Lumley, 1990; Magee, 1992).

Rhomboids (Both Minor and Major)

These two muscles actually function as one muscle. There is a diagonal pull of the muscle that yields both elevation and adduction actions, but the muscle acts only on the medial border of the scapula (Jenkins, 1998). The rhomboids downward rotation of the scapula offsets the undesired force of teres major and contributes to depression of the shoulder. Rhomboids major and minor connect the scapula with the vertebral column and they lie under the trapezius. The upper portion of the muscle is rhomboid minor while the lower portion is rhomboid major (Gench et al., 1995; Hinkle, 1997; Jenkins, 1998; Smith et al., 1996) (Figure 5-17). *Palpation*: The muscles can best be palpated when trapezius is relaxed. Have a subject place his or her hand at small of the back. The therapist then places fingers under medial border of scapula. If subject raises hand just off the small of the back, the rhomboid major contracts as downward rotator and pushes the fingers out from medial border (Esch, 1989; Lumley, 1990; Magee, 1992).

Depressors of the Scapula

Trapezius, Part 4

There is a diagonal force vector with the origin of this muscle lower than insertion so there are two component forces: one directed downward for depression and the other toward the spine for adduction (Gench et al., 1995) (Figure 5-18).

Pectoralis Minor

These fibers are directed downward from the attachment on coracoid and their function as a depressor can be easily seen. Pectoralis minor is entirely covered by pectoralis major (Gench et

humeral joint. This force couple is antagonistic to scapular movement and synergistic to glenohumeral moment, where trapezius and serratus anterior produce scapular upward rotation while preventing undesired motion of the deltoid as it elevates the glenohumeral joint (Nordin & Frankel, 1989; Smith et al., 1996).

Levator Scapula

"When the diagonal line of pull of the muscle is resolved, there is a long vertical component and a relatively short horizontal component. The long vertical component enables levator scapula to be an elevator of the scapula" (Gench et al., 1995) (Figure 5-16). *Palpation*: Levator scapula is covered by the upper trapezius and sternocleidomastoid muscles; in elevation of the shoulder girdle, upper trapezius and levator contract together; it is difficult to isolate and palpate this muscle. By placing the forearm behind you in the small of your back and then shrug the shoulder, you will feel

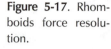

Figure 5-17. Rhomboids force resolution.

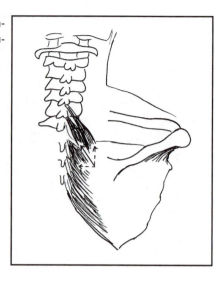

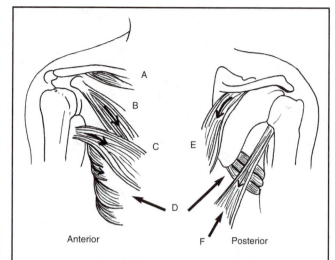

Figure 5-18. Scapular depressors. A. Subclavius; B. Pectoralis minor; C. Pectoralis major (lower portion); D. Serratus anterior; E. Lower trapezius; F. Latissimus dorsi.

al., 1995; Hinkle, 1997; Jenkins, 1998; Smith et al., 1996). *Palpation*: Have the subject place the forearm at small of back, which relaxes pectoralis major. Place a finger just below coracoid process. When the subject lifts the arm off of the back, the tendon of pectoralis minor becomes taut.

Subclavius

Although small, there is a downward force when the line of pull is resolved, making the subclavius a weak depressor (Gench et al., 1995).

Pectoralis

"Inferior fibers of pectoralis major protracts the scapula as it assists in depressing it" (Jenkins, 1998). While the pectoralis major assists the deltoid with flexion of the humerus, the sternal and abdominal portions serve as depressors of shoulder complex (Norkin & Levangie, 1992). Both portions depress the shoulder complex in weight bearing on the hands, while anterior and posterior movement of the humerus and abduction and adduction of the scapula are neutralized (Gench et al., 1995; Hinkle, 1997; Jenkins, 1998; Smith et al., 1996). *Palpation*: This muscle is easily observed and palpated since it is superficial in location and bulk. The upper portion can be seen when the arm is brought obliquely upward toward the head against resistance. The lower portion contracts separately when the arm is adducted in a lower position.

Latissimus Dorsi

Latissimus dorsi is the broadest muscle of the back. It is a thin, sheet-like muscle and it forms the posterior fold of the axilla. Latissimus dorsi and teres major contract when adduction or extension is resisted, as when the subject presses down on the examiner's shoulder. Latissimus dorsi is seen to "retract the scapula as it depresses it" (Jenkins, 1998) and serves to adduct and medially rotate as well as extend the humerus and adduct and depress the scapula (Smith et al., 1996). Some studies say latissimus dorsi is active in abduction and flexion of the arm and may contribute to joint stability because compression of the glenohumeral joint occurs when the arm is overhead (Smith et al., 1996). Latissimus

dorsi attaches to the crest of the ilium so when the arms are stabilized, the distal attachment can aid in lifting the pelvis, as occurs when a client places his or her hands on the armrests of a wheelchair. This is helpful in that the client can do a sitting pushup for pressure relief. This is also useful for clients with injuries to the spinal cord C8 and below because latissimus dorsi is innervated by the thoracodorsal nerve (C6, C7, C8) (Gench et al., 1995; Hinkle, 1997; Jenkins, 1998; Smith et al., 1996).

Protraction (Abduction)

Pectoralis Major

The fibers of the pectoralis major pull downward, inward and forward. Parts of this muscle pull the coracoid medially which enables the scapula to slide laterally along the ribs while the acromion glides forward against the distal end of the clavicle (Gench et al., 1995). Both the clavicular and the sternocostal portions draw the arm medially, which abducts the scapula (Gench et al., 1995; Hinkle, 1997; Jenkins, 1998; Smith et al., 1996) (Figure 5-19).

Serratus Anterior

Referred to as the "saw" muscle because of the multiple digitations, serratus anterior allows one to raise the arm overhead. Since the fibers are nearly horizontal, this is an effective scapular abductor (Gench et al., 1995). *Palpation*: "The lower digitations can be seen and palpated near their proximal attachment on the ribs when arm is overhead; the middle and upper portions can be palpated in the axilla close to the ribs and posterior to pectoralis major if the arm is elevated to horizontal in the plane of the scapula (between flexion and abduction) and then reach forward. When serratus anterior is injured and this motion is attempted, [pathological] winging of the scapula occurs because the scapula fails to

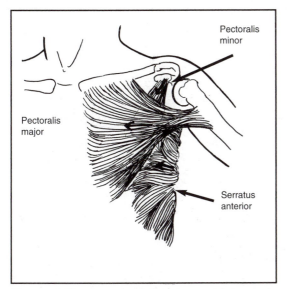

Figure 5-19. Scapular protractors (abductors). Anterior view.

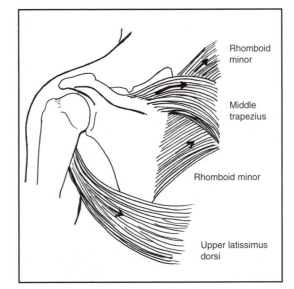

Figure 5-20. Scapular protractors (adductors).

slide forward on the rib and doesn't stay anchored on the thorax" (Gench et al., 1995; Hinkle, 1997; Jenkins, 1998; Smith et al., 1996).

Pectoralis major is cited as a protractor by two authors (Jenkins, 1998; Smith et al., 1996).

Retractors (Adduction)

Rhomboids

The diagonal line of pull of this muscle produces two components, which explains the role in both elevation and adduction actions (Figure 5-20).

Trapezius

The trapezius is a superficial muscle of the neck and upper back, often called the "shawl" muscle. Lower fibers of the trapezius act in upward rotation, adduction, and depression of the scapula, while the middle fibers act in upward rotation and adduction of scapula (Gench et al., 1995; Hinkle, 1997; Jenkins, 1998; Smith et al., 1996). *Palpation*: Have subject abduct shoulder and retract the scapula. If the subject is prone or if the trunk is inclined forward, the muscle works against gravity so the intensity of the contraction increases and the muscle will be more easily identified (Smith et al., 1996). Fibers 2, 3, and 4 function in retraction in the following ways:

- Fiber 2: the fibers are in diagonal direction, which yields two component forces, one of which is directed toward the spine for adduction.
- Fiber 3: fibers are nearly horizontal so this muscle functions only in adduction.
- Fiber 4: diagonal forces with two forces directed down (depression) and toward the spine (adduction) (Esch, 1989; Lumley, 1990; Magee, 1992) (Figure 5-21).

Levator Scapula

This muscle, with a diagonal pull, has a short horizontal component that weakly adducts and long vertical component which elevates (Gench et al., 1995).

Upward Rotation

Trapezius Parts 2,4

Part 2: "This muscle crosses the acromioclavicular joint superior to the sagittal axis of that joint and pulls the acromion toward the neck by pivoting the acromion around its articulation with the clavicle" (Gench et al., 1995, p. 61) (Figure 5-22).

Part 4: "This part of the muscle attaches medially to the acromioclavicular joint and the attachment is from below this joint, so the muscle upwardly rotates by pulling downward on the root or base of the scapular spine" (Gench et al., 1995, p. 60).

Serratus Anterior

These horizontal fibers have a lateral pull on the inferior angle pulling this portion of the medial border laterally and forward to depress the scapula and upwardly rotate the scapula (Jenkins, 1998). "The lower fibers are effective as upward rotators since they exert a lateral pull on the inferior angle" (Gench et al., 1995, p. 64).

Downward Rotation

Rhomboids

Major and minor downward rotation (Figure 5-23) is provided by the lower fibers, which pull medially and upward on inferior angle of the scapula and raise the medial border.

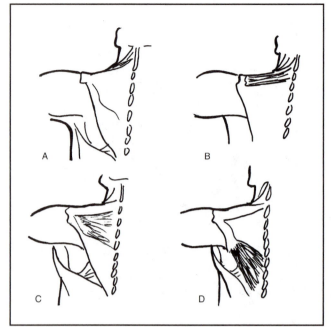

Figure 5-21. Trapezius. A. Part A pulls upward on the clavicle and elevates the scapula. B. Diagonal forces, one of which produces adduction, the other upward rotation; C. Nearly horizontal forces produce adduction; D. Diagonal forces produce depression and adduction, upward rotation.

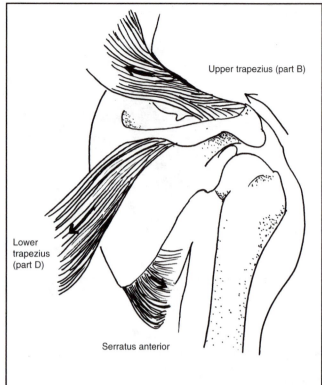

Figure 5-22. Scapular upward rotators.

Levator Scapula

This muscle pulls upward on the vertebral border of the scapula to lower the inferior angle and raise the medial border.

Pectoralis Minor

With a downward pull on the end of the coracoid and the lateral angle, the scapula returns to anatomical position (Gench et al., 1995). Pectoralis major and latissimus dorsi were also identified as downward rotators (Jenkins, 1998) because these muscles pull down on the lateral angle of the scapula.

HUMERUS

Flexors of the Arm

Anterior Deltoid

The deltoid muscle (Figure 5-24) resembles Greek letter Δ in shape and comprises 40% of the mass of the scapulohumeral muscles. The deltoid is responsible for the roundness of shoulder. Its multipennate structure and considerable cross section compensate for small mechanical advantage and less than optimal length tensions. Maintenance of length-tension depends on simultaneous scapular movements and when the scapula is restricted, one can only achieve and barely maintain 90 degrees of glenohumeral abduction (Smith et al., 1996). Full abduction is also dependent upon the rotator cuff muscles because if there are impairments in

these muscles, contraction of the deltoid alone would provide a shrug rather than abduction. The resting length (optimal length-tension) is when the arm is at side whereby the angle of pull is applied as a superior translatory pull on humerus in the plane of the scapula. As a whole, the deltoid abducts the glenohumeral joint while the anterior fibers flex and horizontally adduct the glenohumeral joint. The fibers that run anterior to the frontal axis will flex the humerus and those fibers further from the axis will be the most effective. This muscle is seen by some as the most important flexor of the humerus (Jenkins, 1998). There is too small a rotary component or mechanical advantage to assist with abduction (Gench et al., 1995; Hinkle, 1997; Jenkins, 1998; Smith et al., 1996). *Palpation (anterior):* Move the humerus into a horizontally abducted position and the anterior portion contracts vigorously when horizontal adduction is resisted. *Palpation (middle):* Can be seen when an abducted or adducted position is maintained. *Palpation (posterior):* Seen when hyperextended against resistance or resistance given to horizontal abduction (Esch, 1989; Lumley, 1990; Magee, 1992).

Pectoralis Major–Clavicular Head

Since this muscle crosses the shoulder in front of frontal axis and attaches to the clavicle, it acts as a powerful flexor.

Coracobrachialis

Because of the size and location of the two attachments, this muscle has limited effectiveness; it crosses anterior to the frontal axis so functions in humeral flexion.

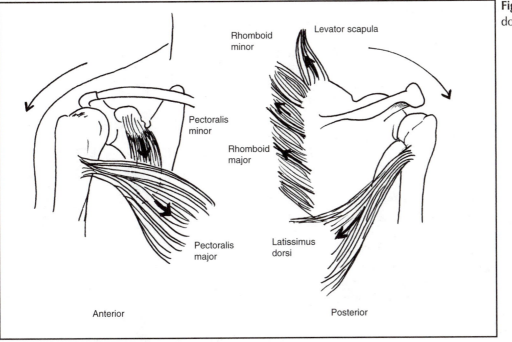

Figure 5-23. Scapular downward rotators.

Rhomboid minor

Levator scapula

Pectoralis minor

Rhomboid major

Pectoralis major

Latissimus dorsi

Anterior

Posterior

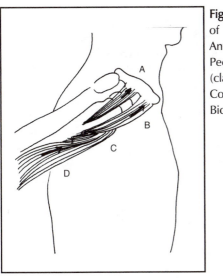

Figure 5-24. Flexors of the humerus. A. Anterior deltoid; B. Pectoralis major (clavicular head); C. Coracobrachialis; D. Biceps brachii.

elbow in extension, thereby putting some stretch on the muscle (Gench et al., 1995). It is important to consider, however, that "complete flexion of the shoulder is impossible when the elbow is extended unless accompanied by medial rotation to diminish the pull of the biceps against front of humerus" (Jenkins, 1998). Biceps can also aid in preventing subluxation of the glenohumeral joint because when the muscle contracts, tension occurs to produce downward and inward force on the head of the humerus, compressing it against the glenoid cavity (Smith et al., 1996).

Extension of the Humerus

Posterior Deltoid

Since the fibers lie posterior to the frontal axis, they function to extend the humerus (Figure 5-25); those fibers further from axis will be more effective in this action and this muscle is capable of extending the humerus back further than other extensors (Gench et al., 1995; Jenkins, 1998).

Coracobrachialis

Because of the size and location of the two attachments, the line of pull of this muscle is quite close to respective axes, and so acts with limited effectiveness to assist other muscles. Not all sources indicate that coracobrachialis is an extensor of the humerus (Gench et al., 1995; Hinkle, 1997; Jenkins, 1998; Smith et al., 1996).

Latissimus Dorsi

This muscle is an excellent extensor because it is located inferior and anterior to the frontal axis and its origin is lower than the insertion.

Palpation: Coracobrachialis is covered by deltoid and pectoralis major. It is possible to palpate this muscle in the distal portion of axillary region if the arm is elevated above the horizontal. Coracobrachialis lies medial and parallel to the tendon of the short head of the biceps, which is seen by supination of forearm and following the short head proximally under muscle where it tapers off (Esch, 1989; Lumley, 1990; Magee, 1992).

Biceps

The line of pull of the biceps fibers is similar to coracobrachialis, and like coracobrachialis, has limited effectiveness as a shoulder flexor. This capacity is enhanced by maintaining the

Pectoralis Major – Sternocostal Fibers

Since the fibers are located anterior to the frontal axis with the origin lower than insertion, these fibers pull downward on the humerus to extend it.

Teres Major

This muscle is located along the axillary border of the scapula and contributes to humeral extension only when resistance is applied to the arm. Teres major also adducts and medially rotates the humerus and is active only in static positions of humerus. The proximal attachment of teres major must be stabilized since unopposed motion would upwardly rotate the scapula (Gench et al., 1995; Hinkle, 1997; Jenkins, 1998; Smith et al., 1996). *Palpate:* Palpate along the inferior aspect of the axillary border of the scapula when prone, with arm hanging over side or in a forward inclined trunk position. If there is internal rotation of the glenohumeral joint, then teres major rises. If you palpate higher on the axillary border and externally rotate, teres minor can be felt as teres major relaxes. Teres major acts in pulling motions when the shoulder is extended or adducted against resistance (Smith et al., 1996).

Triceps – Long Head

Triceps is ineffective as a mover of the humerus because it passes directly over the axis. Since the line of pull passes slightly posteriorly to the frontal axis, triceps contributes to humeral extension. It is possible to increase the effectiveness of triceps in extension by flexing the elbow and thereby putting a stretch on the triceps muscle (Gench et al., 1995).

Abductors of the Humerus

Supraspinatus

Located above the spine of the scapula and hidden by trapezius and deltoid, supraspinatus is an abductor of the glenohumeral joint (Smith et al., 1996). While the supraspinatus fibers are well superior to sagittal axis, there is a pull on head of humerus into glenoid fossa which acts in a complementary way with the deltoid muscle as it initiates abduction (Gench et al., 1995). When the deltoid is paralyzed, supraspinatus alone can bring the humerus through much of range, but it is weak. Supraspinatus also compresses the glenohumeral joint and acts as vertical steerer for humeral head (Smith et al., 1996). *Palpation:* The deepest portion is too deep to palpate, but the more superficial fibers can be felt through the trapezius muscle. Find the spine of the scapula and place your fingers above the spine. Have the subject perform a quick abduction movement in a short range and you will feel momentary contraction of the supraspinatus. You can also test for this by having the subject lie prone with the arm over edge of a table, which causes upward rotation of scapula where one can feel supraspinatus without trapezius.

Deltoid – Middle and Lateral Fibers

As a whole, the deltoid acts as the chief abductor of the glenohumeral joint. The middle portion is the most important as an abductor since most of the anterior and posterior fibers are close to

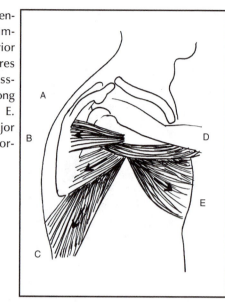

Figure 5-25. Extensors of the humerus. A. Posterior deltoid; B. Teres major; C. Latissimus dorsi; D. Long head of triceps; E. Pectoralis major (sternocostal portion).

axis, which diminishes their effectiveness. In shoulder abduction and flexion, the deltoid contributes half of muscle force for elevation and the contribution increases as abduction increases, with the muscle most active between 90 and 180 degrees. However, the deltoid is most resilient to fatigue at 45 to 90 degrees, so this is the more popular position for arm raising exercises (Hamil & Knutzen, 1995) and is relevant in developing physical abilities in areas of occupation such as combing one's hair or upper extremity dressing.

Biceps Brachii – Long Head

Biceps assists with abduction if the humerus is laterally rotated. It is important to note that lateral rotation of the humerus is always accompanied by complete abduction of the arm to allow the greater tubercle to slide under, and not hit against, the acromion (Jenkins, 1998).

Adductors of the Humerus

Pectoralis Major – Sternal Portions

Since the sternal portions cross inferior to sagittal axis, pectoralis major functions as an adductor muscle (Figure 5-26A, B).

Latissimus Dorsi

Due to its location well inferior to the sagittal axis, latissimus dorsi is a powerful adductor.

Teres Major

"The relationship of the teres major to the three axes of the shoulder is the same as that of the latissimus dorsi and is frequently called the latissimus dorsi's 'little helper'. This conception has been largely in error, however, because the teres major contracts only when resistance has been applied to the arm and only when positions are reached and held in the ranges of movement in adduction, internal rotation and extension" (Gench et al., 1995, p. 75).

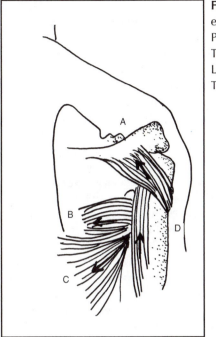

Figure 5-26A. Humeral abductors. A. Posterior deltoid; B. Teres major; C. Latissimus dorsi; D. Triceps (long head).

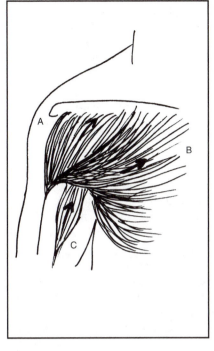

Figure 5-26B. Humeral abductors. A. Anterior deltoid; B. Pectoralis major; C. Coracobrachialis.

Coracobrachialis

This has limited effectiveness and assists with adduction.

Triceps – Long Head

As previously discussed, the triceps is ineffective at the glenohumeral joint and generally is seen to assist with adduction.

Deltoid – Posterior

Deltoid assists with adduction.

Lateral (External) Rotators of the Humerus

Infraspinatus and teres minor are closely related in location and action to externally rotate and adduct the glenohumeral joint. "The infraspinatus and teres minor pass posterior to long axis of the shoulder joint regardless of the position of the humerus to become external rotators and horizontal abductors. That they are not also extensors and adductors or abductors is explained by the fact that they pass directly over both the sagittal and frontal axes of the shoulder" (Gench et al., 1995; Smith et al., 1996). *Palpation*: Some parts are covered by trapezius and posterior deltoid, but most parts are superficial and can be palpated. Have the subject lie prone or stand with the trunk inclined forward and the arm hanging vertically. Find the margin of posterior deltoid and place fingers below deltoid on the scapula near lateral margin. Have the subject externally rotate and these two muscles will rise under the fingers with teres minor next to infraspinatus but farther from spine.

Deltoid – Posterior Fibers

Along with extension and horizontal abduction, the posterior fibers of the deltoid muscle externally rotate the humerus.

Supraspinatus

Due to the distal attachment of posterior portion on the greater tubercle, the line of pull of this muscle is slightly posterior to long axis of the shoulder joint, which makes this muscle an external rotator.

Medial (Internal) Rotators of the Humerus

Subscapularis

Due to the location of this muscle (medial to the long axis and wrapping around anterior the aspect of upper humerus), subscapularis has a medial rotation action.

Pectoralis Major

Since the fibers are anterior relative to the long axis of the glenohumeral joint, the pectoralis major is effective as an internal rotator.

Latissimus Dorsi

The line of pull of this muscle is medial to the long axis when in the anatomical position, so latissimus dorsi medially rotates as it adducts, flexes or extends.

Deltoid – Clavicular Fibers

The clavicular fibers rotate the humerus as it flexes.

Teres Major

Teres major muscle medially rotates with resistance against the arm but is weak for pure medial rotation. Biceps – short head and coracobrachialis muscles have also been indicated as weak medial rotators.

EVALUATION OF THE SHOULDER

Evaluation of the shoulder is complicated by several factors. First, the fact that so many articulations occur at the shoulder and participate in production of a wide variety of movements contribute to the difficulty in evaluation. Evaluation of the acromioclavicular, scapulothoracic, sternoclavicular, and glenohumeral, as well as movement along ribs and thorax, are an essential part of this evaluation.

Second, there are many muscles that add not only to the mobility of the joint but also to the stability. In addition, the function of these muscles varies dependent upon the amount of elevation of the humerus, the load in the distal extremity, the axis of movement, and the position of the scapula. Any interruption in the coordinated synchrony of these muscles and their actions will interfere with shoulder function.

Third, pain is often referred to the shoulder from other areas and the pain experienced in the shoulder region may well be due to lesions and trauma from other structures and organs of the body. For these reasons, the following related problems first must be ruled out prior to attributing the cause of shoulder pain to shoulder girdle joints or muscles:

1. Heart problems: myocardial infarction, angina, pericarditis, which may radiate pain to left shoulder.
2. Lung or diaphragm problems; spontaneous pneumothorax; pulmonary tuberculosis; lung cancer; abscesses; Pancoast tumor, which can relay pain along the same nerve roots of C4 and C5.
3. Chest problems: aortic aneurysm, nodes in the axilla or mediastinum, breast disease, hiatal hernia, which can refer pain to the local area and shoulder.
4. Cervical problems: intervertebral disc herniation or degeneration, facet joint effusion, nerve root irritation, which may also radiate pain to shoulder and scapula.
5. Spinal fracture: cervical or thoracic fracture can radiate pain the shoulder as well as produce local pain.
6. Elbow problems: humeroulnar, humeroradial, or radioulnar joint dysfunction or pathology can also refer pain into shoulder and humerus.
7. Temporalmandibular joint problems due to degeneration or effusion can refer pain down the neck into the shoulder.
8. Rib problems; costovertebral joint or costosternal joint dysfunction.
9. Thoracic spine problems.
10. Abdominal problems: ruptured spleen, pancreas pathology can refer pain to left shoulder; liver pathology and gallbladder disease can refer pain to right shoulder (Hartley, 1995) (Figure 5-27).

It is important to talk with the client to determine specific aspects about the pain that he or she is experiencing. Having the client describe the location, type, and onset of his or her pain can help with the identification of possible causes. Differentiate stiffness from pain and elicit information from the client about the sensations he or she may be experiencing, such as grating, clicking, or snapping sensations.

By observing how the person moves both actively and passively, an understanding of synchronous action of the integrated parts of the shoulder girdle can be determined. Compensatory movements can be observed as clients substitute these motions for impaired function. Information can be obtained as to the stability and symmetry of joint structures.

In particular, look for symmetry at the shoulder level, changes in soft tissue, scapular alignment, observe for scapular winging or tipping that is not related to normal movements at the acromioclavicular joint, and look for normal scapular movements and distraction. General posture and symmetry can influence shoulder motion, and diagnosis by differential tension is used when specific positions are used to determine specific areas of pathology.

By having a client engage in activities relative to areas of meaningful occupation, observation of active, coordinated patterns of movement and substitution as well indications as to how painful the motion is can be obtained. A sense of the client's cooperation is gained as well as a sense of the amount of functional loss and degree of involvement by watching the client move actively.

An assessment of the passive ROM would provide different information about the shoulder joint. When moved passively, there is a pulling of the joint capsule and antagonist ligaments and muscles. If there is pain prior to end range, this may be indicative of acute inflammation. If there is pain as you approach the end range, this may be a subacute condition where there is inflammation but not acute inflammation at this time. The caution at this point is that subacute inflammation can become acute if treatment is too aggressive. If the client does not complain of pain until overpressure at end of range, this is considered a chronic condition where the irritation is minimal unless overpressure is applied. Again, if treatment is too aggressive, chronic inflammation can worsen to subacute or acute levels. The application of overpressure, while not a specific test to identify specific impaired joint structures, is helpful in determining if the end feel of the joint is pathological or physiologically normal.

Capsular pattern problems occur in characteristic proportions and have effects throughout the entire upper extremity. In the shoulder, the greatest limitations that occur due to capsular impairments are seen in limitations in external rotation, then in abduction, followed by impairments in internal rotation and flexion. In the elbow, limitations in both flexion and extension occur, although usually seen more in flexion. Pronation and supination are unaffected. There is an equal amount of limitation in wrist flexion and extension.

SUMMARY

- The shoulder is a complex joint with multiple articulations that enable movement in all planes and axes.
- The sternocostal and vertebrocostal joints enable full shoulder flexion and abduction due to gliding of ribs on sternum and on vertebra.

- The suprahumeral articulation is a functional joint serving in a protective capacity preventing trauma from above, upward dislocation of the humerus, and in limiting abduction of the humerus.
- The scapulothoracic joint is also a functional joint that provides a movable base for the humerus, permitting wide ranges of movement of scapula and thorax. This joint also provides stability in the glenohumeral joint during overhead activities.
- The glenohumeral articulation is an incongruous joint since the bony surfaces are not in direct contact for most movements. Stability is achieved by the joint capsule and muscles of the joint as well as ligaments. Surface motion is mainly rotational but also includes some rolling and gliding. Shoulder motion, especially elevation, is governed by force couples, with the interaction of the deltoid muscle and oblique rotator cuff muscles a good example. Since this is a ball and socket joint, all motions are possible.
- The acromioclavicular joint is also considered to be an incongruent joint and the weak joint capsule is reinforced by ligaments and muscles adding to the stability of the joint. Movements at this joint include rotation of the scapula, tipping, and winging.
- The sternoclavicular joint is the only true articulation of the shoulder girdle with the trunk. Motions possible at this joint include elevation and depression and protraction and retraction. These motions demonstrate a reciprocal movement pattern between the sternoclavicular and the acromioclavicular joints.
- All of the joints work together smoothly and synchronously with scapulohumeral rhythm. Generally a ratio of 2:1 is accepted as the degree of contribution of the glenohumeral articulation and the contributions of the scapulothoracic articulations.
- Shoulder flexion/extension, abduction/adduction occur in phases with differing levels of contribution of different joints during different phases.
- Many muscles contribute to the movement and stability of the shoulder. How much contribution a specific muscle makes to a particular movement is dependent upon the axis and plane of motion, the position of the humerus, what other muscles are involved, the resolution of angle of pull of the muscle fibers, and the size of the muscle.
- Evaluation of the shoulder would include an assessment of pain; observation for changes in soft tissue, symmetry and alignment; active and passive ROM, and the client's participation in areas of occupation.

References

Caillet, R. (1980). *The shoulder in hemiplegia*. Philadelphia: F. A. Davis Co.

Esch, D. L. (1989). *Musculoskeletal function: An anatomy and kinesiology laboratory manual*. Minneapolis: University of Minnesota.

Flowers, K. (1998). Shoulder anatomy and biomechanics. Paper presented at the Ohio Occupational Therapy Association, Columbus, OH.

Gench, B. E., Hinson, M. M., & Harvey, P. T. (1995). *Anatomical kinesiology*. Dubuque, IA: Eddie Bowers Publishing, Inc.

Goss, C. M. (Ed.) (1976). *Gray's anatomy of the human body* (29th ed.). Philadelphia: Lea and Febiger.

Greene, D. P., & Roberts, S. L. (1999). *Kinesiology: Movement in the context of activity*. St. Louis, MO: C. V. Mosby Co.

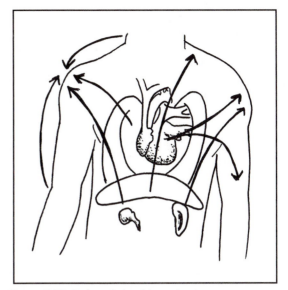

Figure 5-27. Referred shoulder pain sites.

Hamil, J., & Knutzen, K. M. (1995). *Biomechanical basis of human movement*. Baltimore: Williams & Wilkins.

Hartley, A. (1995). *Practical joint assessment: Upper quadrant: A sports medicine manual* (2nd ed.). Philadelphia: C. V. Mosby Co.

Hinkle, C. Z. (1997). *Fundamentals of anatomy and movement: A workbook and guide*. St. Louis, MO: C. V. Mosby Co.

Jenkins, D. B. (1998). *Hollingshead's functional anatomy of the limbs and back* (7th ed.). Philadelphia: W. B. Saunders Co.

Kisner, C., & Colby, L. A. (1990). *Therapeutic exercise: Foundations and techniques* (2nd ed.). Philadelphia: F. A. Davis.

Konin, J. G. (1999). *Practical kinesiology for the physical therapist assistant*. Thorofare, NJ: SLACK Incorporated.

Lumley, J. S. P. (1990). *Surface anatomy: The anatomical basis of clinical examination*. New York: Churchill Livingstone.

Magee, D. J. (1992). *Orthopedic physical assessment*. Philadelphia: W. B. Saunders Co.

Nordin, M., & Frankel, V. H. (1989). *Basic biomechanics of the musculoskeletal system* (2nd ed.). Philadelphia: Lea and Febiger.

Norkin, C. C., & Levangie, P. K. (1992). *Joint structure and function: A comprehensive analysis* (2nd ed.). Philadelphia: F. A. Davis Co.

Perry, J. F., Rohe,, D. A., & Garcia, A. O. (1996). *Kinesiology workbook*. Philadelphia: F. A. Davis Co.

Saidoff, D. C., & McDonough, A. L. (1997). *Critical pathways in therapeutic intervention: Upper extremity*. St. Louis, MO: C. V. Mosby.

Smith, L. K., Weiss, E. L., & Lehmkuhl, L. D. (1996). *Brunnstrom's clinical kinesiology* (5th ed.). Philadelphia: F. A. Davis Co.

Bibliography

Basmajian, J. V., & DeLuca, C. J. (1985). *Muscles alive* (5th ed.). Baltimore: Williams and Wilkins.

Baxter, R. (1998). *Pocket guide to musculoskeletal assessment*. Philadelphia: W. B. Saunders Co.

Burstein, A. H., & Wright, T. M. (1994). *Fundamentals of orthopaedic biomechanics*. Baltimore: Williams and Wilkins.

Hole, J. D. Jr. (1978). *Human anatomy and physiology.* Dubuque, IA: William C. Brown Co. Publishers.

Lehrman, R. L. (1998). *Physics the easy way* (3rd ed.). Hauppauge, NY: Barron's Educational Series, Inc.

LeVeau, B. F. (1992). *Williams and Lissner's biomechanics of human motion* (3rd ed.). Philadelphia: W. B. Saunders Co.

Loth, T., & Wadsworth, C. T. (1998). *Orthopedic review for physical therapists.* St. Louis, MO: C. V. Mosby Co.

MacKenna, B. R., & Callender, R. (1990). *Illustrated physiology* (5th ed.). New York: Churchill Livingstone.

Nicholas, J. A., & Hershman, E. B. (1990). *The upper extremity in sports medicine.* St. Louis, MO: C. V. Mosby Co.

Palastanga, N., Field, D., & Soames, R. (1989). *Anatomy and human movement: Structure and function.* Oxford: Heinemann Medical Books.

Watkins, J. (1999). *Structure and function of the musculoskeletal system.* New York: Human Kinetics.

The Elbow

Chapter 6

The elbow joint and motion of the forearm are important in enabling proper positioning of the hands and fingers in space and permitting height and length adjustments to be made. Rotation of the forearm helps to place the hand closer to the face and to position the arm to enable the most adventitious length-tension relationships in muscles. The elbow joint assists the shoulder with force distribution and in stabilizing the upper extremity for power and fine coordination.

The elbow joint is not one joint but actually three: the humerus articulates with the radius (humeroradial or radiohumeral) and the ulna (humeroulnar or ulnohumeral), and the ulna and radius articulate with each other (the superior/proximal radioulnar articulation). The elbow joint has been classified as a compound uniaxial hinge joint (Gench, Hinson, & Harvey, 1995; Nordin & Frankel, 1989), as a multiarticulating biaxial joint (Hamil & Knutzen, 1995), and as a "composite trochoginglymoid joint" (Nordin & Frankel, 1989). The articulations of the humerus with the ulna and radius are uniaxial hinge/ginglymus joints, whereas the articulation of the ulna with the radius is a uniaxial pivot/trochoid joint. The articulations together provide two degrees of freedom at the elbow with the movements of flexion and extension and of pronation and supination.

The elbow joint is an inherently stable joint due to the bony configuration as well as to ligamental support. The bony support is attributed to the articulation of the trochlea of the humerus with the trochlear fossa of the ulna and the head of the radius with the capitulum of the humerus. The amount of contact of the bony surfaces of the elbow increases from full extension to full flexion, which puts the radius in more contact with the capitulum, providing greater stability for the joint, especially in flexion. The elbow is more stable when in flexion than in extension because there is more contact of the bony surfaces. The lateral part of the olecranon process is not in contact with the trochlea during full flexion, and in full extension, the medial part of the olecranon process is not in contact with the trochlea. However, in full extension, there is no contact between the capitulum and the radial head.

The joint capsule is continuous for all three articulations and the capsule is fairly large, loose, and weak, which allows for free movements. Anteriorly and posteriorly the capsule is protected by muscles, but medially and laterally it is reinforced by ligaments (Nordin & Frankel, 1989; Hartley, 1995). The medial and lateral collateral ligaments provide a stabilizing force to medial and lateral stresses of the joint (Figure 6-1A-C).

The *medial collateral ligament* has three parts: anterior, posterior, and oblique. The anterior collateral ligament is considered the primary stabilizer to valgus stress in elbow flexion from 20 to 120 degrees. The posterior collateral ligament occasionally blends with the medial portion of the joint capsule and is less significant in valgus (outward) stability than the medial collateral ligament. Oblique collateral fibers run between the olecranon and the ulnar coronoid process and assist in valgus stability and in keeping the joints in approximation (Nordin & Frankel, 1989).

The anconeus muscle stabilizes against varus (inward) stress with the lateral collateral ligament. The lateral collateral ligament also provides reinforcement for the humeroradial articulation and assists in providing resistance to distraction of the joint surfaces (Norkin & Levangie, 1992). In addition, at the proximal radioulnar joint, the *annular ligament* allows pronation/supination as the interosseous membrane binds ulna and radial shafts together.

BONES OF THE ELBOW

Humerus

Epicondyle

These are the distal enlargements of the humerus (Figure 6-2). When the forearm is externally rotated, the medial epicondyle lies close to the body and the lateral epicondyle points to the back. The medial epicondyle is known as the flexor epicondyle since many of the wrist and fingers attach here. Likewise, the lateral epicondyle is known as the extensor epicondyle (Smith, Weiss, & Lehmkuhl, 1996).

Ulna

Olecranon Process

This is the "point" of the elbow or the upper and posterior aspect of elbow, which is easily felt when the forearm is flexed to 90 degrees. The ulnar nerve runs in this area, which, when compressed, produces the tingling sensation and is referred to as the funny bone.

Figure 6-1A. Elbow ligaments. Annular ligament.

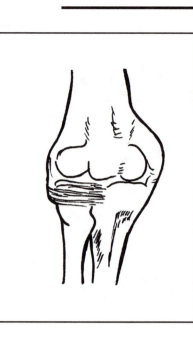

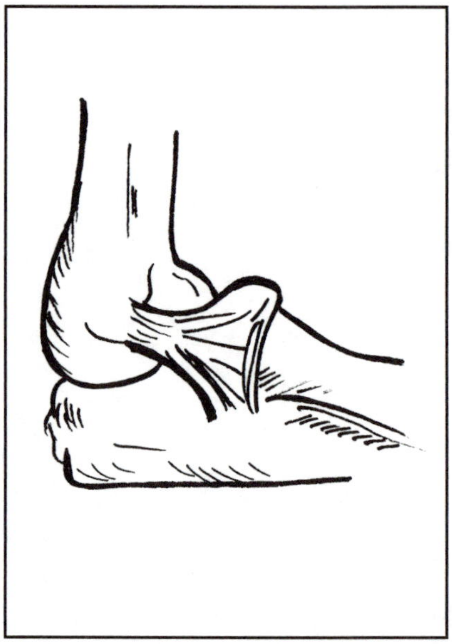

Figure 6-1B. Lateral ligament.

Figure 6-1C. Medial collateral ligament (anterior, posterior, oblique).

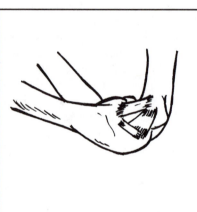

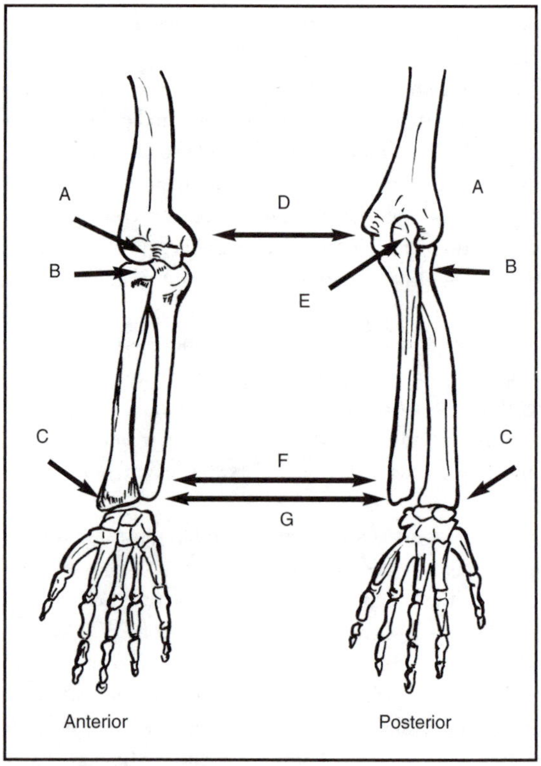

Figure 6-2. Palpable bony structures of elbow and forearm. A. Lateral epicondyle of humerus; B. Head of radius; C. Styloid process of radius; D. Medial epicondyle of humerus; E. Olecranon process; F. Head of ulna; G. Styloid process of ulna.

Anterior

Posterior

Body

On the dorsal surface of the forearm you can palpate the shaft of the ulna from the olecranon process to the distal end or head.

Head

This is the rounded projection on the dorsal surface of the forearm (down by the wrist).

Styloid Process of Ulna

This is a small projection on the medial aspect of the head of the ulna. With your subject's forearm in pronation, place one finger on the styloid and ask the subject to supinate; note the changing position of the styloid as the ulna rotates (Caillet, 1996; Smith et al., 1996).

Radius

Head

With the elbow in extension, palpate the dorsal surface just distal to the lateral epicondyle of humerus. Supinating and pronating the forearm will help in identifying this structure (Smith et al., 1996).

Styloid Process

This is located on the lateral aspect of the wrist proximal to the first metacarpal.

Shaft

You can feel the radial shaft on the lateral side of the forearm in the lower half of the forearm.

Tubercle of Lister

The tubercle of lister is located on the dorsum of the radius, about 1 inch laterally from the head of the ulna. The tendon of extensor pollicis longus lies on the ulnar side of this prominence.

Nonpalpable Structures

- Olecranon fossa
- Neck of radius
- Radial tuberosity
- Trochlear notch
- Capitulum of humerus
- Coronoid process of ulna (Smith et al., 1996)

ARTICULATIONS

Of the three articulations of the elbow, it is the humeroulnar and the humeroradial joints that produce flexion and extension of the elbow.

Humeroradial Joint

This joint includes the articulation of the capitulum of distal humerus with the head of radius.

Orthokinetics

The humeroradial joint is an uniaxial ginglymus hinge joint that allows for flexion and extension of the elbow in a sagittal plane around a frontal axis. This joint has 1 degree of freedom and the resting position is with the elbow extended and the forearm fully supinated. The position of greatest stability, the close packed position, is with the elbow flexed to 90 degrees and supinated to 5 degrees. The muscles primarily producing movement at this joint are the biceps, brachialis, and pronator teres.

Arthrokinematics

Flexion and extension of the humeroradial joint occurs as the concave head of radius rotates with the convex capitulum of the humerus (Kisner & Colby, 1990). As the elbow flexes and extends, the concave radial head slides in the same direction as the bone motion (Kisner & Colby, 1990) (Table 6-1).

Humeroulnar Joint

The humeroulnar joint is the articulation of the trochlea of the distal humerus and the trochlear notch (fossa) of the proximal ulna. Posterior displacement of the elbow is prevented by the coronoid process of the ulna and by the humeroradial articulation.

Osteokinematics

Like the humeroradial joint, the humeroulnar joint is a uniaxial hinge joint permitting the motions of flexion and extension in the sagittal plane around a frontal axis. The resting position of this joint is with the elbow flexed to 70 degrees and the forearm supinated to 10 degrees. The close packed position is extension with the forearm in supination. The primary muscles acting at the humeroulnar joint are the brachialis, triceps, and anconeus.

Arthrokinetics

Since the trochlea at the distal end of the humerus is convex and it articulates with the concave trochlear fossa on proximal ulna, the concave fossa slides in the same direction in which the ulna moves. There is also a slight medial and lateral sliding of the ulna (Kisner & Colby, 1990) (see Table 6-1).

Superior (Proximal) Radioulnar Joint

This is the articulation of the head of the radius with the radial notch of the proximal ulna. The joint is encircled by the annular ligament and the radial head rotates around the annular ligament on the capitulum. In neutral position, the radius and ulna lie parallel to each other, but in pronation, the radius crosses over the ulna diagonally. There is also an interosseous membrane that connects the ulna and radius as well as serves as a surface for attachment of deeper muscles.

Osteokinematics

The proximal radioulnar joint provides the second of the 2 degrees of freedom possible at the elbow joint by enabling pronation and supination at this uniaxial pivot/trochoid joint. This joint plays no part in producing the movements of flexion or extension

Table 6-1.

PHYSIOLOGIC MOTION OF THE ELBOW

Physiological Movement of the Humeroradial Joint	Direction of Slide of the Radius on Capitulum	Physiologic Motion of the Radius	Direction of Slide of the Distal Radius on the Ulna
		When you pronate	The radial head moves posteriorly (dorsal)
Flexion	Anterior	When you supinate	The radial head moves anteriorly (volar)
Extension	Posterior		
Physiological Movement of the Ulna	Direction of Slide of the Ulna on the Trochlea	Physiologic Motion of the Radius	Direction of Slide of the Distal Radius on the Ulna
Flexion	Distal/anterior	Pronation	Anterior (volar)
Varus angular with elbow flexion	Lateral	Supination	Posterior (dorsal)
Extension	Proximal/posterior		
Valgus angulation with elbow in extension	Medial		

at the elbow or in providing additional stability to the joint. The resting position of the proximal radioulnar joint is 35 degrees of supination and 70 degrees of elbow flexion. The position of greatest stability (close packed position) is in 5 degrees of supination. The primary muscles involved at the radioulnar joint are the supinator and the pronator quadratus.

Arthrokinetics

With pronation and supination of the forearm, the direction of slide of the proximal radius on the ulna is opposite to the motion. This is because the convex rim of the radial head articulates with the concave radial notch on the ulna. With rotation of radius, the convex rim moves opposite to the bone motion (Kisner & Colby, 1990) (see Table 6-1).

Inferior (Distal) Radioulnar Joint

This joint is at the distal end of the forearm near the wrist where the ulnar notch of radius articulates with the head of the ulna. This is an extremely stable joint due to the articular disk, the interosseus between the radius and ulna and the pronator quadratus muscle.

Osteokinematics

Like the proximal radioulnar joint, the distal radioulnar joint is a uniaxial pivot joint. In order to produce pronation and supination, the distal end of the radius must be free to move about the ulna at its distal end as well as at the proximal portions (Jenkins,

1998). Rotation of the lower end of the radius around the head of the ulna occurs at the distal radioulnar joint. The resting position is in 10 degrees supination, and close packed position is in 5 degrees supination.

Arthrokinetics

The articulating surface of the radius slides in the same direction as the bone motion because the concave ulnar notch on the distal radius articulates with the convex portion of the head of the ulna (Kisner & Colby, 1990) (see Table 6-1).

MOVEMENTS AT THE ELBOW JOINT

Flexion and Extension

The flexion and extension movements that occur at the humeroradial and humeroulnar joints are primarily gliding motions until the last 5 to 10 degrees, when the surface joint motion changes to rolling. The rolling in *flexion* occurs when the coronoid process of the ulna comes into contact with the floor of the numeral coronoid fossa. During flexion, there is distal (inferior) glide of the ulna in the trochlea. Supination and adduction of the ulna in the trochlea and distal movement and pronation of the radius on the humerus also occurs at the same time (Hamil & Knutzen, 1995). The capsule limits flexion more than extension and total range of elbow flexion ranges from 135 to 146 degrees.

The rolling that occurs in *extension* takes place when the olecranon of the ulna is received by the floor of the numeral olecranon fossa (Esch, 1989; Norkin & Levangie, 1992). The movements occurring during elbow extension are: proximal glide of the ulna on the humerus, pronation and abduction of the ulna on the humerus, and distal movement and pronation of the radius on the humerus (Hamil & Knutzen, 1995, p. 196). In addition, 10 to 15 degrees of hyperextension of the elbow may occur and may be due to a shortened olecranon process or to lax ligaments.

The joint axis for flexion and extension goes through the middle of the trochlea and the capitulum, which bisects the longitudinal angle of the forearm. It is possible to feel this axis by grasping the elbow from side to side distal to the lateral and medial epicondyle. Due to the shape of the trochlea, with the trochlea extending further distally than does the capitulum, the extended forearm angles laterally and is not brought into a straight line with the humerus (Hinkle, 1997). This lateral deviation of the forearm is called the *carrying angle* or *cubical angle*. With the elbow extended and the forearm supinated, the carrying angle in males is 5 to 10 degrees, with slightly larger lateral deviation angle of 10 to 15 degrees in females. Due to this angle, the axis of movement is not horizontal but downward and medial. While it has been suggested that the purpose of the carrying angle is to prevent objects that are held in the hand from coming into contact with the body and that the wider angle in women is to accommodate the female pelvis, a definitive function of this angle has not been identified (Hamil & Knutzen, 1995). If muscles are located posterior to this axis, the muscles are extensors; if the muscles are anterior to the axis, they are flexor muscles.

Pronation and Supination

During pronation and supination, the distal and proximal radioulnar joints work together to enable the head of the radius to spin, roll, and glide in the radial notch. The axis line for pronation and supination goes through the center of the head of the radius proximally and through the center of the head of the ulna distally (Smith et al., 1996). Therefore, the axis is oblique to the longitudinal axis center of the radius and ulna (Norkin & Levangie, 1992). The muscles that cross anterior to this axis are pronators; those crossing posterior to the joint axis are supinators (Gench et al., 1995) (Figure 6-3).

It is important to realize that although the radius rotates over the ulna, the ulna moves too. The ulna moves laterally during pronation and medially during supination. The joint capsule equally limits pronation and supination.

KINETICS

According to Norkin and Levangie (1992), there are six factors that influence motion at the elbow. These are:
1. Location of muscles.
2. Position of elbow and adjacent joints.
3. Position of forearm.
4. Magnitude of applied force.

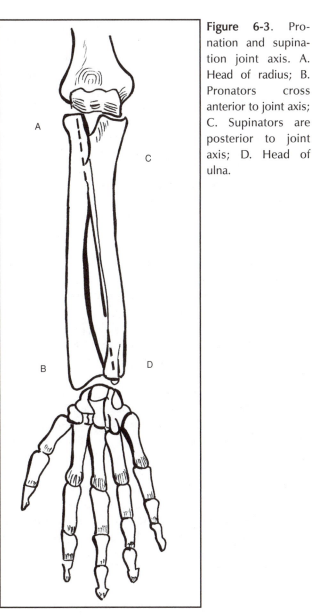

Figure 6-3. Pronation and supination joint axis. A. Head of radius; B. Pronators cross anterior to joint axis; C. Supinators are posterior to joint axis; D. Head of ulna.

5. Types of muscle contraction.
6. Speed of motion.

The location of the muscles has a direct relationship with the motion possible at the joint. For example, pronators cross the joint axis anterior to the axis, whereas supinators cross posteriorly to the joint axis of rotation. Location of muscles as well as the position of the forearm and other joints helps to determine the line of pull of the muscles, which influences the power of the force generated by the muscle due to length-tension relationships. In addition, some of the forearm muscles are active only when the movement is unresisted or when there is external load and only in certain positions. For example, pronator quadratus will pronate the forearm regardless of forearm position or amount of flexion of the elbow, whereas pronator teres contributes to pronation where there is an external load or when rapid pronation is required.

The nervous system utilizes efficient economy of energy when determining which muscles will produce specific movements. Unskilled movements waste energy because muscles that are not needed also contract. As skill increases, the selection of muscles improves, and the gradation of contraction becomes more refined, which results in smoother movements (Smith et al., 1996). The number of muscles is determined by the effort needed and the nervous system prefers to have only one muscle perform the task if possible. For example, if flexion of the elbow and supination of the forearm is the desired motion, biceps would be a good choice since the biceps muscle both flexes the elbow and supinates the forearm. The two actions could also be done by brachialis and supinator, but at the expense of energy required to produce contractions of two muscles rather than just one (Smith et al., 1996). Likewise, if only flexion without supination or pronation was the required motion, biceps would be wasteful because the supination function of biceps would need to be neutralized by pronator muscles.

Small loads applied to the hand dramatically increase the elbow joint reaction force. In studies by Nicol, it was shown that a common activity, such as supporting oneself when pushing up out of a chair, generates loads of more than twice the body weight, which may challenge the view that the elbow is not a load bearing joint (Norkin & Levangie, 1992).

At the elbow joint there are two muscles that are multi-joint muscles; i.e., muscles that cross two or more joints. The biceps is a multi-joint muscle that can develop active insufficiency when the elbow is in full flexion while the shoulder is in full humeral flexion and the forearm is supinated. This puts the biceps muscle in a shortened position, resulting in marked loss of force and some leverage loss. Triceps, also a multijoint muscle, is actively insufficient when the elbow is in full extension with the shoulder in extension (shortened position). The significance of this in intervention is to provide activities or adaptations that will not cause muscle shortening over the multiple joints, resulting in decreased strength and force production.

INTERNAL KINETICS/MUSCLES

The location of muscles, position of the forearm, elbow, and adjacent joints, as well as the angle of the pull of muscle fibers, all contribute to the actions of the muscles of the elbow joint.

Flexors of the Forearm

Biceps Brachii

This fusiform, spurt (mobility) muscle is a multijoint muscle whose contraction produces shoulder flexion and elbow flexion (Figure 6-4). The force components of the pull of the biceps muscle can vary in length so that at full extension, biceps is accompanied by a strong stabilizing component, while at full flexion there is a strong dislocating component. It is for this reason that the biceps is most efficient as an elbow flexor when in 90 degrees of flexion, since the only component is an angular one (Gench et al., 1995) and the moment arm is greatest between 90 and 100 degrees of elbow flexion.

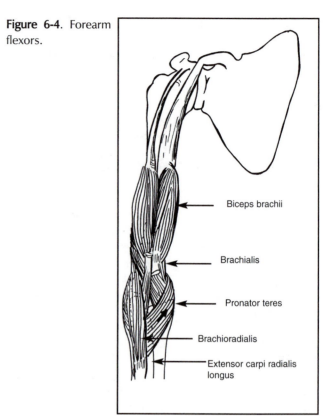

Figure 6-4. Forearm flexors.

Biceps brachii

Brachialis

Pronator teres

Brachioradialis

Extensor carpi radialis longus

The biceps creates an isolated, unopposed contraction when there is simultaneous flexion of shoulder, elbow, and supination. The biceps does not function in slow flexion with the arm pronated, but functions in slow flexion with the forearm supinated as well as in fast flexion with and without an external load. As the speed of the movement increases, and as the load increases, the biceps may act even in pronation. When the elbow is flexed with the forearm in pronation, the biceps is nearly inactive (Greene & Roberts, 1999). An example of how to use the actions of the biceps in a therapeutic situation is provided by Greene and Roberts (1999):

> When Mary Smith arrived at Maple Grove Skilled Care Facility, she held her right arm [elbow] flexed tightly against her body. She refused to let any nurses or aides move her arm through passive range of motion, so the nursing supervisor contacted the occupational therapy department. The occupational therapy assistant who went to see Mary explained that putting her arm through range of motion probably would help her not to feel so stiff and sore all of the time.
>
> The occupational therapy assistant promised to try some new techniques that would make range of motion less painful than it had been in the past. First, the OT assistant gave Mary's right arm a gentle rubdown to gain Mary's trust and then slowly pronated her forearm to inhibit the biceps. The OT assistant explained to Mary that in the past, medical practitioners may have attempted to extend her elbow with her palm up in supination, a position associated with increased activity in the biceps. By pronating the forearm first, the OT assistant inactivated

the biceps and made elbow extension easier and more comfortable. The OT assistant continued to explain that elbow extension in pronation stretches the tight biceps tendon even further because both of the biceps' antagonistic movements—extension and pronation—occur simultaneously (p. 89-90).

The biceps also often works eccentrically in protective capacity to slow down the rate of elbow extension. An example of the biceps working eccentrically would be when a person who is on a ladder slips and the fall necessitates a quick, forced extension of the elbow. The biceps is contracting while lengthening to slow the fall (Konin, 1999). *Palpation:* With the forearm in supination and the elbow flexed, the tendon of insertion can be felt anterior to the elbow joint (Jenkins, 1998). When one "makes a muscle" by bending the elbow, it is the biceps muscle that is seen (Esch, 1989; Lumley, 1990; Magee, 1992).

Brachioradialis

This fusiform, shunt (stability) muscle has its distal attachment farther from the elbow than other elbow flexors. This means that the force arm and moment arm are increased. Since the proximal attachment is closer to the axis and the muscle lies close to the joint axis, there is a small angular component at the distal attachment when compared to a larger stabilizing component. Since brachioradialis tends to pronate as it flexes, the angular component can be increased by placing the forearm in neutral (midposition between pronation and supination), which will lead to a stronger contraction (Gench et al., 1995). Brachioradialis is active during rapid flexion or when an external load is lifted during slow flexion, adding speed and power to elbow flexion. *Palpation:* Brachioradialis is seen when the elbow is flexed to 90 degrees and the forearm is placed in neutral. When resistance is applied to the wrist, brachioradialis contracts. Above the elbow, brachioradialis lies between the triceps and brachialis muscles. At and just below the elbow, brachioradialis forms the lateral border of the antecubital fossa (Gench et al., 1995; Smith et al., 1996).

Brachialis

Since this fusiform, one-joint, spurt (mobility) muscle crosses the elbow closer to the flexion and extension axis than brachioradialis and biceps, it is less favorably located to produce force. The moment arm is greatest at about 100 degrees of elbow flexion, so the greatest torque is produced in this position (Smith et al., 1996). However, the distal attachment is on the ulna rather than the radius, which means that arm position is inconsequential to flexion and extension (Gench et al., 1995). The brachialis is considered the primary flexor of the elbow, and as such, is always a flexor regardless of whether there is an external load and whether or not the rate of movement is fast or slow. An appropriate nickname is "workhorse of elbow", as this muscle has the greatest work capacity of the elbow flexors. In addition, brachialis has been identified as contributing to pronation and supination, but the contribution is weak. Brachialis also works well eccentrically but better concentrically (Gench et al., 1995; Hinkle, 1997; Jenkins, 1998; Smith et al., 1996). *Palpation:* Brachialis can be palpated just lateral to the biceps when resistance is applied to the wrist (Gench, Hinson &

Harvey, 1995). If the examiner places the palpating fingers laterally and medially to the biceps and flexes the elbow with minimal effort, contraction of brachialis may be felt. Quick contraction in a small range will result in a stronger contraction by this muscle (Esch, 1989; Lumley, 1990; Magee, 1992; Smith et al., 1996).

Pronator Teres

This muscle lies quite close to axis throughout the range of motion, making it inefficient as an elbow flexor, and it may actually serve to neutralize the supination action of biceps rather than actually flex the elbow. Pronator teres may not be able to flex the extremity alone against gravity (Jenkins, 1998). *Palpation:* Pronator teres forms the medial margin of the antecubital fossa and the fibers can be identified when the forearm is pronated while the elbow is flexed. When resistance is applied to the forearm in this position, pronator teres can easily be identified. Place one finger on the humeral medial epicondyle and one on the midpoint of the radius and a ridge of muscle will be seen running obliquely between the two fingers (Gench et al., 1995; Smith et al., 1996). More distally, the pronator crosses to the radial side and is covered by brachioradialis. If the forearm is pronated with little effort, pronator teres will contract (Esch, 1989; Lumley, 1990; Magee, 1992).

Extensor Carpi Radialis Longus

Due to the anterior location and origin on the humeral epicondyle, both extensor carpi radialis longus and pronator teres may assist with elbow flexion. However, since extensor carpi radialis longus arises too low on the humerus, attaches too close to the flexion axis, and produces a short moment arm, this muscle fails to be too important in flexion of the forearm. (Greene & Roberts, 1999; Hinkle, 1997).

Extensor Carpi Radialis Brevis

Due to this muscle crossing the elbow anterior to the axis, this muscle may serve to assist in elbow flexion (Gench et al., 1995).

Flexor Carpi Radialis, Palmaris Longus, Flexor Carpi Ulnaris

These muscles were also identified as having assistive actions with elbow flexion (Gench et al., 1995; Lumley, 1990; Smith et al., 1996).

Extensors of the Forearm

Triceps

The triceps muscle has three heads, with the medial head being the primary extensor of the forearm (Figure 6-5). The size of the muscle as well as the angle of attachment on olecranon give triceps power in spite of poor leverage (Gench et al., 1995). Triceps has twice the size of shortening range than anconeus and five times the cross section. The long head of the triceps is affected by positions of the shoulder because this portion crosses both the shoulder and elbow joints. This long head can become actively insufficient when the elbow and shoulder are both extended because this shortens the muscle over both joints. The middle and lateral heads of the triceps muscle are not affected by shoulder position. All three heads of the triceps muscle extend the elbow when there is heavy resistance or when quick extension is required.

Frequently, the triceps muscle works eccentrically, as when one lowers the body to the floor with the elbows flexed and the triceps lengthen (Gench et al., 1995; Hinkle, 1997; Konin, 1999; Loth & Wadsworth, 1998; Smith et al., 1996). *Palpation*: The lateral head can be palpated between the posterior deltoid and the lateral epicondyle. It appears separated from the deltoid by a groove. The long head can be palpated between the axilla and the olecranon process. This is the contour at the lower portion of the arm. The medial head is located beneath the long head and is difficult to palpate. It is best palpated in its distal portion near the medial epicondyle. By placing the dorsum of the wrist on the edge of a table and applying resistance downward, the medial head may be felt contracting (Esch, 1989; Lumley, 1990; Magee, 1992; Smith et al., 1996).

Anconeus

This small, triangular muscle is active in initiating and maintaining extension and in joint stabilization. Since it is very close to the axis and is small, it is weak in these actions (Jenkins, 1998). Thompson and Floyd (1994) stated that the chief function of anconeus was to pull the synovial membrane out of the way of the advancing olecranon process during extension of the elbow (p. 55). *Palpation*: By placing the thumb and index finger on the olecranon process and lateral epicondyle, one can feel the base of this equilateral triangular muscle (Gench et al., 1995). Extensor carpi ulnaris lies close to anconeus and while the two muscles may appear as one, identification can be made by keeping in mind the direction of the line of muscle pull varies and that anconeus lies more proximally and is very short (Esch, 1989; Lumley, 1990; Magee, 1992; Smith et al., 1996).

Pronators of the Forearm

Pronator Quadratus

A rhomboidal or quadrangular muscle, pronator quadratus muscle is considered to be the primary pronator (Figure 6-6). Due to the size of the muscle and the pull of the fibers, this muscle is a pronator of the radioulnar joint without help and in movements that are slow and unresisted. With the triceps muscle, it extends and pronates the elbow. The action of pronator quadratus can be seen in using a screwdriver to remove a screw and in throwing a screwball in baseball (Gench et al., 1995; Hamil & Knutzen, 1995; Hinkle, 1997; Jenkins, 1998; Smith et al., 1996). *Palpation*: Since it is too deeply located, palpation is not possible (Gench et al., 1995).

Pronator Teres

This muscle lies anterior to the axis at the proximal radioulnar joint and has a long angular component. Due to its strength and efficiency, pronator teres does not participate in pronation in slow or unresisted motion but instead contracts during rapid pronation or in pronation against resistance. It is considered to be a secondary pronator (Norkin & Levangie, 1992). If pronator teres were to

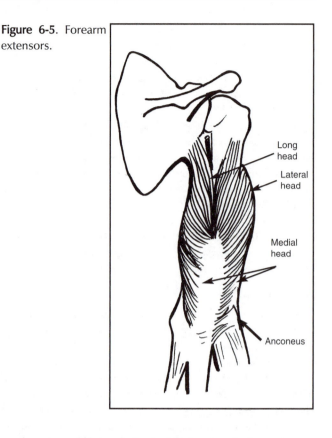

Figure 6-5. Forearm extensors.

Long head

Lateral head

Medial head

Anconeus

act alone, it would bring the back of the hand to the face as it contracts (Smith et al., 1996) (Figure 6-7).

Brachioradialis

While primarily a flexor, the brachioradialis muscle is also a weak pronator. The brachioradialis directs a force volar to the joint axis, pulling the radius toward the ulna in pronation (Greene & Roberts, 1999). In other words, brachioradialis acts in pronation from a position of supination with the ability to pronate decreasing as the forearm rotates to neutral.

Flexor Carpi Radialis

Flexor carpi radialis assists with pronation because the tendon passes obliquely across the wrist (Jenkins, 1998).

Palmaris Longus, Extensor Carpi Radialis Longus

These muscles may assist with pronation (Gench et al., 1995; Hinkle, 1997; Jenkins, 1998; Smith et al., 1996).

Supinators of the Forearm

Supinator

The supinator muscle (Figure 6-8) is in the best position to supinate the radioulnar joint when the elbow is extended and this position puts the muscle on more stretch than other positions (Gench et al., 1995). Two common examples of how this muscle may be seen are turning a screwdriver or throwing a curve ball in baseball. The primary function of this muscle is supination of the

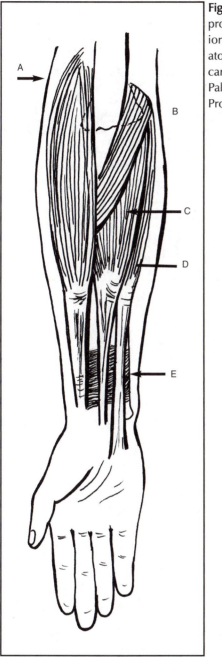

Figure 6-6. Forearm pronators. A. Brachioradialis; B. Pronator teres; C. Flexor carpi radialis; D. Palmaris longus; E. Pronator quadratus.

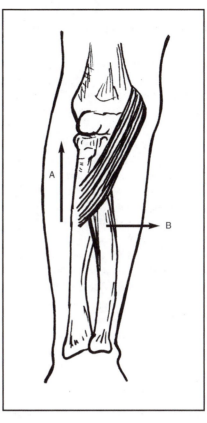

Figure 6-7. Pronator teres force resolution. A. Stabilizing component; B. Angular component.

forearm and it contracts when supination occurs slowly and without resistance. Supinator requires assistance from biceps with resisted motion (Gench et al., 1995; Hinkle, 1997; Jenkins, 1998; Smith et al., 1996). *Palpation*: Supinator is located deeply and is difficult to palpate (Gench et al., 1995).

Biceps

Biceps is the strongest and most efficient supinator, especially when the elbow is flexed to 90 degrees. Biceps is four times more efficient than the supinator muscle in this flexed position and only twice as effective as the supinator muscle with the elbow extended and supinated (Gench et al., 1995). Triceps is needed to counter-

act the flexor action of biceps when the muscle is recruited as a supinator. Biceps assists with rapid, unresisted supination with the elbow flexed or with any supination against resistance (Gench et al., 1995; Hinkle, 1997; Jenkins, 1998; Smith et al., 1996).

Brachioradialis

In addition to flexing the elbow, brachioradialis can function as both a pronator and a supinator. As the forearm pronates, the brachioradialis directs a force on the dorsal side of the axis and supination of the forearm occurs (Greene & Roberts, 1999). Brachioradialis can supinate the forearm from a position of pronation, with the ability to supinate decreasing as the joint moves toward neutral (Thompson & Floyd, 1994).

Abductor pollicis longus, extensor pollicis brevis, extensor indicus proprius, and flexor carpi ulnaris were also identified by some sources as assistive supinators (Jenkins, 1998; Smith et al., 1996).

ASSESSMENT OF THE ELBOW

While there is normative data available for ROM for elbow flexion/extension, pronation, and supination, variance from these norms should be considered for intervention only when the limitations prevent the client from successful engagement in work, play, or self-care. Most activities of daily living require 30 to 130 degrees of elbow extension and flexion and only 50 degrees of pronation or supination.

An assessment of the elbow would include gathering information about the client's level of pain. Determining the location of the pain can help to identify the cause of the pain. For example, if the pain is localized it may be indicative of bursitis or epicondylitis.

Ask the client when the pain was first noticed, when it occurs, and if there was an immediate onset of pain or if the onset was gradual. Differentiating the type of pain the client is experiencing as well as eliciting descriptions about sensations being felt is also helpful.

The assessment of swelling is important at the elbow and specific details about the time the swelling started and where the swelling is located should be gathered from the client.

How well the person can move the joint and the quality of movement is vital to understanding how the limitations will interfere with functional activity. Assessment of ROM (both active and passive) and strength are usually needed, as is a determination about sensory involvement. Observe how the person uses the elbow and arm in activities. Does the client seem willing to move the joint and does the client use the arm automatically in activities and without discomfort? Does the client support one arm or use one arm more than the other? Look at how well the wrist, elbow, and shoulder all work together and observe for lack of symmetry or muscle imbalance.

SUMMARY

- The elbow joint consists of the articulations between the ulna, radius, and humerus.
- The elbow joint is actually made up of three articulations: humeroulnar, humeroradius, and superior radioulnar joints.
- The superior radioulnar joint does not contribute to the uniaxial hinge motions of flexion and extension at the elbow joint.
- The superior and inferior radioulnar joints produce pronation (crossing of radius and ulna) and supination (ulna and radius parallel).
- Stability of the elbow is provided by the ligaments surrounding the joint and the interlocking of the distal humerus, proximal radius, and proximal ulna (Nordin & Frankel, 1989, p. 259).
- Flexors of the elbow (biceps, brachialis, brachioradialis) are, as a group, most efficient in pronation and when the elbow is flexed (also the position of greatest stability).
- Extensors of the elbow (triceps, anconeus) are most efficient when the elbow is flexed to 20 to 30 degrees.
- Contact areas of the radius and ulna on the humerus change as one moves in flexion and extension. Only in full flexion is there contact between the radius and capitulum of the humerus.
- Posterior displacement of the elbow is prevented by the coronoid process of the ulna and the humeroradial articulation.
- The proximal radioulnar joint offers no additional stability to the elbow joint; it only allows pronation/supination.
- Assessment of the elbow should include how the client moves, the amount of edema, and the client's pain. Observation of how the client uses the elbow in activities is an important aspect of evaluation.

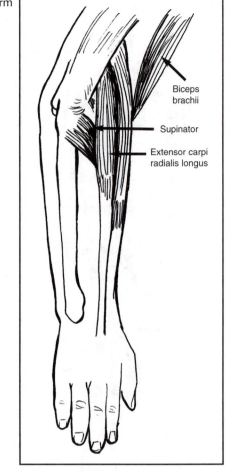

Figure 6-8. Forearm supinators.

Biceps brachii

Supinator

Extensor carpi radialis longus

REFERENCES

Calliet, R. (1996). *Soft tissue pain and disability* (3rd ed.). Philadelphia: F. A. Davis Co.

Esch, D. L. (1989). *Musculoskeletal function: An anatomy and kinesiology laboratory manual*. Minneapolis, MN: University of Minnesota.

Gench, B. E., Hinson, M. M., & Harvey, P. T. (1995). *Anatomical kinesiology*. Dubuque, IA: Eddie Bowers Publishing, Inc.

Greene, D. P., & Roberts, S. L. (1999). *Kinesiology: Movement in the context of activity*. St. Louis, MO: C. V. Mosby.

Hamil, J., & Knutzen, K. M. (1995). *Biomechanical basis of human movement*. Baltimore: Williams & Wilkins.

Hartley, A. (1995). *Practical joint assessment: Upper quadrant: A sports medicine manual* (2nd ed.). Philadelphia: C. V. Mosby.

Hinkle, C. Z. (1997). *Fundamentals of anatomy and movement: A workbook and guide*. St. Louis, MO: C. V. Mosby.

Jenkins, D. B. (1998). *Hollingshead's functional anatomy of the limbs and back* (7th ed.). Philadelphia: W. B. Saunders Co.

Kisner, C., & Colby, L. A. (1990). *Therapeutic exercise: Foundations and techniques* (2nd ed.). Philadelphia: F. A. Davis.

Konin, J. G. (1999). *Practical kinesiology for the physical therapist assistant*. Thorofare, NJ: SLACK Incorporated.

Loth, T., & Wadsworth, C. T. (1998). *Orthopedic review for physical therapists.* St. Louis, MO: C. V. Mosby.

Lumley, J. S. P. (1990). *Surface anatomy: The anatomical basis of clinical examination.* New York: Churchill Livingstone.

Magee, D. J. (1992). *Orthopedic physical assessment.* Philadelphia: W. B. Saunders Co.

Nordin, M., & Frankel, V. H. (1989). *Basic biomechanics of the musculoskeletal system* (2nd ed.). Philadelphia: Lea and Febiger.

Norkin, C. C., & Levangie, P. K. (1992). *Joint structure and function: A comprehensive analysis* (2nd ed.). Philadelphia: F. A. Davis Co.

Smith, L. K., Weiss, E. L., & Lehmkuhl, L. D. (1996). *Brunnstrom's clinical kinesiology* (5th ed.). Philadelphia: F. A. Davis Co.

Thompson, C. W., & Floyd, R.T. (1994). *Manual of structural kinesiology* (12th ed.). St. Louis, MO: C. V. Mosby.

BIBLIOGRAPHY

Basmajian, J. V., & DeLuca, C. J. (1985). *Muscles alive* (5th ed.). Baltimore: Williams & Wilkins.

Baxter, R. (1998). *Pocket guide to musculoskeletal assessment.* Philadelphia: W. B. Saunders Co.

Burstein, A. H., & Wright, T. M. (1994). *Fundamentals of orthopaedic biomechanics.* Baltimore: Williams & Wilkins.

Goss, C. M. (Ed.). (1976). *Gray's anatomy of the human body* (29th ed.). Philadelphia: Lea and Febiger.

Hinojosa, J., & Kramer, P. (1998). *Evaluation: Obtaining and interpreting data.* Bethesda, MD: American Occupational Therapy Association.

MacKenna, B. R., & Callender, R. (1990). *Illustrated physiology* (5th ed.). New York: Churchill Livingstone.

Nicholas, J. A., & Hershman, E. B. (1990). *The upper extremity in sports medicine.* St. Louis, MO: C. V. Mosby.

Palastanga, N., Field, D., & Soames, R. (1989). *Anatomy and human movement: Structure and function.* Oxford: Heinemann Medical Books.

Perry, J. F., Rohe, D. A., & Garcia, A. O. (1996). *Kinesiology workbook.* Philadelphia: F. A. Davis Co.

Saidoff, D. C., & McDonough, A. L. (1997). *Critical pathways in therapeutic intervention: Upper extremity.* St. Louis, MO: C. V. Mosby.

Watkins, J. (1999). *Structure and function of the musculoskeletal system.* New York: Human Kinetics.

The Wrist

Chapter 7

The wrist is a multiarticulating, complex biaxial joint made up of two compound joints. The wrist allows for change in location and orientation of the hand relative to the forearm, and in placing the hand in space, permits fine gradations of prehension as well as powerful grasp. The wrist makes a dynamic contribution to a skill or movement or to stabilization (Hamil & Knutzen, 1995) and contributes to expression and nonverbal communication. The wrist serves a kinetic function in transmitting loads and forces from the hand to the forearm and from the forearm to the hand, as well as providing stability for the hand. These positional adjustments are essential for augmenting fine motor control of fingers and in allowing optimal length-tension of long finger muscles so maximal finger movement can be attained (Nordin & Frankel, 1989).

Because this is a complex joint with many articulations, the joints do not act in isolation. The position of one joint affects the action of others. For example, if the wrist is flexed, the interphalangeal (IP) joints cannot flex fully due to the insufficiency of finger flexors as they cross both joints. The interplay of structures has implications not only for joint and muscle actions, but also is an influence in pathology of the hand and wrist.

ANATOMY

The wrist joint is capable of much mobility and has great structural stability (Smith, Weiss, & Lehmkuhl, 1996). This highly complex area consists of 15 bones, 17 joints, and an extensive ligamental system (Figure 7-1A, B). The joint is formed by articulations of the hand and wrist and has four articular surfaces:

1. Distal surfaces of the radius and the articular disk.
2. Proximal surfaces of scaphoid, lunate, and triangular bones (the pisiform serves no significant part of movement of the hand).
3. An S-shaped surface formed by the inferior surfaces of the scaphoid, lunate, and triangular carpal bones.
4. The reciprocal surface of upper surfaces of the carpal bones of second row (Goss, 1976).

These four surfaces form the two joints of the wrist: the proximal portion is what is commonly thought of as the wrist joint and is called the *radiocarpal joint*; and the distal portion forms the *midcarpal joint*.

Konin (1999) adds an additional functional articulation of the wrist called the *ulnarcarpal* (ulnar-meniscal-triquetrum or ulnomeniscocarpal). This articulation is a meniscal type structure or triangular fibrocartilage complex (TFCC) located between the distal ulna and the proximal part of the triquetrum bone. This joint acts as a shock absorber and binds the distal radioulnar joint. It has similar mechanics to the glenoid labrum of the shoulder and menisci of knee. Notice, too, that the ulna has no contact with the carpal bones because they are separated by this fibrocartilaginous disk; this allows the ulna to glide on the disk for pronation and supination without influence or interference of the carpal bones. The distal end of the ulna can be surgically removed without any impairment of wrist motion because the ulna doesn't influence wrist motion at this articulation.

When the hand is in a resting position, it assumes a slight ulnar and palmar posture (Caillet, 1996) because the dorsal surface is much longer than palmar. The distal end of the radius is concave and usually reaches further distally on the radial side than the ulnar side, although 60% have equal length. The curvature of the proximal carpal row is greater than the opposing curve of the radioulnar surface. These discrepancies permit greater excursion of flexion/extension than of radioulnar motion. There is a greater degree of flexion as compared to extension and of ulnar abduction as compared to radial due to angulation of the distal articular surface of the radius, and also due to the fact that dorsal wrist ligaments are more slack than palmar (Caillet, 1996).

Since no muscle forces are applied directly to the bones of the proximal row and this row serves as a link between the radial and distal carpals, it is considered an intercalated segment. When compressive forces are applied to the wrist, the middle segment tends to collapse and move in the wrong direction. This would happen at the wrist except for the intercarpal bridge formed by scaphoid and ligaments (Norkin & Levangie, 1992).

The wrist joint is very stable due to the proximal radiocarpal and distal midcarpal joints, which act together as a double hinge (Nordin & Frankel, 1989). In addition to the bony support, wrist stability is maintained by an extensive system of ligamental support. Not only do the wrist ligaments provide additional support at the wrist but they also contribute to passive motion.

Primary stability of the joint comes from the radial and ulnar collateral ligaments. The joint is enclosed by a strong but loose

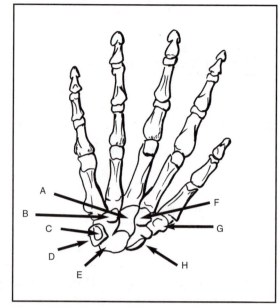

Figure 7-1A. Bones of the wrist. Palmar view. A. Capitate; B. Hamate; C. Pisiform; D. Triquetral; E. Lunate; F. Trapezoid; G. Trapezium; H. Scaphoid.

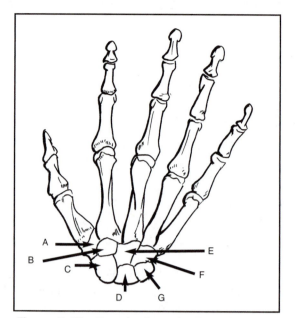

Figure 7-1B. Dorsal view. A. Trapezium; B. Trapezoid; C. Scaphoid; D. Lunate; E. Capitate; F. Hamate; G. Triquetral.

joint capsule and reinforced by the dorsal radiocarpal, palmar radiocarpal, palmar ulnocarpal, and intercarpal ligaments and flexor and extensor retinaculum (Nordin & Frankel, 1989).

On the dorsal surface, the major wrist ligament is the dorsal radiocarpal ligament, which maintains the contact between lunate and radius and becomes taut with full flexion (Norkin & Levangie, 1992). The radial and ulnar collateral ligaments provide significant passive control of radiocarpal motion in the frontal plane. The ulnar collateral ligament becomes taut with radial abduction/deviation, whereas the radial collateral is taut with ulnar deviation.

On the palmar surface, the volar radiocarpal ligament is the most important ligament for motion and stability (Norkin & Levangie, 1992). This ligament has three distinct portions that are named for their attachments: 1) radiotriquetral ligament, which is the strongest and most distinct; 2) the radiocapite ligament; and 3) the radioscaphoid, which aid motion and stability by checking movement of joint surfaces and maintaining joint integrity (Norkin & Levangie, 1992). The radiocarpal ligaments ensure that the carpals follow the radius throughout forearm rotation. In pronation, the dorsal radiocarpal ligament moves with the radius and the motion tightens the dorsal ligaments. Supination tightens the palmar ligaments and the palmar radiocarpal ligament carries the wrist with the radius.

The articular disk adds stability to the joint by maintaining a mechanical relationship that binds the distal ends of radius and ulna as well as the carpal bones and ulna. With the disk intact, the radius takes on 60% of the axial load and the ulna takes on 40%.

If the disk is injured, the radius takes on 95% of the axial load (Gench, Hinson & Harvey, 1995).

The intercarpal ligaments fortify the hand for any impact imposed on knuckles (such as striking with a closed fist), whereas the ulnocarpal ligament, scaphotrapezial ligament, and scapholunate ligaments all help to prevent separation of the carpals to which they attach, ultimately preventing wrist instability.

A carpal arch is formed on the palmar surface of the wrist. A superficial ligament spans the arch and maintains it and is the flexor retinaculum or transverse carpal ligament. This ligament has a proximal and distal band. The proximal band becomes taut when flexor carpi ulnaris contracts and when the hand is held firmly in an ulnar flexed position. This is located at the distal skin crease of the wrist and forms the border on the palmar side of the carpal tunnel. The distal band is always taut and acts as a pulley for flexor tendons (Gench et al., 1995).

There is a concavity formed by the arched carpal bones that is spanned by the transverse carpal ligament; this is known as the *carpal tunnel*. The tendons of flexor digitorum profundus, flexor digitorum superficialis, flexor carpi radialis, flexor pollicis longus, and the medial nerve run through this tunnel. The transverse carpal ligament restricts bowing of the long finger flexor tendons when the wrist is flexed, protects the median nerve, and is the site of origin for thenar and hypothenar muscles (Gench et al., 1995).

There is an extensor retinaculum that goes across the dorsal surface of the wrist and forms a roof for extensor tendons. Fibers of the retinaculum insert on the pisiform and triquetrum on the ulnar

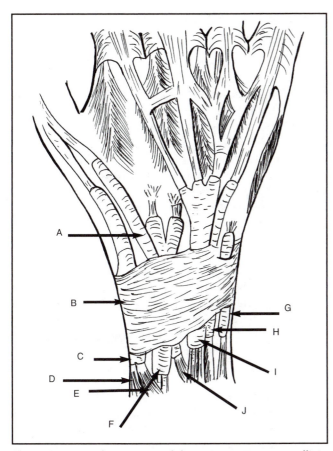

Figure 7-2. Dorsal structures of the wrist. A. Extensor pollicis longus; B. Extensor retinaculum; C. 1st dorsal compartment; D. Abductor pollicis longus; E. Extensor pollicis brevis; F. 2nd dorsal compartment (ECRL, ECRB); G. 6th compartment (Extensor carpi ulnaris); H. 5th compartment (Extensor digiti minimi); I. 4th compartment (Extensor digitorum and extensor indicis).

side, and on the radial side, the retinaculum blends with flexor retinaculum. This acts as a pulley mechanism for extensor tendons.

Each extensor tendon is surrounded by synovial sheath and these form into six compartments that contain the following:

- First: radial nerve, tunnel for abductor pollicis longus, extensor pollicis brevis.
- Second: extensor carpi radialis longus, extensor carpi radialis brevis.
- Third: extensor pollicis longus.
- Fourth: extensor indicis, extensor digitorum.
- Fifth: extensor digiti minimi.
- Sixth: extensor carpi ulnaris (Figure 7-2).

Palpable Bony Structures

Head of Ulna

This can be grasped from side to side at its narrowest portion. This is the rounded projection proximal to the index finger and on dorsum of the wrist. In a pronated position, this eminence can be seen beneath the skin. If the fingertip is placed on the highest part and the forearm is supinated, the head of the ulna can no longer be palpated because during supination, the distal portion of the radius rotates around the head of the ulna (Smith, Weiss, & Lehmkuhl, 1996).

Styloid Process of Ulna

This is a small projection on the medial aspect of the head of the ulna and it feels smaller and sharper than the head of the ulna. It may be palpated in pronation or supination. If the extensor carpi ulnaris tendon interferes with palpation, slide the index finger over this tendon in a palmar direction and the styloid will be more accessible (Smith et al., 1996).

Styloid Process of Radius

This is located at the lateral aspect of the wrist, proximal to first metacarpal, and it extends more distally than the styloid process of the ulna. Note that the radial styloid extends further distally than ulnarly.

Tubercle of Radius or Lister's Tubercle

This tubercle is located on the dorsum of the radius, about 1 inch laterally from the head of the ulna. The extensor pollicis longus tendon lies on the ulnar side of this prominence and the tubercle serves as a landmark for locating many tendons in this region (extensor carpi radialus brevis [ECRB], extensor indicus proprius [EIP], and the extensor digitorum [ED] to the index finger).

Carpal Bones

There is considerable passive accessory motion possible in the wrist with the forearm and wrist relaxed. If the distal radius and ulna are stabilized with one hand, and the other hand is placed around the proximal carpal row, the carpals can move easily in dorsal, volar, medial, and lateral translatory glides and be distracted several millimeters (Smith et al., 1996).

Capitate

This bone is in the central position in the wrist in line with the middle finger. It is best approached from dorsum and is seen as a slight depression. The capitate serves as the axis for deviation motions of the wrist (Smith et al., 1996).

Scaphoid (Navicular)

This can be palpated distally to styloid process of the radius. When in ulnar deviation, the bone becomes prominent and can be palpated, but while in radial deviation, the bone recedes. This is the most commonly fractured bone of the carpals, which is important because this bone is vital to wrist motions. The scaphoid supports the weight of the arm and transmits forces received from the hand to the bones of the forearm (Caillet, 1996). The scaphoid and trapezium make up the floor of anatomic snuff box (fovea radialis).

Trapezium (Greater Multangular)

This bone can be palpated proximal to the first carpometacarpal of the thumb and distal to the scaphoid.

Lunate

The lunate is distal to Lister's tubercle and proximal to the capitate. It is prominent as the wrist is passively flexed and recedes as the wrist is passively extended. This is the most frequently dislocated carpal bone.

Pisiform

This is a pea-shaped bone on the palmar side of wrist near the ulnar border. It can be grasped and moved from side to side and is the point of attachment of the tendon of flexor carpi ulnaris.

Trapezoid (lesser multangular), triquetrum (triangular), and hamate are more difficult to identify except when one is using relationships to other (more easily palpated) carpal bones. For example, the triquetrum bone is just below ulnar styloid (Magee, 1992; Esch, 1989; Hamil & Knutzen, 1995; Smith et al., 1996).

Anatomical Snuff Box

This is an indentation that forms on the dorsum of the hand when the thumb is actively extended. The tendons between EPL and EPB form the medial and lateral borders with the scaphoid bone inside snuff box. The radial styloid is on the lateral aspect when in anatomical position and moving medially over the radius is Lister's tubercle. The ulnar styloid is on the medial aspect (Hinkle, 1997).

Radiocarpal Joint

This is the joint that is commonly referred to as the wrist. It is made up of the distal end of the radius and the distal surface of radioulnar articulating disk, connecting with the proximal row of carpal bones (scaphoid, lunate, and triangular/triquetrum bones). The radius articulates with scaphoid and lunate, while the lunate and triquetrum articulate with the disk, not the ulna (MacKenna & Callender, 1990). The distal radius and the disk form an elliptical, biconcave surface and the superior articulating surfaces of scaphoid, lunate, and triangular/triquetrum form a smooth biconvex surface (Goss, 1976; MacKenna & Callender, 1990). The disk binds the radius and the ulna together at their distal ends and separates the distal ulna from the radiocarpal joint.

Osteokinetics

The radiocarpal joint is a biaxial, condyloid synovial joint with 2 degrees of freedom capable of producing flexion and extension, abduction and adduction, and circumduction of the wrist. This is a true condyloid joint with all motions except rotation. Circumduction is produced by the consecutive sequential combination of movements of adduction, extension, abduction, and flexion. No rotation is possible, but the effect of rotation is achieved by pronation and supination of the forearm. The motion at this joint is primarily gliding produced by movement of the proximal row of carpal bones on the radius and the radioulnar disk.

Arthrokinetics

Since the convex surface of carpals move on the concave distal radius, the glide of carpals is in a direction opposite to the movement of the hand (Kisner & Colby, 1990) (Table 7-1).

Midcarpal Joints

The midcarpal joints are formed as a compound articulation between the proximal and distal rows of carpal bones (with the exception of pisiform bone). On the radial (lateral) side, the scaphoid articulates with the trapezoid and triquetrum (triangular) bones. The scaphoid is essentially a convex surface on which the concave surfaces of the trapezoid and triquetrum slide. The central portion consists of the head of capitate and superior part of hamate articulating with the deep cavity formed by scaphoid and lunate (Goss, 1976). This forms a type of ball and socket joint where some axial rotation may be possible (Nordin & Frankel, 1989).

The ulnar (medial) side of the joint is the articulation of the hamate with the triangular/triquetrum bone. The articulating surface of the hamate is in essence convex as it slides on the concave articulating surface of the triquetrum.

Flexion and extension motions are possible at this joint, as is some rotation. The trapezium and trapezoid on the radial side and the hamate on the ulnar side glide forward and backward on the scaphoid and triangular, while the head of capitate and the superior surface of hamate rotate in the cavity of the scaphoid and lunate (Goss, 1976). This joint is inherently stable because it is bound by the dorsal and palmar, and ulnar and radial ligaments.

Osteokinetics

This joint is mostly described as a condyloid joint, although it was also cited as a sellar (saddle shaped) joint (Gench et al., 1995). The excursion of the articulating surfaces favor the range of extension over flexion and radial deviation over ulnar, which is opposite to what occurs at the radiocarpal joint (Nordin & Frankel, 1989).

Arthrokinetics

The concave-convex relationship descriptions seem to apply in the case of the midcarpal joints, but the relationships between these bones are actually more complex than is readily apparent. The relationship of the motion with direction of movement of the distal carpal bones in respect to proximal carpals is shown in Table 7-1.

Intercarpal Joints

The intercarpal joints are those articulations between the individual bones in the proximal and distal rows of carpal bones. It is the articulation of the scaphoid, lunate, and triangular (triquetrum) bones, which form gliding joints and are connected by dorsal, palmar, and interosseus ligaments as well as the articulation of the bones of the distal row (trapezium, trapezoid, capitate, hamate), which also form gliding joints and are connected by dorsal, palmar, and interosseus ligaments. The intercarpal joints are bound by intercarpal ligaments and are capable of slight movements.

Pisotriquetral Joint

This is a separate joint and it does not take part in other intercarpal movements. The articulation is the pisiform with the triquetrum (triangular) bone. This is capable of slight movement due to ligamental connections.

Table 7-1.

PHYSIOLOGIC MOTION OF THE WRIST

Motion	Direction of Movement of Carpals on Radius
Flexion	Dorsal (posterior)
Extension	Volar (anterior/palm)
Radial deviation	Ulnar
Ulnar deviation	Radial

Motion	Direction of Movement of Distal Carpals in Respect to Proximal Carpals
Flexion	Capitate and hamate dorsal (posterior)
	Trapezium and trapezoid volar (palmar)
Extension*	Capitate and hamate volar
	Trapezium and trapezoid dorsal
Radial deviation*	Capitate and hamate ulnar
	Trapezium and trapezoid dorsal
Ulnar deviation	Capitate and hamate radial
	Trapezium and trapezoid volar

*greater movement

Reprinted with permission from Kisner, C. & Colby, L. A. (1990). *Therapeutic exercise: Foundations and techniques*. Philadelphia: F. A. Davis Co.

MOVEMENTS AT THE WRIST

Movements at the wrist include flexion, extension, abduction, adduction, and circumduction (see Appendix D). The amount of movement varies considerably from person to person, varies due to the position of the forearm, and can even vary from one hand to the other of the same person (Jenkins, 1998). Movement of carpal row upon the radius and triangular ligament is gliding with translatory movement produced concomitantly with wrist movements (Hamil & Knutzen, 1995). As the hand flexes in palmar direction, the carpal row glides dorsally; in radial abduction, the proximal carpal row glides in ulnar direction, but this must be accompanied by an elastic capsule and lax ligaments. The proximal row of carpal bones are more mobile than the distal.

The function that occurs at the wrist depends on the muscles relative to the axes of motion. The wrist does not move in a direct plane but along a plane between radial extension (deviation) and ulnar flexion (deviation) and an opposite plane of ulnar extension and radial flexion due to direction of muscles and their tendons acting on the wrist (Caillet, 1996).

The amount of motion depends also on the shape of the articulating surfaces. The surface of the radioulnar articulation is less concave across than anterioposteriorly. Plus, the curvature of the proximal carpal row is greater than the opposing curve of the radioulnar surface. "Due to these discrepancies, greater excursion of flexion/extension motion occurs than radioulnar motion. The greater degree of flexion as compared to extension and of ulnar abduction as compared to radial is due to the angulation of the distal articular surface of the radius and to the fact that dorsal wrist ligaments are more slack than are the palmar ligaments" (Caillet, 1996, p. 3).

The proximal carpals form a convex surface that moves the concave surface of the distal radius and radioulnar disk. The glide of proximal carpal row occurs in a direction opposite to the movement of the hand. For example, in wrist flexion the carpals slide dorsally on the radius and disk, while in wrist ulnar deviation, the carpals slide radially (Nordin & Frankel, 1989).

Grip strength is influenced by position of the wrist. Hamil & Knutzen (1995) cited a study by Nordin and Frankel that found that when the wrist is in 40 degrees of hyperextension (extension), grip was more than three times greater than if the wrist was in 40 degrees of wrist flexion (p. 181). In addition, wrist flexion has more than twice the work capacity of extension, and radial deviation slightly exceeds ulnar deviation in work capacity (Baxter, 1998).

Flexion and Extension

The axis for wrist flexion and extension of the wrist occurs in the sagittal plane, frontal or side-to-side axis through the wrist just

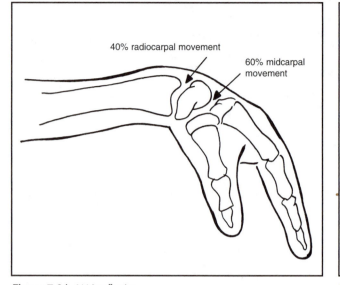

Figure 7-3A. Wrist flexion.

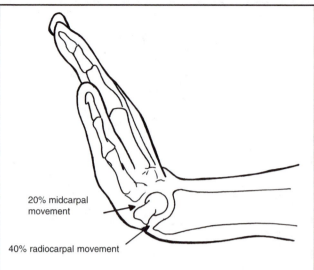

Figure 7-3B. Wrist extension.

distal to styloid process of radius and ulna through the capitate carpal bone. Smith et al. (1996) indicate that the axis migrates distally when moving from full flexion to extension, which is caused by translatory and rotational movements of the lunate and scaphoid. These movements change the height of the bones of the wrist, which is necessary to maintain tension on the ligaments. Muscles that lie anterior to the wrist's flexion/extension axis are wrist flexors, whereas muscles lying posterior to the axis are wrist extensors.

There is a different amount of movement at the different joints of the wrist as the distal carpi glide on the proximal carpal row to produce flexion and extension. In flexion, the greatest degree of movement occurs at the radiocarpal joint, a significant amount of movement at the intercarpal joint, and less movement at the midcarpal joints. In extension, the movement of the midcarpal joints is the most significant, and secondary movement is achieved at the radiocarpal joint (Figure 7-3A, B).

Flexion of the wrist is produced when the carpals slide dorsally on the radius and the disk. It has been estimated that 60% of the flexion motion occurs at the midcarpal and 40% at the radiocarpal joint. The movement of flexion is often accompanied by slight ulnar deviation and supination, and the primary wrist flexors are flexor carpi radialis, flexor carpi ulnaris, and palmaris longus. End feel for wrist flexion is firm secondary to tautness of the dorsal radiocarpal ligament and dorsal joint capsule.

Wrist extension also has a firm end feel secondary to the tautness of the palmar radiocarpal ligament and palmar joint capsule. The motion of extension is initiated by the distal carpals, with the capitate at center as the axis. It has been estimated that 67% of the movement of extension occurs at this radiocarpal joint. Ligaments draw the capitulum and scaphoid together in a close packed position, which increases the extensor force and unites the carpals, which now will act as a single unit. Midcarpal motion, estimated at 33% at this midcarpal joint, occurs with distal carpals gliding on proximal carpals (lunate and triquetrum), which are relatively

fixed. Full wrist extension requires a slight spreading of distal radius and ulna, and if these two bones were grasped together, complete wrist extension would not be possible (Smith et al., 1996). Wrist extension is usually accompanied by slight radial deviation and pure extension (without deviation) is dependent upon the ulnar and radial extensors working together for balance. The most powerful extensors are the extensor carpi radialis longus, extensor carpi radialis brevis, and extensor carpi ulnaris. These muscles are active in activities requiring wrist extension or stabilization against resistance, especially if pronated, as occurs when doing the backhand stroke in racquet sports (Hamil & Knutzen, 1995).

Ulnar and Radial Deviation

Ulnar and radial deviation (Figure 7-4) are terms that are synonymous with ulnar flexors and extensors and wrist adduction and abduction. This motion occurs in the frontal/coronal plane at the anterioposterior/sagittal axis, with the axis of motion through the capitate at a right angle to the palm (Nicholas & Hershman, 1990). Motion that occurs lateral to this front-to-back axis is radial deviation (abduction) and motion medial to this axis is ulnar deviation (adduction). There is more movement in ulnar deviation than radial because the radial styloid process comes into contact with the scaphoid in radial deviation, which prevents further motion and causes the normal hard end feel. Ulnar and radial deviation is greatest if the wrist is neutral regarding wrist flexion or extension. If the wrist extends, very little deviation occurs because the carpals are drawn into a locked, close packed position. In wrist flexion, further movement is not possible because the bones are already splayed and the joint is in its loose packed position (Norkin & Levangie, 1996).

In radial deviation, the proximal carpal row moves ulnarly on the radius and the radioulnar disk, while the distal row of carpal bones is displaced radially. If movement occurred in a single plane (frontal), the distal row would swing radially during radial devia-

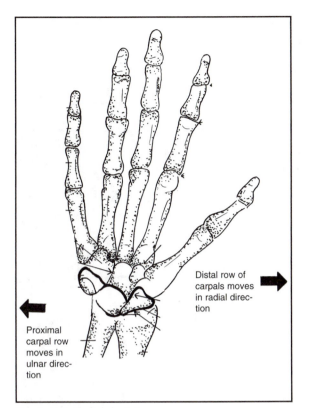

Figure 7-4. Radial deviation.

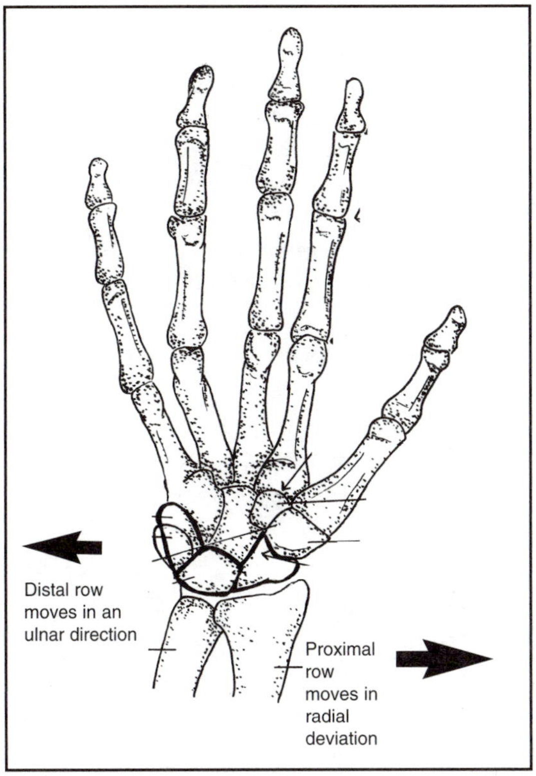

Distal row of carpals moves in radial direction

Proximal carpal row moves in ulnar direction

Figure 7-5. Ulnar deviation.

Distal row moves in an ulnar direction

Proximal row moves in radial deviation

tion to push the scaphoid into the radial styloid. Instead, what happens is that there is a shift in the position of the scaphoid. The distal portion of scaphoid rotates toward the palm and the proximal row exhibits some flexion due to the scapholunate ligament. The capitate glides ulnarly toward the proximal row, causing close packed congruity between surfaces. Most of the motion occurring in radial deviation occurs at the midcarpal joints, and primary radial deviators are extensor carpi radialis longus, extensor carpi radialis brevis, and flexor carpi radialis.

Ulnar deviation occurs similarly to radial deviation, with the triquetrum moving much like the scaphoid in radial deviation. The triquetrum glides distally on the hamate and extends, which brings the lunate into an extended position and rotates toward the palm. The capitate rotates a small amount by rotating around the vertical axis while slightly gliding around the medial and lateral portions of the joint. This produces movement toward the radial side and functionally disengages the capitate from the proximal row. The scaphoid also moves into some extension and the distal carpal bones move ulnarly. Most of the motion of ulnar deviation occurs at the radiocarpal joint, with very little contribution of the movements of the bones of the midcarpal articulations. Ulnar deviation or adduction is produced primarily by the flexor carpi ulnaris and extensor carpi ulnaris working together synergistically to produce a movement neither could produce alone. Ulnar abduction has a firm end feel due to tension on the radial collateral ligament and the radial portion of joint capsule. In ulnar deviation, radiocarpal movement predominates (Figure 7-5).

INTERNAL KINETICS

Many of the wrist muscles work together to cancel one action of one muscle to produce a unique motion with another. This can be seen with the radial and ulnar wrist extensors, which work together to produce deviation. Flexor carpi radialis and extensor carpi radialis longus work together to cancel the flexion and extension actions of each other and to produce radial deviation. Similarly, flexor carpi ulnaris and extensor carpi ulnaris function antagonistically in flexion and extension but synergistically in ulnar deviation. Other synergistic actions occur when flexor carpi radialis and flexor carpi ulnaris work together to hold the wrist in neutral or flexion needed when one performs delicate work or when extensor carpi radialis longus and brevis and extensor carpi ulnaris work together to produce a powerful grip and maintain wrist extension even when the fingers tightly grasp an object. These are but a few of the muscular combinations that occur to provide sufficient wrist positioning for optimal and diverse hand function and the transmission of forces from the hand to the forearm.

Flexors at the Wrist

The following muscles flex the wrist because they lie anterior to side to side axis (Figure 7-6). Flexor carpi radialis, flexor carpi ulnaris, and palmaris longus are the primary flexors, with flexor carpi ulnaris considered the strongest of the three. All three of these muscles are fusiform and are most powerful with the wrist in flexion or in stabilization of the wrist against resistance (Thompson & Floyd, 1994).

Flexor digitorum profundus, flexor digitorum superficialis, and palmaris longus are multijoint muscles and their capacity to produce effective forces at the wrist is dependent upon a synergistic stabilizer to prevent full excursion of more distal joints. If these muscles attempt to act over both the wrist and more distal joints, they will become actively insufficient (Gench et al., 1995; Hinkle, 1997; Jenkins, 1998; Norkin & Levangie, 1992; Smith et al., 1996).

Flexor Carpi Ulnaris

Flexor carpi ulnaris is a superficial muscle on the palmar aspect of the ulna. It crosses the wrist anterior to the flexion/extension axis and to ulnar side of the deviation axis, so this muscle flexes and ulnarly deviates. This muscle is active in activities requiring a stronger, sustained power grip such as using a hammer or in the stroke of an axe (Gench et al., 1995). This muscle is considered the strongest wrist flexor, especially due to the tendon encasing the pisiform bone, which adds mechanical advantage and decreases tendon tension (Gench et al., 1995; Hinkle, 1997; Jenkins, 1998; Norkin & Levangie, 1992; Smith et al., 1996). *Palpation*: This muscle lies close to the ulnar border of the forearm and the tendon may be palpated between the ulnar styloid process and proximal to the pisiform bone with wrist flexion resisted (Gench et al., 1995; Smith et al., 1996). Pinch fingertips together or flex the wrist and palpate proximal to the pisiform (Gench et al., 1995).

Flexor Carpi Radialis

While a primary flexor of the wrist, flexor carpi radialis is only 60% as strong as flexor carpi ulnaris. This muscle crosses the wrist anterior to the flexion/extension axis and to the radial side, and assists with radial deviation as well as flexing the wrist (Gench et al., 1995; Hinkle, 1997; Jenkins, 1998; Norkin & Levangie, 1992; Smith et al., 1996). *Palpation*: When resistance is applied with the wrist in flexion and radial deviation, the flexor carpi radialis muscle is located on the radial side, in a superficial position in the lower part of the forearm. Palmaris longus is in the central location, while flexor carpi radialis is located radially to palmaris longus. The muscle cannot be followed to its distal attachment (Gench et al., 1995; Smith et al., 1996).

Palmaris Longus

Palmaris longus is a small fusiform muscle that varies widely in structure and is actually absent in 10 to 15% of people (Gench et al., 1995; Thompson & Floyd, 1994). This muscle is generally seen as a contributor to wrist flexion, but since palmaris longus crosses the wrist farther from the flexion/extension axis than flexor carpi ulnaris or flexor carpi radialis and is small, it produces weak flexion even with its long force arm. Due to its insertion in the flexor retinaculum, palmaris longus contributes to the cupping motion of the hand. *Palpation*: While applying resistance in wrist flexion, the centrally located tendon is palmaris longus (Smith et al., 1996). It can also be seen and palpated when the thumb is opposed to the small finger with the wrist flexed. Palmaris longus, if present, will be between the flexor carpi radialis and flexor carpi ulnaris (Gench et al., 1995).

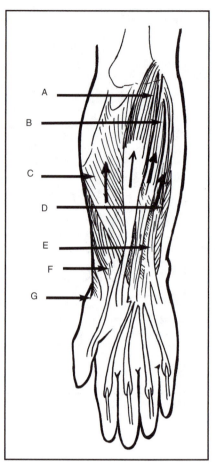

Figure 7-6. Wrist flexors. A. Flexor carpi radialis; B. Palmaris longus; C. Flexor digitorum superficialis; D. Flexor digitorum profundus; E. Flexor carpi ulnaris; F. Flexor pollicis longus; G. Abductor pollicis longus.

Flexor Digitorum Superficialis (Flexor Digitorum Sublimis)

This muscle has four tendons on the palmar aspect of the hand that insert into each of the four fingers. Flexor digitorum superficialis crosses the wrist, metacarpophalangeal, and proximal IP joints anterior to the flexion/extension axis. The action of flexor digitorum superficialis is vital in gripping activities because it acts with the flexor digitorum profundus to flex the digits (Gench et al., 1995; Hinkle, 1997; Jenkins, 1998; Norkin & Levangie, 1992; Smith et al., 1996). *Palpation*: With the fist closed tightly and wrist flexion simultaneously resisted, one or more of these tendons may become apparent between palmaris longus and flexor carpi ulnaris. The tendons may be seen to move within their sheaths as the fingers are flexed to make a fist (Gench et al., 1995). Flexor digitorum superficialis is located underneath flexor carpi radialis and palmaris longus and runs from the medial epicondyle to the center of the palmar side of the wrist. It is not possible to palpate the proximal attachment because the muscle is widespread, but one can observe it in the distal forearm and wrist (Smith et al., 1996).

Flexor Digitorum Profundus

This deep muscle, covered by flexor digitorum superficialis, flexor carpi ulnaris, palmaris longus, flexor carpi radialis, and pronator teres, assists with wrist flexion when the digits are kept extended. Flexor digitorum profundus flexes the metacarpophalangeal (MCP), proximal interphalangeal (PIP), and distal inter-

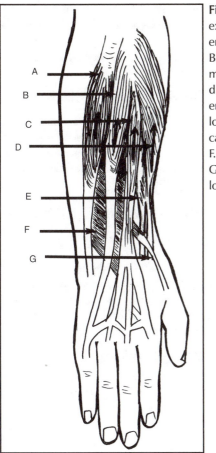

Figure 7-7. Wrist extensors. A. Extensor carpi ulnaris; B. Extensor digiti minimi; C. Extensor digitorum; D. Extensor carpi radialis longus; E. Extensor carpi radialis brevis; F. Extensor indicis; G. Extensor pollicis longus.

Flexor Pollicis Longus

This penniform muscle lies deep on the radial side of the forearm, where it assists with wrist flexion due to the palmar location in the wrist and plays an important role in grip activities (Thompson & Floyd, 1994). Some authors disagree with the role of this muscle in wrist flexion because it lies too close to both wrist axes and the power of the muscle is already spent as it flexes the thumb (Gench et al., 1995; Goss, 1976). *Palpation*: the tendon can be palpated on the palmar surface of the thumb between the MCP and IP joints as the IP joint is flexed (Gench et al., 1995).

Abductor Pollicis Longus

This muscle crosses the wrist directly above the axis of flexion/extension but "bowstrings" during wrist flexion, allowing it to contribute to wrist flexion. *Palpation*: The superficial tendon can be palpated as it crosses the wrist on the palmar side of extensor pollicis brevis when the thumb is forcefully abducted (Gench et al., 1995).

Extensors at the Wrist

Extensor carpi radialis longus, extensor carpi radialis brevis, and extensor carpi ulnaris are the most powerful wrist extensors and are active in activities requiring wrist extension or stabilization against resistance, especially if pronated (as occurs in the backhand stroke in racquet sports) (Figure 7-7). These three muscles act on the elbow so joint position is important. ECRL and ECRB cause flexion at the elbow and so can be enhanced as a wrist extensor with extension of the elbow, whereas ECU is an elbow extensor and is enhanced as a wrist extensor with the elbow in flexion (Hamil & Knutzen, 1995).

Extensor Carpi Ulnaris

Extensor carpi ulnaris is active in wrist extension and frequently in wrist flexion, too, and adds stability to the less stable position of wrist flexion (Gench et al., 1995; Hinkle, 1997; Jenkins, 1998; Norkin & Levangie, 1992; Smith et al., 1996). When the forearm pronates, the crossing of the radius over the ulna leads to a smaller moment arm of extensor carpi ulnaris, so this muscle is less effective as a wrist extensor and is more effective as an extensor when the forearm is supinated. *Palpation of the tendon*: The tendon can be palpated between the head of the ulna and the prominent tubercle on the base of the 5th metacarpal. The tendon becomes prominent if the wrist is extended with the fist closed and is even more prominent if the wrist is simultaneously abducted ulnarward. The tendon is also easily palpable when the thumb is extended and abducted. *Palpation of the muscle*: The muscle can be palpated 2 inches (5 cm) below the lateral epicondyle of the humerus as the wrist is forcefully extended where it lies between anconeus and extensor digitorum, and it can be followed distally along the dorsoulnar aspect in the direction toward the head of the ulna (Gench et al., 1995; Smith et al., 1996).

phalangeal (DIP) joints, but is dependent upon wrist position for length-tension relationships in these actions. The length-tension relationship is favorable for flexor digitorum profundus when the wrist is extended and the fist can be closed. As the wrist moves toward greater flexion, flexor digitorum superficialis is recruited to aid in closure of the fist. Forceful fist closure elicits high activity levels of flexor digitorum superficialis, flexor digitorum profundus, and the interossei (Smith et al., 1996). The line of pull is to the palmar side of the flexion/extension axis of each joint and the only action is flexion, which progresses sequentially from the most distal joint (DIP joint) to the most proximal (wrist joint). The strength of the contraction lessens progressively so that flexor digitorum superficialis contributes only weakly to wrist flexion (Gench et al., 1995). *Palpation*: The contracting muscle belly may be palpated provided tension is minimal in the more superficial muscles. To achieve relaxation of the overlying muscles, the subject is seated with the forearm supinated or resting in the lap while the wrist is extended by the weight of the hand. Then ask the subject to close the fist fully with moderate effort and profundus may be felt under the fingers in the region between pronator teres and flexor carpi ulnaris about 2 inches below medial epicondyle of humerus (Smith et al., 1996). Stabilize the PIP joint in extension and flex the DIP joint (Gench et al., 1995).

Extensor Carpi Radialis Longus

Extensor carpi radialis longus lies posterior to the side/side axis so it extends the wrist and is most effective as a wrist extensor when the elbow is also extended. Extensor carpi radialis longus has increased activation when in either radial deviation or in a position supported against ulnar deviation, or when forceful finger flexion is performed (Norkin & Levangie, 1992). *Palpation of the muscle*: This muscle may be palpated just superior to the elbow as the wrist is forcefully extended with the fist closed. *Palpation of the tendon*: The tendon is prominent during wrist extension on the dorsoradial aspect of the wrist located on the radial side of the capitate bone but on the ulnar side of the tubercle of radius. If the subject places a lightly closed fist on a table or in the lap with the forearm pronated and the subject alternately closes and relaxes the fist, the rise and fall of the tendon may be felt and the muscle belly identified in the forearm close to brachioradialis. It may improve the accuracy of identification of the extensor carpi radialis longus muscle by identifying the extensor pollicis longus muscle first, which is seen when the thumb is in extension (Gench et al., 1995; Smith et al., 1996).

Extensor Carpi Radialis Brevis

This muscle crosses well posterior to the flexion/extension axis so it extends the wrist. While extensor carpi radialis brevis is in a central location on the forearm, it is covered by the extensor carpi radialis longus muscle. Its tendon is crossed by the tendons of the abductor pollicis longus and extensor pollicis longus, which makes identification of the extensor carpi radialis brevis tendon difficult. *Palpation*: While the tendon protrudes less than extensor carpi radialis longus, it can be felt on the dorsum of the wrist in line with the third metacarpal during fisted wrist extension (Gench et al., 1995; Smith et al., 1996).

Extensor Digitorum (Extensor Digitorum Communis)

Extensor digitorum, a fusiform muscle, crosses the wrist, MCP, PIP, and DIP joints. If all of these joints are extended simultaneously, then the extensor digitorum will be contracted to its shortest length and can be only weakly responsive at the wrist as an extensor (Gench et al., 1995). *Palpation*: With the wrist extended and fist closed, the prominent tendon of extensor carpi radialis longus can be palpated at the base of the second metacarpal. If you maintain the wrist in this position and extend the fingers, the four tendons of the extensor digitorum can be seen and palpated on the dorsum of the hand (Smith et al., 1996).

Extensor Digiti Minimi and Extensor Indicis (Extensor Indicis Proprius)

Extensor digiti minimi and extensor indicis are capable of wrist extension after continued contraction, but wrist extension action is credited more to the extensor digitorum muscle. If the MCP and IP joints are held in flexion, then extensor indicis is an effective wrist extensor. *Palpation of extensor digiti minimi*: Located on the ulnar side of extensor digitorum, the tendon can be palpated and observed on the dorsum of the hand when the small finger is extended against resistance, especially at the 5th MCP joint (Gench et al., 1995). *Palpation of extensor indicis*: The tendon is superficial and can be observed on the ulnar side of and parallel to the tendon of extensor digitorum as it approaches the base of the index finger (Gench et al., 1995).

Extensor Pollicis Brevis, Extensor Pollicis Longus

While specified as contributors to wrist extension due to the location dorsal to the joint axis by some sources (Hamil & Knutzen, 1995), these muscles do not contribute much to wrist function (Thompson & Floyd, 1994).

Radial Deviation/Abductors at Wrist

Flexor Carpi Radialis

Even though this muscle is located to the radial side of the deviation axis, it is not significantly effective as a radial deviator in isolated contractions due to the longer moment arm for flexion than for deviation. However with palmaris longus, flexor carpi radialis does contribute to radial deviation (Figure 7-8).

Extensor Carpi Radialis Longus

Since this muscle is located on the radial side of the deviation axis, it serves to abduct the wrist. Since this muscle has a longer moment arm for deviation than for extension, it is more effective as a deviator than as an extensor.

Extensor Carpi Radialis Brevis

The extensor carpi radialis brevis muscle is located close to the deviation axis, so it provides scant contribution to deviation (Gench et al., 1995).

Abductor Pollicis Longus

This muscle lies on the radial side of deviation axis and assists with wrist abduction.

Extensor Pollicis Brevis

This muscle is located so that there is a favorable line of muscle action for radial deviation regardless of the position of the thumb (Gench et al., 1995). Other sources feel that since the muscle crosses directly over the axis, this muscle is not involved in adduction or abduction (Burstein & Wright, 1994).

Extensor Pollicis Longus

This muscle lies to the radial side of the deviation axis and serves to abduct the wrist, in addition to its contribution to wrist extension.

Adductors at the Wrist

Flexor Carpi Ulnaris

Flexor carpi ulnaris crosses farther away from the axis than flexor carpi radialis, so it is more effective in ulnar deviation than flexor carpi radialis is in radial deviation.

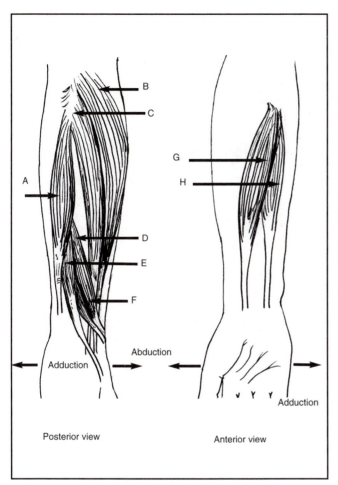

Figure 7-8. Wrist adductors and abductors. A. Extensor carpi ulnaris; B. Extensor carpi radialis longus; C. Extensor carpi radialis brevis; D. Abductor pollicis longus; E. Extensor pollicis longus; F. Extensor pollicis brevis; G. Flexor carpi radialis; H. Flexor carpi ulnaris.

Extensor Carpi Ulnaris

Since this muscle crosses the axis posteriorly and ulnarly, it extends and ulnarly deviates the wrist. Due to the muscle's flare at the base of the 5th metacarpal, it increases the angle of the muscle's attachment and helps to stabilize the head of the ulna during wrist movements. It is a stronger ulnar deviator when the forearm is pronated (Gench et al., 1995).

Extensor Indicis

This is considered a weak adductor since the muscle crosses on the ulnar side of the adduction/abduction axis.

WRIST ASSESSMENT

While the wrist is important in positioning the hand in space and for prehension, very little pure wrist motion is necessary for everyday activities. Even with a significant loss of motion in the wrist, adjacent joints can be used to compensate for diminished movement of the wrist. Most activities of daily living require 10

degrees flexion to 15 degrees extension as minimal requirements for ROM (Nicholas & Hershman, 1990).

Assessment of the wrist includes looking at the skin for blisters or lacerations and observing for any abnormal formations or nodules. Edema may be seen in local swollen ganglions (synovial hernia in tendonous sheath or joint capsule), usually on the dorsum of the hand, or there could be inflammation of the tendon or its synovial sheath. Diffuse swelling usually is seen on the dorsal surface of the hand because there is more room for expansion (Hartley, 1995). While swelling is difficult to observe in the wrist, edema will limit joint movement. Edema of the wrist is dangerous because it can congest the carpal tunnels and restrict extensor tendon compartments (Hartley, 1995).

Pain may be limited to tenderness in areas that the client can pinpoint, likely due to injury to more superficial structures. There may be referred pain in the deeper structures, such as in the more deeply located muscles and ligaments, in the bursae, or in bones (especially the scaphoid or radius) (Hartley, 1995). Questions about when the pain occurs, where it is, and what activities aggravate the pain are necessary in recommending activities for intervention.

Observation of the use of the wrist and hand during activities and an assessment of ROM (both passive and active) and wrist strength are also vital to wrist assessment.

SUMMARY

- The radiocarpal joint is made up of the radius and carpal bones.
- The wrist includes three joints: radiocarpal, midcarpal, and intercarpal joints.
- Movements at the radiocarpal and midcarpal joints occur at the same time and are involved in the motions of flexion and extension.
- Adduction/abduction of the wrist (also known as ulnar and radial deviation) are accomplished when the capitate and scaphoid carpal bones move in radial deviation; triquetrum/triangular in ulnar deviation.
- Circumduction is a combined sequence of movement of adduction, extension, abduction, and flexion.
- Many muscles work together at the wrist to produce movement that a single muscle alone would not be able to produce.
- Assessment of the wrist includes consideration of the movement produced, pain, edema, and functional use of the wrist in activities.

REFERENCES

Baxter, R. (1998). *Pocket guide to musculoskeletal assessment.* Philadelphia: W. B. Saunders Co.

Burstein, A., & Wright, T. M. (1994). *Fundamentals of orthopaedic biomechanics.* Baltimore: Williams & Wilkins.

Calliet, R. (1996). *Soft tissue pain and disability* (3rd ed.). Philadelphia: F. A. Davis Co.

Esch, D. L. (1989). *Musculoskeletal function: An anatomy and kinesiology laboratory manual.* Minneapolis: University of Minnesota.

Gench, B. E., Hinson, M. M., & Harvey, P. T. (1995). *Anatomical kinesiology*. Dubuque, IA: Eddie Bowers Publishing, Inc.

Goss, C. M. (Ed.) (1976). *Gray's anatomy of the human body* (29th ed.). Philadelphia: Lea and Febiger.

Hamil, J., & Knutzen, K. M. (1995). *Biomechanical basis of human movement*. Baltimore: Williams & Wilkins.

Hartley, A. (1995). *Practical joint assessment: Upper quadrant: A sports medicine manual* (2nd ed.). Philadelphia: C. V. Mosby.

Hinkle, C. Z. (1997). *Fundamentals of anatomy and movement: A workbook and guide*. St. Louis, MO: C. V. Mosby.

Jenkins, D. B. (1998). *Hollingshead's functional anatomy of the limbs and back* (7th ed.). Philadelphia: W. B. Saunders Co.

Kisner, C., & Colby, L. A. (1990). *Therapeutic exercise: Foundations and techniques* (2nd ed.). Philadelphia: F. A. Davis Co.

Konin, J. G. (1999). *Practical kinesiology for the physical therapist assistant*. Thorofare, NJ: SLACK Incorporated.

MacKenna, B. R., & Callender, R. (1990). *Illustrated physiology* (5th ed.). New York: Churchill Livingstone.

Magee, D. J. (1992). *Orthopedic physical assessment*. Philadelphia: W. B. Saunders Co.

Nicholas, J. A., & Hershman, E. B. (1990). *The upper extremity in sports medicine*. St. Louis, MO: C. V. Mosby Co.

Nordin, M., & Frankel, V. H. (1989). *Basic biomechanics of the musculoskeletal system* (2nd ed.). Philadelphia: Lea and Febiger.

Norkin, C. C., & Levangie, P. K. (1992). *Joint structure and function: A comprehensive analysis* (2nd ed.). Philadelphia: F. A. Davis Co.

Smith, L. K., Weiss, E. L., & Lehmkuhl, L. D. (1996). *Brunnstrom's clinical kinesiology* (5th ed.). Philadelphia: F. A. Davis Co.

Thompson, C. W., & Floyd, R. T. (1994). *Manual of structural kinesiology* (12th ed.). St. Louis, MO: C. V. Mosby.

BIBLIOGRAPHY

Basmajian, J. V., & DeLuca, C. J. (1985). *Muscles alive* (5th ed.). Baltimore: Williams & Wilkins.

Greene, D. P., & Roberts, S. L. (1999). *Kinesiology: Movement in the context of activity*. St. Louis, MO: C. V. Mosby.

Loth, T., & Wadsworth, C. T. (1998). *Orthopedic review for physical therapists*. St. Louis, MO: C. V. Mosby Co.

Lumley, J. S. P. (1990). *Surface anatomy: The anatomical basis of clinical examination*. New York: Churchill Livingstone.

Melvin, J. L. (1982). *Rheumatic disease: Occupational therapy and rehabilitation* (2nd ed.). Philadelphia: F. A. Davis Co.

Palastanga, N., Field, D., & Soames, R. (1989). *Anatomy and human movement: Structure and function*. Oxford: Heinemann Medical Books.

Palmer, M. L., & Epler, M. E. (1998). *Fundamentals of musculoskeletal assessment techniques* (2nd ed.). Philadelphia: J. B. Lippincott.

Perry, J. F., Rohe, D. A., & Garcia, A. O. (1996). *Kinesiology workbook*. Philadelphia: F. A. Davis Co.

Saidoff, D. C., & McDonough, A. L. (1997). *Critical pathways in therapeutic intervention: Upper extremity*. St. Louis, MO: C. V. Mosby.

Trombly, C. A. (Ed.) (1995). *Occupational therapy for physical dysfunction* (4th ed.). Baltimore: Williams & Wilkins.

Watkins, J. (1999). *Structure and function of the musculoskeletal system*. New York: Human Kinetics.

The Hand

Chapter 8

The hand is amazingly complex, intricately constructed, and vital to daily life activities. Capable of complex movements, the hand is a vital connection and mechanism for interaction with the environment. Not only does the hand provide mobility for the proximal joints to move the hand in large areas of space and to reach nearly all parts of the body, but the hand participates in fine motor grasp and pinch, tactile exploration of the environment, and in nonverbal communication with others.

ANATOMY

The hand consists of five digits or four fingers and one thumb (Figure 8-1A, B). Each of the digits has a carpometacarpal (CMC) articulation and a metacarpophalangeal (MCP) joint. The fingers have two interphalangeal (IP) joints while the thumb has only one. There are nineteen bones distal to the carpal bones of the wrist that make up the hand: five metacarpal bones, five proximal phalanges, five middle phalanges, and four distal phalanges (Norkin & Levangie, 1992). The metacarpals can be palpated on the dorsum of the hand as can the proximal, middle, and distal phalanges.

Mobility within the hand is variable. The distal row of carpals and their articulation with the metacarpals of the index and long fingers are relatively fixed due to the intercarpal ligaments and distal carpal bones. The thumb is the most mobile digit, followed (in order from most to least) by the phalanges of the index, long, ring, and small fingers and then the fourth and fifth metacarpals.

Many ligaments operate within the hand to provide stability and to permit mobility. A heavy fibrous aponeurosis that covers the center of the palm is called the *palmar fascia*. This tissue receives the insertion of the palmaris longus muscle and it merges with the flexor retinaculum at its distal edge. The palmar aponeurosis thickens at the wrist and with the carpal arch and flexor retinaculum becomes the carpal tunnel, through which the long flexor tendons and median nerve pass. Distally, the palmar aponeurosis gives slips to each finger.

At the wrist, there are two synovial sheaths that provide a surface for free movement for the flexor tendons. One synovial sheath is for flexor pollicis longus and the other for flexor digitorum superficialis and flexor digitorum profundus (Figure 8-2).

The hand has a concave appearance even when the palm is fully opened. This is due to the arches in the hand produced by the carpal bones and ligaments. There are two transverse arches and one longitudinal arch in the hand. The *proximal transverse arch* (or *carpal transverse arch*) is curved due to the shape of the carpal bones, with the flexor retinaculum (transverse carpal ligament) as the "roof" of the arch (Magee, 1992). This becomes the carpal tunnel. There is much variability in the shape of this arch due to the mobility of the bones that make up the arch.

The *longitudinal arch* runs from the wrist to the fingertips, with the apex of the arch along the row of metacarpal heads. The carpal bones, metacarpal bones, and phalanges make up this arch, with the metacarpal bones providing the stability. The length of the arch is greatest at the second metacarpal and shortest at the fifth metacarpal. Greene and Roberts (1999) caution that if the shorter length of the longitudinal arch on the ulnar side is not considered when making splints, the splint may extend too far distally, blocking flexion of the fourth and fifth MCP joints (p. 101) (Figure 8-3).

Weakness or atrophy of intrinsic hand muscles will lead to loss of arches, which are most noticeable with medial and ulnar nerve damage resulting in the development of the ape hand deformity. The palmar arches provide the function of palmar cupping, which enables the hand to conform to the object being held. Maximum surface contact is made, increased stability produced, and additional sensory input provided in this cupped hand position.

The two transverse arches are connected by the longitudinal arch. In finger flexion, the longitudinal arch curls in a pattern called an *equiangular spiral* or *logarithmic spiral*. This is a spiral pattern that comprises a series of isosceles triangles with angles of 36 degrees and is a biologically natural pattern, as seen in flowers and in the shell of the nautilus. It is again important to recognize the importance of maintaining these arches when splinting to enable normal hand function.

Visually, the hand and wrist have many creases that are easily seen. In the palmar view, the *proximal skin crease*, located at the wrist, is the upper limit of the synovial sheaths of flexor tendons. The *middle skin crease* is an indication of the location of the radiocarpal joint, and the *distal skin crease* is the location of the upper margin of flexor retinaculum. The *radial longitudinal skin crease*

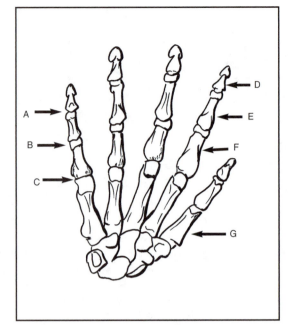

Figure 8-1A. Bones of the hand. Palmar aspect. A. DIP joint; B. PIP joint; C. MCP joint; D. Distal phalange; E. Middle phalanges; F. Proximal phalange; G. Metacarpal.

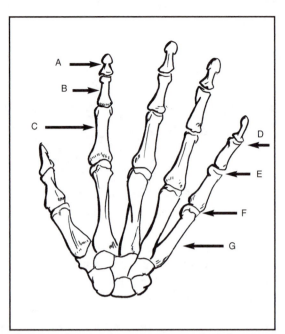

Figure 8-1B. Dorsal aspect. A. Distal phalange; B. Middle phalanges; C. Proximal phalange; D. DIP joint; E. PIP joint; F. MCP joint; G. Metacarpal.

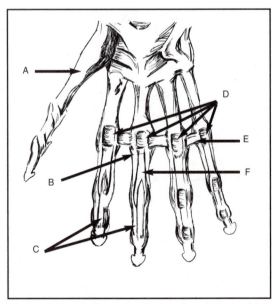

Figure 8-2. Ligaments and sheaths of the palmar aspect of the hand. A. Sheath for flexor pollicis longus; B. Cut portion of flexor sheath; C. Flexor digitorum profundus; D. Palmar ligaments; E. Deep transverse metacarpal ligament; F. Flexor digitorum superficialis.

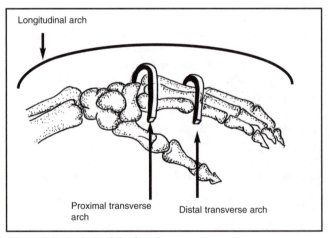

Figure 8-3. Arches of the hand.

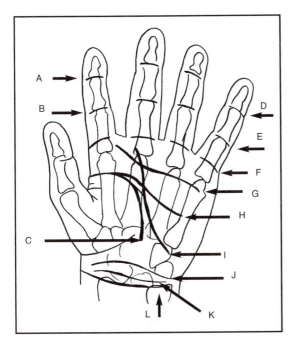

Figure 8-4. Palmar creases of the hand. A. DIP joint; B. PIP joint; C. Thenar crease; D. Distal digital crease; E. Middle digital crease; F. Proximal digital crease; G. Distal palmar transverse crease; H. Proximal palmar transverse crease; I. Middle palmar crease; J. Distal crease of wrist; K. Middle crease of wrist; L. Proximal crease of wrist.

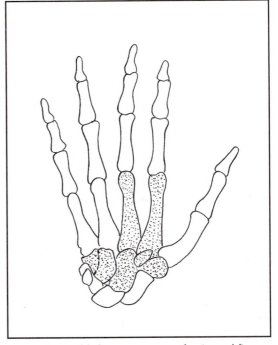

Figure 8-5. Stable bony segments of wrist and fingers.

(thenar crease) encircles the thenar eminence and is sometimes referred to as the life line. The *proximal transverse line* of the palm runs across shafts of metacarpal bones (sometimes called the head line) and the *distal transverse line* of the palm lies over the head of the second to fourth metacarpals (commonly called the love line). The *proximal skin crease of fingers* is 2 cm distal to the MCP joints, the *middle skin crease of fingers* indicates the location of the proximal IP joints, and the *distal skin crease of fingers* lies over the distal interphalangeal (DIP) joints (Greene & Roberts, 1999) (Figure 8-4).

CARPOMETACARPAL JOINT OF THE FINGERS

The (CMC) joint is the articulation of digits two through five with the distal row of carpal bones, as well as the articulation of each metacarpal bone with the base of the adjacent metacarpal bone. Specifically, the second metacarpal bone articulates primarily with the trapezoid and partially with the trapezium and the capitate and with the base of the third metacarpal. The third metacarpal articulates with the capitate and the second and fourth metacarpals. The fourth metacarpal articulates with the capitate and the hamate bones and with the side of the third and fifth metacarpal bones. The fifth metacarpal articulates with the hamate and the ulnar side with the fourth metacarpal bone. They are united by the dorsal, palmar, and interosseous ligaments.

The ligaments primarily control the amount of movement and range of motion (ROM) of the CMC joint (Norkin & Levangie, 1992). The *dorsal ligaments* are the strongest and most distinct ligaments of this joint. They connect the carpal and metacarpal bones on the dorsal surface. The *palmar ligaments* perform a similar function on the palmar surface of the hand. The *interosseous ligament* is short and thick in appearance and is limited to one part of the CMC articulation—that of connecting the inferior angles of the capitate and hamate with the third and fourth metacarpal bones (Goss, 1976). The *transverse metacarpal (intermetacarpal) ligament* is a narrow, fibrous band connecting the palmar surfaces of the heads of the second through fifth metacarpal bones. This ligament functions to prevent abduction and adduction at the CMC joint (Nordin & Frankel, 1989).

The CMC joint provides the most movement for the thumb and the least amount of movement for the fingers (Hamil & Knutzen, 1995). The most movement of the CMC joint is the metacarpal bone of the little finger, followed by the metacarpal bone of the ring finger. The metacarpal bones of the index and middle fingers are almost immovable, so the ROM increases from the radial side to the ulnar side, which enables the hand to curve anteriorly or to cup the hand. The relative immobility of the second and third metacarpals enables us to hold tools more firmly and enhances the function of the radial wrist flexors and extensors (FCR, ECRL, ECRB), serving as a fixed axis about which the first, fourth, and fifth metacarpals can move. This provides an increased lever arm without the loss of tension resulting from excessive ROM (Norkin & Levangie, 1992) (Figure 8-5).

Movements at the CMC joints of the fingers are of the uniaxial gliding plane synovial type, although one author suggests it is a modified saddle joint (Gench, Hinson, & Harvey, 1995).

Movements produced are flexion and extension, which can be seen when the hand is cupped or flattened. There is approximately 25 to 30 degrees in the fifth metacarpal, 10 to 15 degrees in the fourth, and minimal movements in the second and third metacarpals.

Muscles contributing to the movement at the CMC joints of the fingers are radial wrist muscles (flexor carpi radialis, extensor carpi radialis longus, extensor carpi radialis brevis, extensor carpi ulnaris) and flexor digitorum superficialis and flexor digitorum profundus.

When the metacarpals flex (as when cupping the hand), the metacarpals slide on the carpals in a volar (palmar or anterior) direction, whereas when the hand is flattened in extension, the metacarpals slide on the carpals in a dorsal or posterior direction (Kisner & Colby, 1990).

CARPOMETACARPAL JOINT OF THE THUMB

This articulation is formed at the juncture of the trapezium and base of the first metacarpal. It is surrounded by a thick but loose joint capsule that is reinforced by radial, ulnar, volar, and dorsal ligaments as well as an intermetacarpal ligament that holds the bases of the first and second metacarpals together. This prevents extreme movement of radial and dorsal displacements of the base of the first metacarpal (Nordin & Frankel, 1989). The laxity of the joint capsule allows 15 to 20 degrees of rotation and the metacarpal can be distracted up to 3 mm from the trapezium.

Since there are both convex and concave bone surfaces, this is a biaxial sellar (saddle-shaped) joint. Due to the shape of the articular surfaces, there is a great amount of movement possible to include abduction and adduction, flexion and extension (2 degrees of freedom).

The orientation of the axis of motion in the thumb differs from the axes at other joints. The two axes of motion are offset from the cardinal planes of motion and are not perpendicular to the bones or to each other (Gench et al., 1995) (Figure 8-6). Flexion and extension occur in the plane of the palm, with the axis oriented to the front and back in relation to the palmar and dorsal hand surfaces; that is, the motion is parallel to the palm (Goss, 1976; Greene & Roberts, 1999). This axis goes through the trapezium but at a right angle to the palm (Gench et al., 1995). Adduction and abduction occur in the plane at right angles to the palm, with the axis in a side-to-side orientation rather than front to back (Goss, 1976; Greene & Roberts, 1999). This axis is at the base of the first metacarpal and slants toward the base of the ring finger (Gench et al., 1995).

In addition to flexion and extension, and adduction and abduction, a combination movement called opposition and reposition occurs. Flexion and abduction combine to produce opposition where the first metacarpal rotates on the trapezium to permit placement of the pad of the thumb on the pads of one or more fingers. This produces a cone-shaped path that Brand (1999) calls circumduction. Reposition or retroposition is returning to the original position in a combination of extension and adduction. Other terms

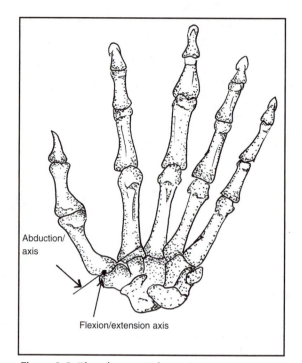

Figure 8-6. Thumb axes. Palmar view.

for opposition are thumb rotation, thumb pronation, and for reposition occasionally supination of the thumb is used (Figures 8-7 and 8-8).

Flexion and extension occur in the frontal plane with the convex trapezium articulating on the concave metacarpal base so the surface slides in the same direction as the angulating bone (Table 8-1). Adduction and abduction movements occur in the sagittal and frontal axis and because the trapezium is concave and the metacarpal convex, the surface slides in an opposite direction of the articulating bone (Kisner & Colby, 1990).

METACARPOPHALANGEAL JOINT OF THE FINGERS

The metacarpal bones articulate into shallow cavities of the proximal ends of the first phalanges (with the exception of the thumb) at the MCP joints (Goss, 1976). Each joint has a palmar and two collateral ligaments. The *palmar ligaments* are thick, dense, multilayered, and fibrocartilagenous, and located between the collateral ligaments to which they are connected. Also referred to as the *volar plate*, these palmar ligaments are loosely united to the metacarpal bones but firmly attached to base of first phalanges. In this way, the palmar ligaments help to not only reinforce the joint capsule but also to provide a surface for contact in extension and to prevent excessive hyperextension (Norkin & Levangie, 1992).

The *collateral ligaments* are strong and they run along the sides of the joints. The dorsal surface is covered by the extensor tendons with tissue that connects the deep surfaces of the tendons to bones. The collateral ligaments are slack in extension, although some authors disagree and say that parts provide stability throughout the

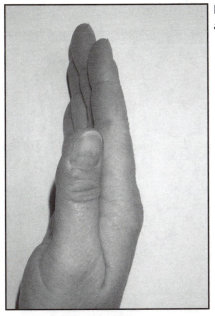

Figure 8-7A. Thumb adduction.

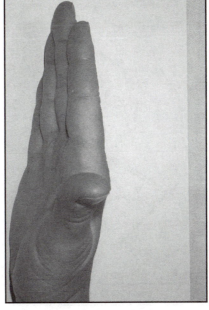

Figure 8-7B. Thumb extension.

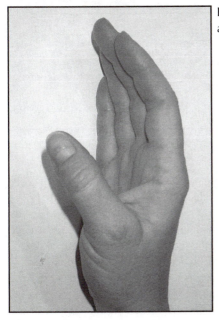

Figure 8-7C. Thumb abduction.

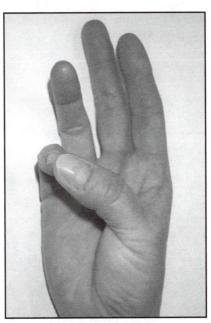

Figure 8-7D. Thumb opposition.

Table 8-1.

PHYSIOLOGIC MOVEMENT OF THE MCP JOINT

Physiological Motion of First Metacarpal	*Direction of Slide of Base of Metacarpal*	*Physiological Motion of First Phalanx*	*Direction of Slide of First Phalanx*
Flexion	Ulnar	Flexion	Volar
Extension	Radial	Extension	Dorsal
Adduction	Volar	Abduction	Away from center of hand
Abduction	Dorsal	Adduction	Toward center of hand

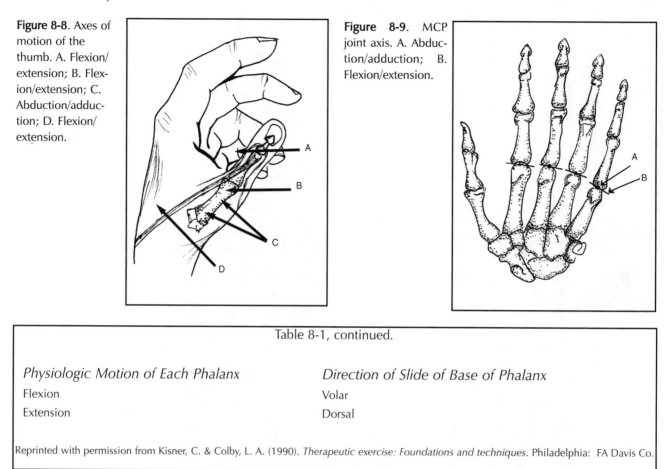

Figure 8-8. Axes of motion of the thumb. A. Flexion/extension; B. Flexion/extension; C. Abduction/adduction; D. Flexion/extension.

Figure 8-9. MCP joint axis. A. Abduction/adduction; B. Flexion/extension.

Table 8-1, continued.

Physiologic Motion of Each Phalanx	Direction of Slide of Base of Phalanx
Flexion	Volar
Extension	Dorsal

Reprinted with permission from Kisner, C. & Colby, L. A. (1990). *Therapeutic exercise: Foundations and techniques*. Philadelphia: FA Davis Co.

range (Norkin & Levangie, 1992). The laxity in extension allows some passive axial rotation of the proximal phalanx. Since the ligament is taut with flexion, this prevents abduction and adduction because there is a longer distance between the points of attachment when these joints are flexed than extended. Abduction and adduction can occur only when the joints are extended. This enables mechanical stabilization of the MCP joint (Smith, Weiss, & Lehmkuhl, 1996).

The MCP joint is a unicondylar diarthrodial biaxial joint with three planes of movement (Nordin & Frankel, 1989), with flexion, extension, abduction, adduction, and slight rotational movements possible. The axis for flexion and extension is side-to-side through the joints or transverse through the metacarpal head (Figure 8-9). The location of the axis permits as much as 95 to 110 degrees of flexion in the little finger and approximately 70 to 90 degrees in the index finger. This illustrates that there is less mobility in the index and middle fingers at this joint, which enables these joints to provide stabilization while allowing more mobility in the little and ring fingers to provide greater grasping capabilities on the ulnar side of the hand. Passive hyperextension of the MCP joint is often used as a measure of generalized body flexibility, and values for hyperextension can vary.

Brand and Hollister (1999) describe the adduction/abduction axis as a cone that runs forward from the metacarpal head with an

inclination distally of approximately 30 degrees above a right angle (p. 52). Abduction and adduction can occur in this axis that passes from the palmar to dorsal surfaces when the fingers are extended because the tip of the finger is a long distance from the joint axis, thereby permitting this motion. When the fingers are flexed, the tips of the fingers are on the axis of rotation so no further lateral movement can occur. For example, when the hand holds a hammer in a power grip, the thumb aligns with the longitudinal axis, providing maximal strength and stabilization against lateral forces. In full flexion, the phalange is parallel to the longitudinal axis putting the joint into the most stable, close packed position (Figure 8-10). The physiological motion is shown in Table 8-1.

METACARPOPHALANGEAL JOINT
OF THE THUMB

The articulation of first metacarpal bone and proximal phalange produces a condyloid joint that acts like a ginglymous (hinge) joint. Goss (1976) states this is a "ginglymoid" joint, Hamil and Knutzen (1995) say this is a hinge joint, while Norkin & Levangie (1992) and Kisner & Colby (1990) indicate this is a condyloid joint. Movements include flexion/extension, abduction/adduction, circumduction, and opposition with an insignifi-

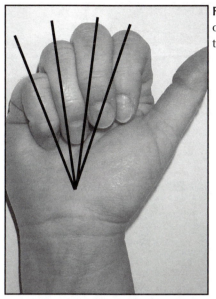

Figure 8-10. Motion of finger flexion toward the palm.

cant amount of passive motion possible. As with the other metacarpals, the head is convex and fits into the concave base of the first phalange, so arthrokinematically the MCP joint of the thumb slides, as do the phalanges as previously discussed regarding the MCP joints of the fingers.

Motion at the MCP joint of the thumb is more restricted than at the fingers. The joint capsule and ligaments of the thumb at this joint are similar to the other MCP joints with the addition of two sesamoid bones that act as additional reinforcement for thumb stability.

INTERPHALANGEAL JOINTS

The articulation of the IP joints with each other and proximally with the phalanges produces two IP joints for digits two through five and one IP joint for the thumb. The thumb IP is structurally and functionally identical to the DIP joints of the fingers (Norkin & Levangie, 1992).

There are two collateral ligaments and a palmar (volar plate) ligament with a similar arrangement as those of the MCP joint.

Flexion and extension movements in the sagittal plane around a coronal axis are more extensive between the proximal and middle phalanges than between the middle and distal joints. In addition, flexion is considerable while extension is limited by the ligamental tautness. Since there is a larger proximal articular surface than distal, there is very little hyperextension and practically no passive hyperextension at the proximal interphalangeal (PIP) joint. The joints are closely congruent during movement, which adds stability to these joints. There is greater ROM going from radial to ulnar joint, permitting more opposition in the ulnar fingers by angling these fingers toward the thumb so one can get a tighter grip on objects from the ulnar side. This reinforces the idea that digits one and two are primarily functional in prehension and precision movements while digits three through five are used for power. Notice how many tools have handles that are narrower at

the ring and little fingers and wider at the radial side along the base of the long and index fingers. These also are concepts to be remembered in making adaptations to tools and utensils.

With flexion of the phalanx, the base of the phalanx slides in a volar direction, while during extension, the base of the phalanx slides dorsally because the distal end of each phalanx is convex and the articulating surface at the proximal end of each phalanx is concave (Kisner & Colby, 1990) (see Table 8-1).

INTERMETACARPAL JOINTS

An additional five joints are formed among the five metacarpal bones, which produce slight gliding motions. These joints are bound together by palmar, dorsal, and interosseous ligaments.

INTERNAL KINETICS

Flexors of the Fingers

The *flexor apparatus* is made up of the flexor digitorum superficialis (sublimis) and the flexor digitorum profundus. The flexor digitorum profundus tendon inserts into the base of the distal phalanges of the digits after passing through the openings in the flexor digitorum superficialis tendons just opposite to the first phalanges. The flexor digitorum superficialis splits into four tendons and passes under the flexor retinaculum in the palm of the hand. At the base of the first phalange, each tendon divides into two slips to allow passage of the flexor digitorum profundus tendon. Three quarters of the superficialis fibers continue to the middle phalanx to insert and one quarter of the fibers cross under flexor digitorum profundus to insert into the proximal phalange.

The flexor tendons are restrained by tendon sheaths and retinaculum that keep the tendons close to the bones and to the planes of motion, while maintaining a relatively constant moment arm rather than producing "bowstringing" of the tendons. There are five dense annular pulleys and three thinner cruciform pulleys that allow for smooth curves and no sharp bends in the tendon excursions (Nordin & Frankel, 1989) (Figure 8-11A, B).

Flexion of the DIP joint produces flexion of the PIP joint because flexion of the DIP is produced by flexor digitorum profundus with a simultaneous flexor force produced by the muscle as it crosses the PIP. Norkin and Levangie add that when the DIP joint begins flexing, the terminal tendon and lateral bands stretch over dorsal aspect of DIP, which pulls the extensor hood (from which the lateral bands arise) distally. This causes the central tendon of the extensor expansion to relax, creating a flexor force at the PIP joint. Active (FDP) and passive forces (release of the central tendon) occur when the lateral bands migrate volarly. The coupling of the flexor action at the DIP and PIP joint can be overridden as some people can actively flex the DIP while the PIP extends (1992). To achieve full flexion of all joints, the long finger flexors must override the extension components of the lumbricals and interossei, which is easier if in some wrist extension (Hamil & Knutzen, 1995) (Figure 8-12).

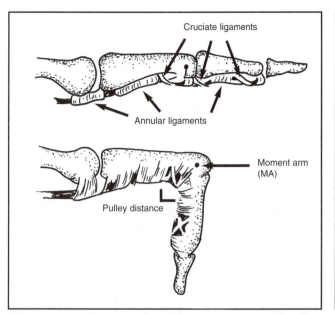

Figure 8-11A. Flexor tendon pulley system. Normal pulley mechanism.

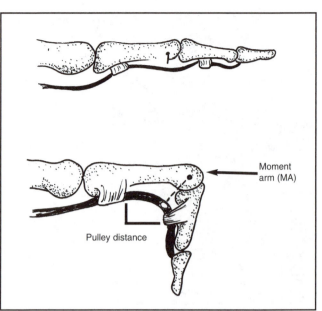

Figure 8-11B. Pathological pulley system.

Flexor Digitorum Superficialis

The largest of the flexor muscles of the forearm, this muscle crosses the wrist, MCP, and PIP joints anterior to the flexion-extension axis, so this muscle flexes these joints and assists with extension at the wrist. Flexor digitorum superficialis (FDS) is capable of flexing each finger individually at the proximal, but not distal, IP joints. *Palpation*: In its location underneath flexor carpi radialis and palmaris longus, it is difficult to palpate at the more proximal location because the attachment is widespread. Movement of the tendon can be seen and palpated on the palmar surface of the wrist in the space between the flexor carpi radialis and flexor carpi ulnaris tendons as the fingers flex to make a firm fist with the wrist flexed (Gench, et al., 1995; Smith et al., 1996).

Flexor Digitorum Profundus

Due to the line of pull to the palmar side of the flexion-extension axis, the muscle acts in flexion of PIP, DIP, MCP, and finally at the wrist with the strength of the contraction lessening progressively. This is because the muscle gradually shortens and can therefore contribute only weakly to wrist flexion. There is a single muscle belly so contraction of the muscle causes movements in all fingers simultaneously. As an example, flex the long finger; notice that the ring finger also moves as would the index and small fingers if not for the neutralizing effects of extensor indicis and extensor digiti minimi. *Palpation*: Flexor digitorum profundus (FDP) lies deep and is covered by flexor digitorum superficialis, flexor carpi radialis, flexor carpi ulnaris, palmaris longus, and pronator teres. A contracting muscle belly can be palpated if tension is minimal in the more superficial muscles. Have the subject supinate the forearm and rest the hand in the lap while the wrist is extended by weight of the hand. Have the subject close the fist fully and the profundus may be felt under the fingers in the region between

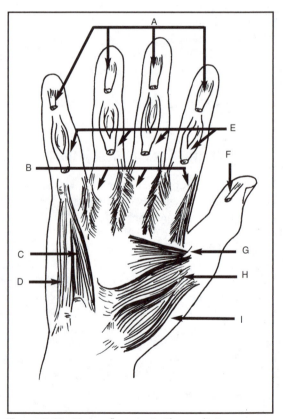

Figure 8-12. Finger flexors. A. Flexor digitorum profundus; B. Interossei; C. Flexor digiti minimi brevis; D. Abductor digiti minimi; E. Flexor digitorum superficiales; F. Flexor pollicis longus; G. Abductor pollicis; H. Flexor pollicis brevis; I. Abductor pollicis brevis.

pronator teres and FCU about 2 inches (5 cm) below medial epicondyle of the humerus (Gench et al., 1995; Smith, et al., 1996).

FDS and FDP

FDP is more active than FDS in finger flexion. FDS works alone in finger flexion only when flexion of the DIP joint is not required. When simultaneous PIP and DIP flexion is required, FDS acts as reserve, joining FDP when greater force is needed or when finger flexion with wrist flexion is required (Smith et al., 1996).

FDP and FDS are dependent on wrist position for an optimal length-tension relationship. Finger flexor effectiveness would be reduced by 1/4 without the counterbalancing effect of extensor muscles (ECRB or ED) since wrist flexion would occur, reducing tension at the more distal joints. The wrist extensors also serve to stabilize the wrist as well as provide optimal length-tension relationships for these long finger flexors.

Flexor Digiti Minimi Brevis

This muscle lies parallel to and on the radial side of abductor digiti minimi. While superficially located, it is easily confused with abductor digiti minimi. Crossing on the palmar side of the flexion/extension axis, flexor digiti minimi brevis (FDMB) flexes the fifth MCP joint.

Opponens Digiti Minimi/Opponens Digiti Quinti

The proximal fibers of opponens digiti minimi (ODM) flex the fifth CMC joint while the distal fibers adduct. It is this combination of flexion and adduction that produces opposition if both contract simultaneously, actually drawing the fifth metacarpal forward, which deepens the hollow of the hand (Gench et al., 1995; Smith et al., 1996). *Palpation*: This muscle lies beneath abductor digiti minimi and flexor digiti minimi brevis in hypothenar eminence, so it is not palpable.

Palmar Interossei

Although somewhat farther from the flexion/extension axis than are the dorsal interossei, the palmar interossei are more effective as flexors. Both the lumbricals and palmar interossei are located on the palmar side of the axis for flexion and extension, and so mechanically are capable of flexion, with the lumbricals more favorably located. The role of the interossei in flexion and adduction at the MCP joint is thought to be from passive stretch (Smith et al., 1996). *Palpation*: The three palmar interossei are located deep in the palm beneath lumbricales and dorsal interossei, so these are very difficult muscles to palpate (Gench, et al., 1995; Smith et al., 1996).

Dorsal Interossei

These four muscles lie between the metacarpals but are very difficult to palpate except for the first dorsal interossei. The dorsal interossei serve to flex the MCP joints of the second, third, and fourth digits (Gench et al., 1995).

Lumbricales

The four lumbricals are not active in MCP flexion unless the IP joints are extended. The lumbricals do not participate in grip and rarely contract synchronously with the FDP (Smith et al., 1996). *Palpation*: While one source says that the lumbricals are too deep to palpate, others state that these muscles may be palpated on the radial side of long finger flexors and are best visible in the claw hand position of MCP hyperextension and IP flexion (Smith et al., 1996).

Abductor Digiti Minimi

Located superficially on the ulnar border of the hypothenar eminence, this muscle is closer to the flexion/extension axis than to the abduction/adduction axis, so abductor digiti minimi (ADM) is primarily an abductor with a secondary role as a flexor of the PIP joint when the long extensor is relaxed. *Palpation*: ADM can be palpated next to the fifth metacarpal during resisted abduction of the small finger (Gench et al., 1995).

Flexors of the Thumb

Flexor Pollicis Longus

The most radial of the tendons of the carpal tunnel, flexor pollicis longus (FPL) crosses the IP and MCP joints of the thumb to the palmar side of the flexion-extension axis and acts as a flexor of the IP joint. FPL also crosses to the ulnar side of the CMC axis for flexion-extension, so this muscle also flexes the CMC joint but is not credited with wrist motion because the muscle lies too close to both wrist axes (Gench et al., 1995).

Flexor Pollicis Brevis

Flexor pollicis brevis is a strap-like muscle with long parallel fibers with two heads. The deep head crosses only the MCP joint on the ulnar side and serves to adduct the MCP joint; the superficial head crosses the MCP and CMC. At the CMC joint, flexor pollicis brevis crosses on the palmar side of the flexion-extension axis and is a flexor of the MCP and CMC joints. There is not always a clear distinction between flexor pollicis brevis and opponens pollicis because the muscles become continuous on the ulnar side and both muscles flex the metacarpals on the carpus. Interestingly, the superficial portion is innervated by the median nerve, whereas the deep portion is innervated by the ulnar nerve.

Abductor Pollicis Brevis

Abductor pollicis brevis (APB) lies to the palmar side of the flexion-extension axis and assists with flexion and abduction of the MCP joint of the thumb (Gench et al., 1995). *Palpation*: This is most superficial muscle of the thenar eminence, so it can be palpated in the center of the eminence during resisted abduction of the CMC joint of the thumb.

Adductor Pollicis

Called the "pinching muscle" by Brand (1999), adductor pollicis (AP) is a fan-shaped penniform muscle favorably located on the palmar side of the flexion/extension axis to flex the first CMC joint (Gench et al., 1995). *Palpation*: Even though the muscle is deep in the palm, AP can be palpated between the first and second metacarpal on the palmar surface of the thumb between the MCP and IP joints as the thumb presses against the tip of the index finger. Or, you can ask the subject to hold a piece of paper between the thumb and radial aspect of proximal phalanx of the index finger (Smith et al., 1996; Gench et al., 1995).

Opponens Pollicis

Triangular in shape, the upper portion flexes the CMC joint while the lower portion abducts so the muscle acts to oppose the CMC of the thumb. *Palpation*: While opponens pollicis is located beneath abductor pollicis brevis, it is superficial along the radial border of the thenar eminence next to the first metacarpal and can be palpated when the thumb is pressed firmly against the tip of the long finger (Gench et al., 1995).

Dorsal Interossei

While normally considered a muscle acting on the index finger, the first dorsal interossei is important in stabilization of the thumb CMC joint. The first dorsal interossei pulls ulnarly and distally against the forces of the adductor-flexors that push the metacarpal base dorsally and radially (Brand & Hollister, 1999). *Palpation*: The first dorsal interossei can be palpated in the space between the metacarpal bones of the thumb and index finger when resistance is applied to abduction of the index finger (Gench et al., 1995).

Extensors of the Fingers

The *extensor apparatus* (also called the extensor hood, extensor expansion, extensor mechanism, dorsal aponeurosis, or dorsal finger apparatus) is made up of the extensor digitorum (extensor digitorum communis), connective tissue, and expansion fibers from the dorsal interossei, volar interossei, and lumbricals (Figure 8-13). Extensor digitorum tendons pass through the first dorsal compartment with extensor indicis. At the proximal phalanx, each tendon divides into three components. One portion, the central slip, inserts into the dorsum of the proximal end of the middle phalange. This central slip acts to extend the proximal phalange and to stabilize the proximal finger joint so that the lumbricals and interossei can extend DIP and PIP and laterally move the digit. Two lateral bands pass on either side of the central tendon, cross the proximal phalange, reunite as a single terminal tendon on the distal phalange, then unite with the lumbricals and interossei. Fascia extends laterally from the extensor tendon that forms a hood that encircles the intrinsics (interossei and lumbricals).

As extensor digitorum passes dorsally to the MCP joint, contraction of the muscle creates tension on the extensor hood, which is pulled proximally over this joint and acts to extend the proximal phalange. The intrinsics pass volar/anterior to the MCP joint axis, so a flexor force is created. When all muscles contract simultaneously, the MCP will generally extend because extensor digitorum generates greater torque (Norkin & Levangie, 1992).

Extensor digitorum, the interossei, and the lumbricals produce extensor forces on the PIP joint due to their attachments on the

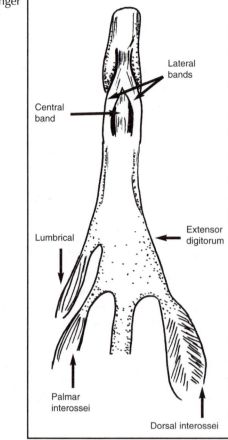

Figure 8-13. Finger extensors.

extensor hood. Extensor digitorum alone cannot produce sufficient tension in either the central slip or lateral bands to overcome the passive forces of flexor digitorum profundus and superficialis. When the extensor digitorum contracts, the forces are distributed along all three phalanges of each finger. If extensor digitorum contracts unopposed, a claw hand position will result (MCP hyperextension and IP flexion) due to the passive pull of the extrinsic flexor tendons (Norkin & Levangie, 1992). The intrinsics (interossei and lumbricals) act as moderators between flexion and extension forces and the lumbricals are said to have a counterclawing bias (Nordin & Frankel, 1989).

The influence of extensor mechanism on DIP and PIP extension is interdependent; that is, when the PIP joint is actively extended, the DIP also extends as a result of the combined active and passive forces applied to the lateral bands and the terminal tendon (Norkin & Levangie, 1992). Extension of the IP joints can occur only if there is tension at the extensor digitorum because this forms a firm base for the interossei and lumbricals to execute their pull (Gench et al., 1995).

Similarly, Nordin and Frankel (1989) state:

> If a finger is flexed at the PIP joint only, the whole trifurcated extensor assembly is pulled distally following the central slip. The slip becomes taut and the lateral bands are slack but are allowed to shift distally over the same distance. Some slack will remain, allowing passive or active flexion of distal phalange but no active extension.

They add that if the DIP is actively flexed, the entire extensors assembly is displaced distally, which relaxes the central slip and increases tension in oblique retinacular ligaments. This creates a tension force at the PIP so flexion of this joint is unavoidable. In addition, simultaneous flexion of MCP, PIP, and DIP forces extensor digitorum to stretch to its fullest and full flexion of the wrist can only occur if fingers are allowed to uncurl. This is important to remember when ROM exercises are being performed.

Extensor Digitorum/Extensor Digitorum Communis

A fusiform muscle on the dorsal surface of the forearm, extensor digitorum extends the MCP, proximal and distal IP joints of the four fingers, and if contraction continues, can extend the wrist. The extension of the IP joints occurs due to the attachment on the extensor hood. Several different sources cite how the function of the extensor digitorum can be utilized in self-defense maneuvers. Since it is not possible to simultaneously and fully flex the wrist, IP, and MCP joints into flexion, by forcing the wrist into flexion a villain will be forced to loosen the grip on any weapon (Gench et al., 1995; Smith et al., 1996; Norkin & Levangie, 1992; Greene & Roberts, 1999). *Palpation*: Extensor digitorum can be palpated except where it is covered by extensor carpi radialis longus. The four tendons can be easily seen and palpated as they cross the second through fifth metacarpal joints and are especially prominent when the MCP joint is fully extended (Gench et al., 1995) or when one finger is extended while the others are flexed into the palm (Smith et al., 1996).

Interossei

The dorsal and palmar interossei extend the IP joints of the index, long, and ring fingers by their attachments to the extensor hood.

Lumbricals

The lumbricals extend the IP joints of the index, long, and ring fingers by their attachments to the extensor hood. The lumbricals have better leverage for extension than do the interossei (Smith et al., 1996). Some authors indicate that the function of the lumbricals is to pull the profundus tendon distally to decrease passive tension and therefore facilitate extension by the extensor digitorum. Other researchers indicate the prevention of hyperextension of the MCP joint by extensor digitorum contractions is an additional function of these muscles (Nordin & Frankel, 1989; Norkin & Levangie, 1992; Smith et al., 1996). Of special note, the lumbricals have a high rate of variability with a low number of muscle fibers per motor unit, indicative of a skilled muscle with a high number of spindles. The lumbricals are richly innervated and it has been hypothesized that the lumbricals may have a specialized proprioceptive function.

Smith et al. (1996) indicate that the line of pull of interossei and lumbricals is dorsal to the joint centers of the IP joints so these muscles are mechanically capable of extension. While the intrinsics are called the primary extensors of IP joints, this is always not true. In unresisted extension, the long extensor and lumbricals only are active. The interossei are not active unless there is forceful or resisted extension (p. 206).

Extensor Digiti Minimi/Extensor Digiti Quinti Proprius

A slender muscle, extensor digiti minimi is located to the ulnar side of the extensor digitorum and acts to extend and abduct the IP joints of the little finger due to the attachment in the extensor hood. Extensor digiti minimi also extends the fifth MCP joint and with continued contractions, contributes to wrist extension. *Palpation*: Extensor digiti minimi is superficially located and slightly proximal to the wrist and can be palpated and observed on the dorsum of the hand at the fifth metacarpal when the small finger is extended against resistance (Gench et al., 1995).

Extensor Indicus/Extensor Indicis Proprius

Extensor indicis extends the MCP joint of the index finger and with the connection to the extensor hood, extends the PIP and DIP joints. With continued contraction, the extensor indicus can contribute to extension of the wrist. If the MCP joint is held in flexion, the ability to extend the IP joint and the wrist is improved. Since extensor indicus inserts on the extensor digitorum tendons of the first and fourth fingers, this adds independence of action to these fingers rather than strength or additional actions (Norkin & Levangie, 1992). *Palpation*: This muscle is superficial and runs on the ulnar side and parallel to the extensor digitorum on the dorsal aspect. It can be seen when one extends the index finger with the other fingers flexed into the palm (Gench et al., 1995; Smith et al., 1996).

Extension of the Thumb

Abductor Pollicis Longus

Since abductor pollicis longus inserts on the radial side of the MCP joint, it acts to pull the thumb into extension at the CMC joint in addition to its actions of abduction of the CMC and radial deviation and flexion of the wrist. The thumb cannot function without the abductor pollicis longus muscle, as is seen in deQuervain's disease (Brand & Hollister, 1999).

Extensor Pollicis Longus

Extensor pollicis longus (EPL) has its own compartment in the retinaculum on the dorsum of the wrist and is located dorsal to the flexion/extension axis, so it extends both the IP and MCP joints of the thumb. *Palpation*: While muscle belly is difficult to palpate, the tendon can be palpated when the thumb is fully extended (Gench et al., 1995).

Extensor Pollicis Brevis

This muscle extends the MCP and CMC joints of the thumb. At the wrist, the tendon passes posterior to the flexion/extension axis and to the radial side of the deviation axis, so extensor pollicis brevis (EPB) extends and radially deviates the wrist. At the CMC joint, it passes on the radial side of the flexion/extension axis so it extends this joint. At the MCP and IP joints, EPB is dorsal to flexion/extension axis, so it extends these joints. EPB is closely associated with abductor pollicis brevis with similar actions at the wrist and CMC joints, and its primary action is extension of the MCP joint. *Palpation*: Beneath and to the radial side of EPL, the EPB tendon is superficial as it crosses the wrist and can be seen during forced extension of thumb. EPB and EPL form the medial and lateral borders of the anatomical snuff box (Gench et al., 1995).

Gench indicates that EPB is different from EPL in three ways (Burstein & Wright, 1994):

1. The tendon of EPL crosses the wrist posterior to the flexion/extension axis to become a wrist extensor; the tendon of EPB crosses directly over the axis and is ineffective as an adductor or abductor.
2. The tendon of EPL passes dorsal to the axis of adduction/abduction of the CMC joint to act as an adductor; the tendon of EPB crosses directly over and is ineffective as an abductor or abductor of CMC joint.
3. EPB does not cross the IP joint of thumb as does extensor pollicis longus, so EPB has no action at that joint (Gench et al., 1995).

Abductors of the Fingers

Abductor Digiti Minimi

This muscle abducts and flexes the MCP joint of the little finger. The muscle's line of pull is more favorably placed for abduction than for flexion because muscle is further from the adduction/abduction axis than from the flexion/extension axis, so this is primarily an abductor with secondary flexion action (Gench et al., 1995).

Dorsal Interossei

The dorsal interossei have relatively long force arms so they act to abduct the second through fourth MCP joints in addition to radial and ulnar deviation of the third metacarpal joint (Gench et al., 1995).

Extensor Digiti Minimi/Extensor Digiti Quinti Proprius

This muscle extends the MCP and the IP joints as well as abducts the little finger.

Abductors of the Thumb

Abductor Pollicis Brevis

While small and weak in size and tension, this muscle is considered by Brand (1999) to be important for opposition and therefore in grasp and pinch. Opponens pollicis is located underneath abductor pollicis brevis so when opponens pollicis contracts, it pushes APB farther from the axis of the CMC joint and increases the moment arm and its effectiveness (Brand & Hollister, 1999). Since this is a fan-shaped muscle, different fibers contribute differently to the muscle action; the most radial portions are abductors of the CMC joint; the most distal are adjacent to FPB and so are flexor-abductors of the MCP joint. The strength of the abductor

pollicis brevis is relatively weak because the action of abduction of the thumb is not one usually done against resistance and this demonstrates that the primary function of this muscle is to position the thumb for action rather than performing the action itself. In action, it is the EPL muscle that most directly opposes APB, not the adductors.

Abductor Pollicis Longus

A stout muscle, abductor pollicis longus abducts and extends the MCP joint and stabilizes the first metacarpal joint. Since the muscle spirals from the dorsal radius to lateral aspect of the first metacarpals, fibers are variable in length and moment arms vary. The name of this muscle doesn't reflect the true action. The tendon pulls the thumb laterally or radially, which is abduction in body terms but not in terms of the thumb. The muscle pulls on the back or extends the thumb so it extends the thumb and abducts it. Stronger than FPL, abductor pollicis longus works to oppose the adductor and short flexor at the CMC joint and allows them to flex the MCP joint (Brand & Hollister, 1999).

Opponens Pollicis

The lower portion of this muscle abducts the CMC joint of the thumb. With the upper portion, which flexes the CMC, this muscle is capable of opposition. There is considerable variation in fiber length and it is capable of producing greater tension than abductor pollicis brevis. The action of opponens pollicis is swinging the thumb in an arch toward the fingers (Gench et al., 1995; Hinkle, 1997; Jenkins, 1998; Nordin & Frankel, 1989; Riley, 1998).

Adductors of the Fingers

Opponens Digiti Minimi/Opponens Digiti Quinti

While the proximal fibers flex the CMC joint of the fifth joint, the distal fibers adduct. By drawing the fifth metacarpal forward, this deepens the hollow of the hand (Gench et al., 1995; Hinkle, 1997; Jenkins, 1998; Nordin & Frankel, 1989; Riley, 1998).

Extensor Indicis

Extensor indicis extends and adducts the MCP joint of the index finger but since it passes just to the ulnar side of the axis, it is weak in adductor action.

Palmar Interossei

Given the medial location to the adduction/abduction axis, the palmar interossei adduct the MCP joints of the index, ring, and little fingers (Gench et al., 1995).

Adductors of the Thumb

Flexor Pollicis Brevis

The deep head of flexor pollicis brevis crosses only the MCP joint and is on the ulnar side of the abduction/adduction axis, so it adducts the MCP joint.

Adductor Pollicis

Adductor pollicis slides the thumb across the palm and bases of finger toward ulnar side as it adducts the CMC joint of the thumb. This muscle is most effective when the joint is fully abducted, which pulls the metacarpal closer to the palm. When the thumb is even with the palm, AP is not effective because the position aligns the muscle with the adduction/abduction axis (Gench et al., 1995).

Extensor Pollicis Longus

Not only an extensor at the CMC and MCP, EPL also acts an adductor at these joints. It is an adductor at the CMC joint because it crosses to the dorsal side of the abduction/adduction axis. (Gench et al., 1995; Bellace, Healy, Bess, Bryon, & Hohman, 2000; Jenkins, 1998).

Flexor Pollicis Longus

While not the primary action, with continued contraction, flexor pollicis longus can adduct the metacarpal joint (Goss, 1976).

In discussing the multiple ways in which the hand moves and the dynamics of the muscles involved, it is often convenient to distinguish between intrinsic and extrinsic muscles. Extrinsic muscles are those that originate outside of a part and act on a part. In the hand, these are often referred to as the "long" hand muscles. Those that are "short" hand muscles are intrinsic muscles, which originate and act upon the part..

Since the hand is capable of such diverse movements, there is much intricacy in the relationships of the many muscles involved. The finger muscles have effects on the wrist and actually have moment arms as long as those of the wrist (Greene & Roberts, 1999). The finger muscles would move both the wrist and joints of the fingers if they were not stabilized. For example, the finger flexors are multijoint muscles and without stabilization at the wrist, these flexors would flex each of the joints they cross. By doing this, the fingers would be unable to fully flex due to active insufficiency of the flexors since they can't fully flex at each of the joints they cross. This inability to fully flex all of the joints crossed by the finger flexors is actually a combination of insufficient excursion and insufficient strength capability.

The insufficient strength production is due to poor length-tension relationships that limit the amount of force that can be produced. By flexing over all of the joints, the flexors are attempting to produce strength in a shortened position at the lower end of the length-tension curve.

Excursion refers to the distance that each tendon slides as the fingers move. Excursion takes place simultaneously in flexor and extensor tendons and this is an important concept in determining muscle forces, fabricating splints, and in rehabilitation as well as in surgical procedures. Measurement of tendon excursion is in relation to angular motion. Nordin and Frankel (1989) state that "when a lever rotates around an axis of an angle, the distance moved by every point on the lever is proportional to its own distance from the axis" and that "every point on the lever moves through a distance equal to its own distance from the axis—its moment arm" (p. 285). Given this, the moment arms and the

excursion are larger in more proximal muscles. For example, flexor superficialis has a longer tendon excursion than does flexor profundus. The excursion of the flexor tendons is larger than the extensors and the excursion of the extrinsic muscles is generally larger than the intrinsic muscles.

When the finger flexors attempt to flex fully over all of the joints they cross, there is insufficient excursion of the flexor muscles. This insufficiency explains teneodesis grasp where passive tension yields finger extension and forces the fingers to release an object. Wrist extension stretched the flexor digitorum profundus, producing finger flexion. Passive tension, not contraction, produces the finger movement. The same is true for the passive insufficiency that develops when the wrist is flexed and passive tension develops to produce finger extension.

There also exists a relationship between adduction and abduction with flexion and extension. In abduction and adduction with the MCP joints extended, the movements are free since the collateral ligaments are loose. When there is flexion at MCP joint, the fingers automatically adduct, which limits the range of abduction because the collateral ligaments become tight. There is a natural tendency to abduct the fingers when they are also extended. Also, when fingers flex one at a time, they point toward the base of the thumb, which is important to remember when applying stretch to fingers (Smith et al., 1996). Another combined action that occurs is that when the fingers flex, the hand is cupped, and the hand is flattened when the fingers extend.

Synergistic relationships exist between the muscles of the wrist and the finger muscles. For example, when the little finger is abducted by means of abductor digiti minimi, the flexor carpi ulnaris contracts to provide countertraction on the pisiform. In order to prevent flexor carpi ulnaris from abducting the wrist in an ulnar direction, abductor pollicis longus contracts.

Synergistic actions occur in the thumb as well. When the thumb is moved in a palmar direction as in flexion, palmaris longus contributes to the movement by tensing the fascia of the palm, while extensor carpi radialis brevis contracts to prevent palmaris longus from flexing the wrist. Another example is the thumb extension. The extensor carpi ulnaris contracts to prevent radial deviation of the wrist by the abductor pollicis longus muscle.

PREHENSION

The hand is capable of many movements and variations in strength or precision. Many efforts have been made to categorize these movement patterns so that consistent use of descriptive terminology can be used. Movements can be produced where the hand as a whole pushes, pulls, or moves an object and where no actual grasp is involved. This would be essentially a nonprehensile movement pattern. Prehension would include reaching, grasping, carrying, and releasing and not just pushing or pulling on the object. The thumb tends to be the defining factor in prehension as to stabilization, control of direction, and power. When the thumb is not functional in the grasp pattern, the prehension is nonmanipulative and essentially one of power. When the thumb and one or more fingers are involved in the action, the pattern is one of manipulative prehension and precision. Often the distinction is made between grasp (or power grip), precision grip, and pinch to differentiate those actions with the thumb and those without.

Gripping an object occurs in four stages. Opening the hand requires simultaneous activity of the intrinsics and long extensor muscles and is considered the first stage. Closing the hand around the object is stage two, requiring flexion of the fingers to grasp it. The third stage involves application of the correct amount of force upon the object based on the weight and size of the object, its surface characteristics, fragility, and use. In stage four, the hand opens to release the object (Magee, 1992).

In prehensile nonmanipulative patterns, three types of power grips are used to seize and hold objects in the hand for objects requiring firm control. The digits position the object against the palm and the thumb is essentially nonfunctional. The joint position brings the hand into line with the forearm with the fingers flexed, wrist in ulnar deviation and extended (Magee, 1992). In the *hook* grip, digits II to V are used as a hook (Smith et al., 1996) to carry objects such as a purse or briefcase where force is sustained for long periods of time. The thumb is nonfunctional and the heel of the hand may provide some counterpressure. The MCP joints are in neutral with the fingers flexed at the PIP and DIP joints. The thumb is in extension. Primarily the muscles involved include flexor digitorum superficialis, flexor digitorum profundus, extensor pollicis longus and brevis, extensor digitorum, and fourth lumbrical and interossei. If a powerful grip is needed, the fingers will flex at all three joints and thumb will be adducted (Jenkins, 1998).

In the second and third types of prehensile nonmanipulative grip, the fingers are used to hold an object in the palm of the hand so that the actual position of the hand varies according to the size, shape, and weight of the object being held. The palm contours to the object and the thumb provides an additional surface for the object by adducting against it. The thumb applies counterpressure to the partially flexed fingers but again is essentially not functional as a manipulative force. *Cylindrical grasp* and *spherical grasp* are considered palmar prehension or power grips. In cylindrical grasp, the thumb is in opposition and fingers are adducted and flexed; this can be visualized by the position of the hand in holding a beverage can. Flexor pollicis longus and the thenar group, adductor pollicis, flexor digitorum profundus, and the fourth lumbrical are active in this grasp pattern. Spherical grasp is seen when one holds a round object such as a ball where the thumb is in opposition with fingers flexed and abducted. Flexor pollicis longus and the thenar group, adductor pollicis, flexor digitorum profundus, and fourth lumbrical are active in this prehension pattern. Some sources state that cylindrical and spherical grasps are merely descriptions of the objects held in the hand and are not distinct grasp patterns. The third type of power grip is the *fist grasp* or digital palmar prehension pattern when the hand grips a narrow object such as a broom handle.

Prehensile manipulative pinch patterns include lateral pinch, palmar pinch, and tip pinch. *Lateral pinch* (also known as key pinch, pad-to-side, subterminolateral opposition, or pulp pinch) is used when a thin object is held in the hand, such as a card or a key. It is the least precise of the manipulative prehension patterns and

is the finest grasp that can be accomplished without active hand musculature via teneodesis action (Norkin & Levangie, 1992). The object is grasped between the palmar surface of the thumb and the lateral side of the index finger (Smith et al., 1996). The thumb is adducted with IP flexion with the index finger flexed and abducted, which involves the flexor pollicis longus and brevis, adductor pollicis, flexor digitorum profundus and superficialis, as well as first dorsal interossei.

Palmar pinch, also known as subterminal opposition or pad-to-pad prehension, occurs when the palmar surfaces of the distal phalanges contact the palmar surface of the thumb. The thumb is in opposition and slight flexion with the fingers in flexion at the MCP and PIP joints. This grip pattern can be seen in picking up and holding a coin between the thumb and fingers or even with larger objects. From a radial view, this grip pattern forms an oval. The muscles involved in this pinch pattern are those in the thenar group, flexor pollicis longus, select interossei, and flexor digitorum superficialis of the involved fingers (flexor digitorum profundus in DIP flexion is also present). If the index and middle fingers meet the opposed thumb, this is called *three jaw chuck*, *three point chuck*, *three fingered or digital prehension*, or the *dynamic tripod*, and can be considered a "precision grip with power" (Magee, 1992, p. 187). This type of grip pattern is seen when one holds a pencil.

Tip pinch is described as the movement of the tip of the thumb against the tip of another finger to pick up a small object such as a pin. From the radial side, the finger and thumb form a circle. As with palmar pinch, the thumb is in opposition with slightly greater flexion and the fingers are flexed at the MCP, DIP, and PIP joints. The same muscles are involved in tip pinch as are in palmar pinch. Tip pinch is also referred to as terminal opposition and tip pinch is involved in activities required fine coordinated movement rather than power.

A study by Smith (1995) shows the frequency of use of the three types of prehension patterns for picking up and holding objects (Table 8-2).

This indicates that palmar prehension is the most commonly used prehension pattern for both picking up and holding objects for use. The frequency of pinch patterns used in daily activities such as buttoning, tying a shoelace, and tracing activities found by McPhee is shown in Table 8-3.

From these studies, it could be stated that different types of pinch are used to pick up and hold objects and that daily activities did not significantly indicate one pinch preference over another.

Other researchers disagree with the distinction of power and prehension, contending that hand function is far more complex than these descriptions portray and that these words limit descriptions of the hand to static positions. Cassanova (1989) proposes a classification system based on the contact of the hand surfaces using anatomical terminology. The fingers would be designated by roman numerals (thumb = I, index = II, middle = III, ring = IV and little = V), and contact areas would be noted as well (such as palmar, surface, or pad).

Appendix E indicates information from two sources relative to hand function descriptions. On the left, the results from Smith's

Table 8-2.			
FREQUENCY OF USE OF PREHENSION PATTERNS			
	Palmar	*Tip*	*Lateral*
Pick up	50%	17%	33%
Hold for use	88%	2%	10%

Adapted from McPhee, S. D. (1987). Functional hand evaluations: A review. *Am J Occup Ther, 41*(3), 158-163.

Table 8-3.	
FREQUENCY OF USE OF PINCH PATTERNS	
Pulp to pulp pinch	20%
Three lateral pinch	20%
Five finger pinch	15%
Fist grip	15%
Cylindrical grip	14%
Three fingered pinch	10%
Spherical grip	4%
Hook grip	2%

Adapted from McPhee, S. D. (1987). Functional hand evaluations: A review. *Am J Occup Ther, 41*(3), 158-163.

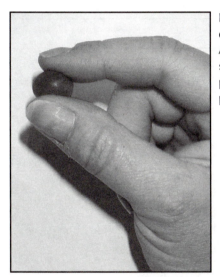

Figure 8-14. I pad distal to II pad distal. Also known as: true square pinch, pulp pinch, and palmar pinch.

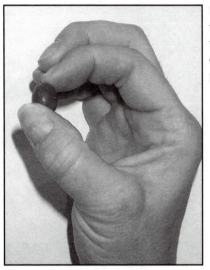

Figure 8-15. I tip to II tip. Also known as: tip to tip, terminal opposition, and tip prehension.

study indicate the inconsistent identification of grasp and pinch patterns. The figures on the right are diagrams and descriptions based on Cassanova's proposed classification system. Tip pinch, for example, actually can include six different hand positions and descriptions if using Cassanova's more precise terminology (Figures 8-14 through 8-29).

ASSESSMENT OF THE HAND

Magee (1992) states that the hand is the terminal part of the upper limb and that many pathological conditions manifest themselves in this structure and may lead the examiner to suspect pathological conditions elsewhere in the body (p. 176). Thick, brittle nails with longitudinal ridges may be evidence of exposure to radiation. Spoon-shaped nails may be the result of dysphasia with atrophy in Plummer-Vinson Syndrome, while clubbing of the nails may be due to chronic respiratory disorders or congenital heart disease. Psoriasis may cause scaling, deformity, or detachment of the nails. Darkened nails or those with lack of growth may be due to arterial diseases (Magee, 1992).

As with other joints, *active* and *passive range of motion* are important assessments of the hand. Observation of the active use of the hand as well as passive movements and joint play provide initial information about the structures of the hand.

Observation and palpation of any abnormal formations should also be noted in the documentation as to location and description. For example, a description may be : "single nodule, freely movable, nontender, .5 cm in diameter located over the dorsum of the ring PIP" (Melvin, 1982, p. 212). Nodules can occur in several conditions including Dupuytren's contracture, which is the progressive fibrosis of the palmar aponeurosis and usually affects the ring and little fingers first. Fibrous nodules can develop in the flexor tendons that can catch on the annular sheath opposite metacarpal head, causing trigger fingers or thumb. Swelling and bony enlargement of the PIP joint may indicate secondary synovitis from rheumatoid arthritis (Bouchard nodes) (Hartley, 1995).

Figure 8-16. I pad distal to II tip. Also known as tip to tip opposition and tip prehension.

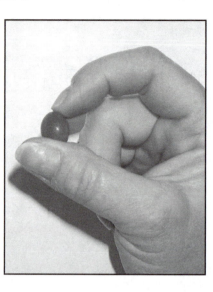

Figure 8-17. I tip to II tip. Also known as coin precision pinch.

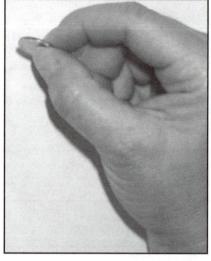

Figure 8-18. Palmar pad to pad/two point.

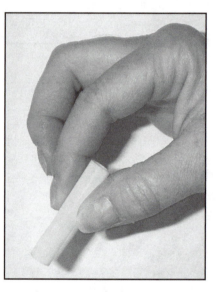

Figure 8-19. I pad distal to II pad distal and middle. Also known as delicate pulp to pulp grip, pad to pad, and subterminal thumb-finger pinch.

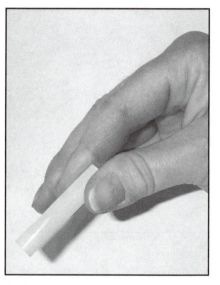

Figure 8-20. I pad distal to II pad distal.

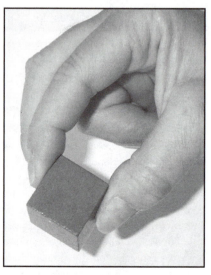

Figure 8-21. Lateral pinch.

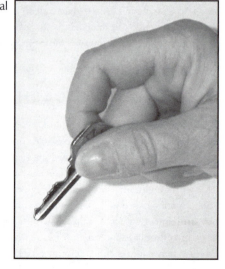

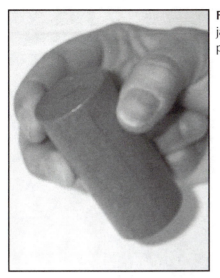

Figure 8-22. Three jaw chuck or three point prehension.

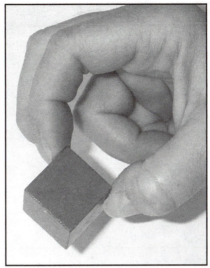

Figure 8-23. I tip to II tip.

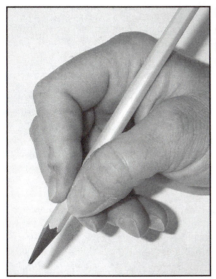

Figure 8-24. I pad distal to web to II pad distal and II radial distal.

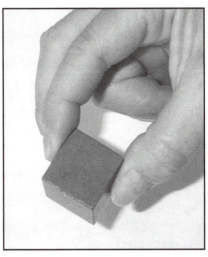

Figure 8-25. I pad distal to II & III pads distal.

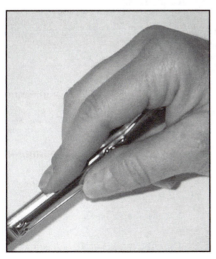

Figure 8-26. I pad distal and palm to II pad distal and III dorsal radial.

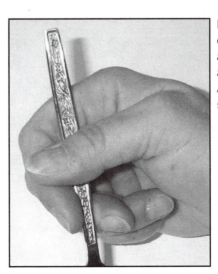

Figure 8-27. I pad distal to II pad distal and radial proximal and III dorsal distal. Also known as tea-spoon finger grip.

Figure 8-28. Dynamic grip. I pad distal to II pad distal and radial proximal to III radial distal.

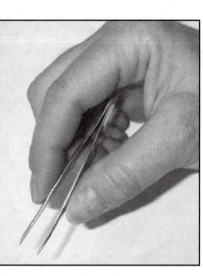

Figure 8-29. Dynamic grip. I pad distal to II pad middle to III radial middle.

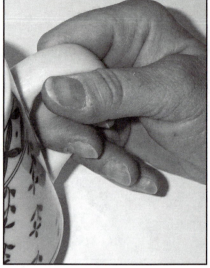

Comparison of both hands usually shows that the dominant hand is slightly larger than the nondominant or nonpreferred hand. Look at the eminences of the hand: muscle wasting of the thenar eminence may be indicative of C6 nerve root problems, whereas wasting of the hypothenar eminence may indicate C8 nerve root damage.

Pain is an important part of the assessment. Determination of pain onset, type, and location is necessary.

Strength may be assessed by individually testing muscles (as in a manual muscle test) or a brief screening can be done (as in a functional motion test). Dynamometers are used to evaluate grasp and pinch meters to measure pinch.

SUMMARY

- The hand is amazingly complex with many articulations between carpal bones, metacarpals, and phalanges. As a result, the following joints are formed: carpometacarpal, metacarpophalangeal, distal interphalangeal, and proximal interphalangeal.
- By observation, one can identify three arches in the hand: two transverse and one longitudinal. Many creases are visible in the hand as well.
- The carpometacarpal joint provides the most movement for the thumb and the least amount for the fingers.
- The thumb is capable of flexion/extension, adduction/abduction, circumduction, and opposition/reposition.
- There is less mobility in the index and middle fingers so that these digits can provide stabilization while permitting greater mobility in the little and ring fingers.
- The interphalangeal joints of the fingers are closely congruent during movement so these are relatively stable joints.
- The flexor apparatus is made up of the flexor digitorum superficialis and flexor digitorum profundus muscles.
- The extensor apparatus or extensor hood comprises the extensor digitorum, connective tissue, fibers from the interossei muscles, and the lumbricals.

- Hand muscles, while many in number, are often distinguished by those that are intrinsic to the hand and those that are extrinsic.
- Synergistic relationships exist between the muscles of the wrist and the finger muscles.
- Prehension is the use of the hand in precise ways. Defining how the hand moves has proved challenging. Grasp usually involves more fingers and often the thumb, whereas pinch usually only involves one or two fingers. Pinch is usually described as tip, palmar, lateral, and pulp. Cassanova has described a more detailed description of grasp and pinch patterns which demonstrates the variety of ways hands are used in everyday activities.
- Evaluation of the hand includes assessment of pain, edema, symmetry, movement, and observation and palpation. In addition, grasp and pinch measurements are taken to determine the strength of the muscles in the hand in addition to strength.

REFERENCES

Bellace, J. V., Healy, D., Bess, M. P., Bryon, T., & Hohman, L. (2000). Validity of the Dexter Evaluation System's Jamar dynamometer attachment for assessment of hand grip strength in a normal population. *Journal of Hand Therapy, 13*(1), 46-51.

Brand, P. W., & Hollister, A. M. (1999). *Clinical mechanics of the hand* (3rd ed.). St. Louis, MO: C.V. Mosby.

Burstein, A. H., & Wright, T. M. (1994). *Fundamentals of orthopaedic biomechanics*. Baltimore: Williams & Wilkins.

Cassanova, J. S., & Gurnert, B. K. (1989). Adult prehension: Patterns and nomenclature. *J Hand Ther*, 231-243.

Gench, B. E., Hinson, M. M., & Harvey, P. T. (1995). *Anatomical kinesiology*. Dubuque, IA: Eddie Bowers Publishing, Inc.

Goss, C. M. (Ed.) (1976). *Gray's anatomy of the human body* (29th ed.). Philadelphia: Lea and Febiger.

Greene, D. P., & Roberts, S. L. (1999). *Kinesiology: Movement in the context of activity*. St. Louis, MO: C.V. Mosby.

Hamil, J., & Knutzen, K. M. (1995). *Biomechanical basis of human movement.* Baltimore: Williams & Wilkins.

Hartley, A. (1995). *Practical joint assessment: Upper quadrant: A sports medicine manual* (2nd ed.). Philadelphia: C.V. Mosby.

Hinkle, C. Z. (1997). *Fundamentals of anatomy and movement: A workbook and guide.* St. Louis, MO: C.V. Mosby.

Jenkins, D. B. (1998). *Hollingshead's functional anatomy of the limbs and back* (7th ed.). Philadelphia: W.B. Saunders Co.

Kisner, C., & Colby, L. A. (1990). *Therapeutic exercise: Foundations and techniques* (2nd ed.). Philadelphia: F. A. Davis.

Magee, D. J. (1992). *Orthopedic physical assessment.* Philadelphia: W.B. Saunders Co.

Melvin, J. L. (1982). *Rheumatic disease: Occupational therapy and rehabilitation* (2nd ed.). Philadelphia: F. A. Davis Co.

Nordin, M., & Frankel, V. H. (1989). *Basic biomechanics of the musculoskeletal system* (2nd ed.). Philadelphia: Lea and Febiger.

Norkin, C. C., & Levangie, P. K. (1992). *Joint structure and function: A comprehensive analysis* (2nd ed.). Philadelphia: F. A. Davis Co.

Riley, M. A. (1998). The effects of medical conditions and aging on hand function. *OT Practice, 3*(6), 24-27.

Smith, R. (1985). Pinch and grasp strength: Standardization of terminology and protocol. *Am J Occup Ther, 39*(8), 531-535.

Smith, L. K, Weiss, E. L., & Lehmkuhl, L. D. (1996). *Brunnstrom's Clinical kinesiology* (5th ed.). Philadelphia: F. A. Davis Co.

BIBLIOGRAPHY

Aaron, D. H., & Jansen, C. W. S. (2000). Hand rehabilitation: Matching patient priorities and performance with pathology and tissue healing. *OT Practice,* 10-15.

Basmajian, J. V., & DeLuca, C. J. (1985). *Muscles alive* (5th ed.). Baltimore: Williams and Wilkins.

Baxter, R. (1998). *Pocket guide to musculoskeletal assessment.* Philadelphia: W. B. Saunders Co.

Caillet, R. (1971). *Hand pain and impairment.* Philadelphia: F. A. Davis Co.

Calliet, R. (1996). *Soft tissue pain and disability* (3rd ed.). Philadelphia: F. A. Davis Co.

Cooper, C., & Evarts, J. L. (1998). Beyond the routine. *OT Practice,* 18-22.

Esch, D. L. (1989). *Musculoskeletal function: An anatomy and kinesiology laboratory manual.* Minneapolis: University of Minnesota.

Fuller, Y., & Trombly, C. (1997). Effects of object characteristics on female grasp patterns. *Am J Occup Ther, 51*(7), 481-487.

Jones, L. A. (1989). The assessment of hand function: A critical review of techniques. *J Hand Surg, 14A*(2), 221-228.

Kellor, M., Frost, J., Silberberg, N., Iversen, I., & Cummings, R. (1971). Hand strength and dexterity. *Am J Occup Ther, 25*(2), 77-83

Konin, J. G. (1999). *Practical kinesiology for the physical therapist assistant.* Thorofare, NJ: SLACK Incorporated.

Loth, T., & Wadsworth, C. T. (1998). *Orthopedic review for physical therapists.* St. Louis, MO: C.V. Mosby Co.

Lumley, J. S. P. (1990). *Surface anatomy: The anatomical basis of clinical examination.* New York: Churchill Livingstone.

MacKenna, B. R., & Callender, R. (1990). *Illustrated physiology* (5th ed.). New York: Churchill Livingstone.

Masaki, K., Leveille, S., Curb, J. D., & White, L. (1999). Midlife hand grip strength as a predictor of old age disability. *JAMA,* 558-60.

Nicholas, J. A., & Hershman, E. B. (1990). *The upper extremity in sports medicine.* St. Louis, MO: C. V. Mosby Co.

Norkin, C., & White, D. J. (1989). *Measurement of joint motion: A guide to goniometry.* Philadelphia: F. A. Davis Co.

Oxford, K. L. (2000). Elbow positioning for maximum grip performance. *J Hand Ther, 13*(1), 33-36.

Palastanga, N., Field, D., & Soames, R. (1989). *Anatomy and human movement: Structure and function.* Philadelphia: Lippincott Williams and Wilkins.

Palmer, M. L., & Epler, M. E. (1998). *Fundamentals of musculoskeletal assessment techniques* (2nd ed.). Philadelphia: J. B. Lippincott.

Petersen, P., Petrick, M., Connor, H., & Conklin, D. (1989). Grip strength and hand dominance: Challenging the 10% rule. *Am J Occup Ther, 43*(7), 444-447.

Perry, J. F., Rohe, D. A., & Garcia, A. O. (1996). *Kinesiology workbook.* Philadelphia: F. A. Davis Co

Rice, M. S., Leonard, C., & Carter, M. (1998). Grip strengths and required forces in accessing everyday containers in a normal population. *Am J Occup Ther, 52*(8), 621-626.

Richards, L. G., Olson, B., & Palmiter-Thomas, P. (1996). How forearm position affects grip strength. *Am J Occup Ther, 50*(2), 133-138.

Saidoff, D. C., & McDonough, A. L. (1997). *Critical pathways in therapeutic intervention: Upper extremity.* St. Louis, MO: C. V. Mosby.

Thompson, C. W., & Floyd, R. T. (1994). *Manual of structural kinesiology* (12th ed.). St. Louis, MO: C. V. Mosby.

Torrens, G. E., Hann J., Webley, M., & Sutherland, I. A. (2000). Hand performance assessment of ten people with rheumatoid arthritis when using a range of specified saucepans. *Disability and Rehabilitation, 22*(3), 123-134.

Toth-Fejel, G. E, Toth-Fejel, G. F., & Hendricks, C. A. (1998). Occupation-centered practice in hand rehabilitation: Using the experience sampling method. *Am J Occup Ther, 52*(5), 381-385.

Trombly, C. A. (Ed). (1995). *Occupational therapy for physical dysfunction* (4th ed.). Baltimore: Williams and Wilkins.

Watkins, J. (1999). *Structure and function of the musculoskeletal system.* New York: Human Kinetics.

The Spine, Pelvis, and Posture

Chapter 9

The vertebral column and ribs serve to protect the spinal cord and internal organs, provide a means for breathing, support the head and extremities, transmit loads between the extremities, and stabilize and mobilize the body for hand function and ambulation (Smith, Weiss, & Lehmkuhl, 1996).

THE SPINE

The spine is formed by 33 vertebral bones that are labeled according to location: 7 cervical, 12 thoracic, 5 lumbar, 5 sacral, 4 coccygeal (Gench, Hinson, & Harvey, 1995). Each vertebra consists of a body, discs, pedicles, spinous process, vertebral arch, and laminae. The body is the largest part of the vertebra and is essentially a cylindrical shape. The intervertebral disks of fibrocartilage attach to the superior and inferior surfaces and this enables each vertebra to articulate with the vertebra above and below it (Gench et al., 1995). There are two pedicles that project dorsally from the body. The pedicles merge with a pair of lamina, creating the vertebral arch with the vertebral foramen in the center. The vertebral arch supports seven processes: four articular, two transverse, and one spinous process. The processes help to increase the leverage for the muscles of the trunk and extremities (Smith et al., 1996).

There are distinct differences in the vertebrae in each of the spinal segments. The differences depend on the purpose and function of each vertebral segment, how movement occurs, and the level of participation in load bearing in which the vertebra is involved (Figure 9-1). While some portions of the spine function more in stability and others in instability, in general the posterior portions of the vertebrae serve to protect the spinal cord and stabilize the spine, while anterior portions function as a shock absorber, to bear weight and loads, and to mobilize the trunk (Smith et al., 1996).

The cervical vertebrae are the smallest of the vertebrae and are different from the thoracic and lumbar vertebrae due to a foramen in each of the transverse processes. The body is generally smaller, oval, and broader than other vertebra. The first three vertebrae are peculiar too. The first cervical vertebra, C1 or atlas, has no body and resembles a bony ring. This vertebra supports the head, has a shorter (and some say no) spinous process but long transverse processes (Gench et al., 1995; Goss, 1976). There are two large concavities on the superior surface that articulate with occipital condyles of skull, allowing flexion and extension around a frontal

axis (Gench et al., 1995). The second cervical vertebra, C2 or the axis, form a pivot around which the first vertebra, carrying the head, rotates. This rotational movement permits extensive range of motion (ROM) around a vertical axis so that we can look side to side by turning our heads. The most conspicuous difference of C2 is the superior extension of the body called the *dens* where it articulates with the atlas. The seventh cervical vertebra is also distinctive in having a long and prominent spinous process. Since this spinous process protrudes further than all other cervical vertebrae, it is easily palpated and useful as a skeletal landmark, especially when describing to clients where their injuries occurred in relation to this landmark.

The thoracic vertebrae are intermediate in size and have four articular facets not found on other vertebrae. These form the articulation with the 12 ribs. Another difference is that the spinous processes project downward, especially T2-T10, which limits the ability of the thoracic spine to hyperextend.

Lumbar vertebrae are the largest of the movable vertebrae, and are important because they support the weight of body. The articular processes provide more of an interlocking articulation with other vertebrae, which limits movement around the long axis (Gench et al., 1995, p. 159). The L5 vertebra articulates distally with the sacrum through the lumbosacral joint, so there is greater movement here than elsewhere in the lumbar spine (Gench et al., 1995).

The fusion of the five sacral vertebrae forms a triangular bone in the dorsal part of the pelvis located like a wedge between the two coxal bones of the hip. The sacrum articulates with the last two lumbar vertebrae proximally and the immovable coccyx distally. The coccyx is formed by three to five rudimentary vertebrae, the last of which is only a nodule of bone.

The spine has four naturally occurring curves: the thoracic and sacrococcygeal curve in a convex direction posteriorly; cervical and lumbar bend in a convex direction anteriorly. The cervical and lumbar curves exist before birth and are called *primary curves*, whereas the thoracic and sacrococcygeal curves are *secondary curves* that develop in infancy and young childhood (Gench et al., 1995) (Figure 9-2). Other curves associated with the spine occur when there is an increase in an anterior curve (lordosis), an increase in the posterior curve (kyphosis), or the existence of a lateral curve (scoliosis).

The movements of the spine are made by the articulations of the vertebral bodies and by the articulations with the vertebral

Figure 9-1. Comparison of vertebrae.

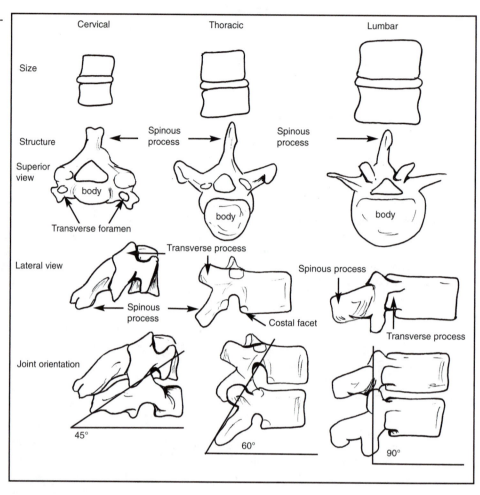

arches. While motion of the spinal column is small within each vertebra, the combined motion of the spine is much more. Flexion, extension, and hyperextension occur in the sagittal plane around multiple axes through nucleus pulposa, and lateral flexion occurs in the frontal plane around sagittal axes, also through nucleus pulposa (Figure 9-3A-C).

Flexion and extension have a range of 110 to 140 degrees, with free movement in cervical and lumbar regions but limited motion in the thoracic area. The axis of rotation moves anteriorly with flexion and posteriorly with extension. Flexion of the whole trunk occurs primarily in the lumbar area for the first 50 to 60 degrees and then more flexion is achieved by forward tilting of the pelvis and backward movement of the sacrum. Similarly, greater extension is achieved by posterior pelvic tilting and anterior sacral movement, followed by lumbar spine extension (Figure 9-4).

Lateral flexion of 75 to 85 degrees occurs mainly in cervical and lumbar and is often accompanied by rotation. Rotation of the spine is described as right or left rotation and occurs in a transverse plane around the long axis from the top of the head through the disks to the sacral region. Rotation of 90 degrees is possible with free movements in the cervical area and with lateral flexion in thoracic and lumbar regions. Rotation is generally more limited in the lumbar region (Gench et al., 1995).

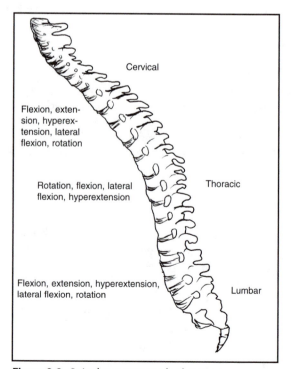

Figure 9-2. Spinal movements by location.

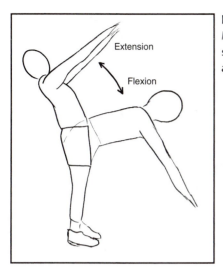

Figure 9-3A. Movements of the spine. Extension and flexion.

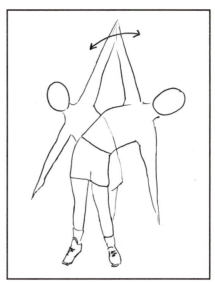

Figure 9-3B. Lateral flexion.

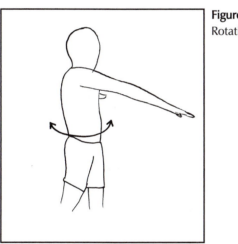

Figure 9-3C. Rotation.

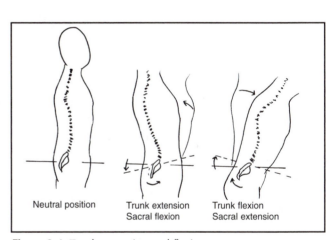

Figure 9-4. Trunk extension and flexion.

While little discussion will be made about the spinal muscles, generally the muscles are anterior or posterior in location. Anterior muscles flex the spine, whereas posterior muscles extend or hyperextend spinal segments. Lateral flexion occurs when one side of each pair of anterior and posterior muscles contracts, and rotation occurs when anterior and posterior muscles contract but only if they do not lie parallel to the long axis (Gench et al., 1995).

The lower extremity comprises the hip and ankle joints as well as multiple joints in the feet. The lower extremities absorb high forces and support the body weight as well as providing a mechanism for movement. The joints and muscles of the lower extremity are important in balance and posture. Every movement made or posture assumed in the lower extremity or trunk is interrelated (Hamil & Knutzen, 1995). Forces from the lower extremity are transmitted through the hips to the pelvis and trunk, and the hips have the function of supporting the head, trunk, and upper extremities (Jenkins, 1998). When considering posture or positioning of a client, the relationship between the trunk and the hip is essential.

THE PELVIC GIRDLE

The hip joint, or coxofemoral joint, is a joint often compared to the glenohumeral joint. Both are ball and socket joints capable of a variety of movements. However, the hip acts more often as a closed chain that is opposite to the open kinetic chain of the shoulder. This demonstrates the different functions of these two ball and socket joints. The shoulder functions to enable the hands to be used to their most efficient capacity, whereas the hip provides stability, balance, and weight bearing to provide postural accommodations and locomotion.

The pelvic girdle is made up of the sacrum, the coccyx, and two coxal (innominate) bones, which comprise the fused ilium, ischium, and pubis. These bones form seven joints: the lumbosacral, sacroiliac (two in number), sacrococcygeal, symphysis pubis, and the hip (two of them). While small amounts of movement are possible at the sacroiliac, symphysis pubis, and sacrococcygeal joints, the ability to have even these small amounts of movement is very important. The pelvic girdle attaches posteriorly to the axial skeleton at the sacroiliac joint. The two coxal bones attach anteriorly to the pubic symphysis and form a strong arch that is slightly movable and is able to transmit the weight of the body to the femur (Jenkins, 1998).

The sacroiliac joint is formed by the articulation between the sacrum and the ilium, which forms a synchondrosis joint. Small amounts of movement are possible at this joint. The amount of movement varies from individual to individual and between the genders. Men have stronger and thicker sacroiliac ligaments so they have less mobile sacroiliac joints, and as many as 3 out of 10 men have fused joints. Men have a higher precedence of developing osteophytes and ankylosis in older age than do females. Females have more mobile sacroiliac joints due to greater ligamental laxity, which increases with monthly cycles of hormones and with pregnancy. The male sacroiliac joint is also more stable. In females, the center of gravity is in the same plane as the sacrum and in males the center of gravity is more anterior, so there is more of a load on the male sacroiliac joint than the female (Hamil & Knutzen, 1995, p. 205).

The hip joint is made up of the convex acetabulum of the pelvic bone and the convex head of the femur. The acetabulum is deepened by a ring of fibrocartilage, the acetabulum labrum, which is located in the lateral aspect of the pelvis. The acetabulum faces laterally, anteriorly, and inferiorly (Kendall & McCreary, 1983, p. 317). The synovial capsule encloses the entire joint and it thickens and forms ligamentous bands (Gench et al., 1995). This strong articular capsule is reinforced by iliofemoral, pubofemoral, and ischiofemoral ligaments (Kendall & McCreary, 1983, p. 317) (Figure 9-5).

The iliofemoral ligament, also known as the Y ligament, covers the hip anteriorly. In standing, the iliofemoral ligament (especially the inferior band) prevents posterior motion of the pelvis on the femur (hyperextension of hip). The pubofemoral ligament is anterior and inferior to the hip (Hamil & Knutzen, 1995, p. 208) and this ligament assists in checking extreme abduction and some external rotation. The ischiofemoral ligament is in a posterior and inferior location. This ligament limits internal rotation. All of these ligaments are slack when the hip is flexed and all ligaments become taut with hyperextension. Abduction is limited by the pubofemoral and ischiofemoral ligaments and adduction is limited by the superior or iliotrochanteric portion of iliofemoral (Y) ligament.

The head of the femur fits deeply in the acetabulum. The femoral head is attached to the femoral neck, which projects anteriorly, medially, and superiorly at an angle of inclination of 125 degrees. This angle of inclination is between the axis of the femoral neck and the shaft of the femur. Angles greater than 125 degrees are called *coxa valga*; angles less than 125 degrees are called *coxa vara* (Kisner & Colby, 1990). Following are the structures that can be palpated.

Ilium

Crests of Ilia

There are two of these, one on each side, and they are easily seen and palpated by placing the thumbs laterally. These two crests

should be level in a standing position and the highest point on the crest is at the level of the spinous process of the fourth lumbar vertebra (Esch, 1989; Smith et al., 1996).

Anterior Superior Spines of Ilia

With the thumbs on the front of the crest, follow downward from the crest and trace the crest to the most anterior point to the rounded anterior superior spines of ilia (ASIS) (Esch, 1989; Smith et al., 1996).

Posterior Superior Iliac Spine

If the crest is followed in a posterior direction about 1.5 inches from the midline, the broad and sturdy posterior superior iliac spine (PSIS) will feel rough. Below each is a depression that is a posterior landmark for the sacroiliac joint.

Sacrum

This is the flat bone at the center of the back between the PSIS (Esch, 1989).

Ischium

Tuberosities of ischia, also called the "sit bones", are easy to locate when sitting on a hard chair or sidelying with hips and knees flexed. These are the large bony prominences at the midline of the buttocks just below the gluteal fold, and they can be palpated when the gluteus maximus and hamstrings are relaxed (Esch, 1989; Sine, Liss, Rousch, Holcomb, & Wilson, 2000).

Femur

Greater Trochanter of the Femur

With the thumb on the crest laterally, reach down on the thigh as far as possible with middle finger, or 4 to 5 inches inferior to the most lateral portion of the iliac crest. These large bony prominences can be felt if one stands on the opposite leg and rotates the femur in internal and external rotation. Also, this is marked by the depression that appears when the thigh is abducted (Esch, 1989).

Osteokinematics

There is a functional relationship between the hips, pelvis, and spine so that with pelvic motion, the angle of the hip and the lumbar spine changes (Kisner & Colby, 1990). Movements of the pelvis include pelvic tilt, pelvic shift, rotation, and lumbar-pelvic rhythm. Due to these pelvic movements, flexion, extension, abduction and adduction, and internal and external rotation of the hip occur.

Movements that tilt the pelvis occur in a sagittal plane around a coronal axis. These movements can occur simultaneously or in a single limb around one axis. *Anterior pelvic tilt* is the forward movement of the pelvis and is produced when the anterior superior iliac spine moves anterior and inferior. The ASIS is then in a position closer to the anterior portion of the femur as pelvis rotates around the transverse axis of hip joint (Kisner & Colby, 1990). The symphysis pubis is more inferior in location and as a result of anterior pelvic tilt, hip flexion and lumbar spine extension (hyperexten-

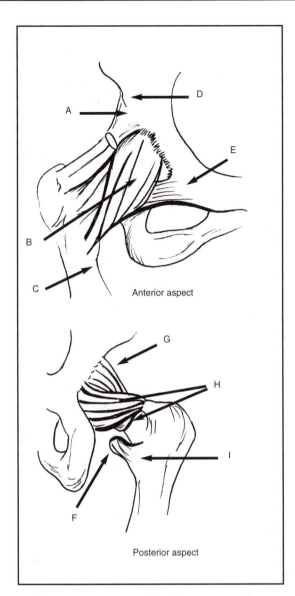

Figure 9-5. Ligaments of the hip. A. Rectus femoris tendon; B. Iliofemoral ligament; C. Lesser trochanter of femur; D. Anterior inferior iliac spine; E. Pubofemoral ligament; F. Psoas tendon; G. Iliofemoral ligament; H. Transverse band and orbicular zone (ischiofemoral ligament); I. Lesser trochanter.

sion) occur. *Posterior pelvic tilt* occurs when the PSIS move posteriorly and inferiorly, bringing the pelvis closer to the posterior aspect of the femur as the pelvis rotates backward around the axis of hip joints (Kisner & Colby, 1990). There is an upward and forward movement of the symphysis. This results in hip extension and lumbar spine flexion.

When one hip is moved into a position that is higher than the other side, this occurs due to *lateral pelvic tilt*. On one side, there is hip hiking and hip adduction; on the other, there is hip drop and hip abduction. This occurs when the lumbar spine laterally flexes

toward the side of the elevated pelvis (Gench et al., 1995; Kendall & McCreary, 1983).

Forward translatory *pelvic shifting* occurs in standing when one is in a relaxed or slouched position, resulting in extension of the hip and extension of LE spinal segments. There is a compensatory posterior shifting of the thorax on the upper lumbar spine with increased flexion of these segments (Kisner & Colby, 1990). This position requires little muscle action and the position is maintained by the iliofemoral ligaments of the hip, anterior longitudinal ligaments of lower lumbar spine, and posterior ligaments of the upper lumbar and thoracic spine (Kisner & Colby, 1990).

Pelvic rotation occurs to the left or right at the lumbosacral joint, resulting in a pivotal movement of hips around the long axis (Gench et al., 1995). This movement generally occurs in a transverse plane around a vertical axis. When one leg is fixed on the ground, the other unsupported leg swings forward or backward. If the leg moves forward, there is forward rotation with the trunk rotating backwards on the stabilized side with the femur on the stabilized side internally rotated. With backward rotation, there is posterior rotation and the femur externally rotates with the trunk moving in the opposite direction (Kisner & Colby, 1990).

The coordinated movement between the lumbar and pelvic segments is known as *lumbar-pelvic rhythm*. Due to this coordinated muscular activity, maximal forward flexion is possible, enabling us to pick up items from the floor and to touch our toes. It is the combined movements of hip flexion, pelvic tilt, and flexion of the lumbar spine seen as an analog to the scapulohumeral rhythm of the upper extremity except there are no proportional contributions of each motion nor a set sequence of occurrence as is true in the shoulder (Norkin & Levangie, 1992). Once the head and upper trunk initiate the flexion movement, the pelvis shifts posteriorly to maintain the center of gravity over the feet. At approximately 45 degrees of forward flexion, the ligaments become taut, the vertebrae become stabilized, and the muscles relax. Anterior pelvic tilt occurs once all vertebral segments have been stabilized.

The posterior ligaments and the pelvis rotate forward. Forward movement continues until the full length of the muscles is reached and is influenced by muscle extensibility in the back and hips (Kisner & Colby, 1990). Similar combined movements of hip abduction, lateral pelvic tilt, and flexion of the lumbar spine occur when one is sidelying and attempting maximal hip abduction. Full abduction would not be possible without the lateral tilting of the pelvis and the lumbar spine.

Movements of the femur in the acetabulum at the hip joint include flexion, extension, abduction, adduction, internal and external rotation, and circumduction. Since the hip is a ball and socket or triaxial joint, it is capable of all movements in three planes and has 3 degrees of freedom.

The axis for flexion and extension is around a coronal axis in a sagittal plane through the head and neck of the femur. Flexion ROM is generally considered to be 0 to 90 degrees with the knee extended and 0 to 120 degrees to 140 degrees with the knee flexed. The difference in ranges is due to the effect of the hamstrings, which restrict the motion when the knee is extended. With hip

Table 9-1. MOTIONS OF THE FEMUR	
Physiologic Motions of the Femur	*Direction of Slide*
Flexion	Posterior
Extension	Anterior
Abduction	Inferior
Adduction	Superior
Internal rotation	Posterior
External rotation	

Table 9-2. MOTIONS OF PELVIS WHEN LOWER EXTREMITY IS FIXED	
Physiologic Motions of the Pelvis	*Direction of Slide of the Acetabulum*
Anterior pelvic tilt	Anterior
Posterior pelvic tilt	Posterior
Lateral pelvic tilt:	
Pelvis elevated	Inferior
Pelvis dropped	Superior
Forward pelvic rotation	Anterior

flexion, anterior pelvic tilt and increased lumbar extension will occur unless the pelvis is stabilized by the abdominal muscles (Kisner & Colby, 1990). The range for hip extension is 0 to 10 degrees to 30 degrees of motion. Posterior pelvic tilt and decreased lumbar extension will also occur with extension.

Abduction and adduction occur in a frontal plane around a sagittal (anterioposterior) axis. The femur can be abducted 0 to 30 degrees to 50 degrees and adduction can occur in a range from 0 to 10 degrees to 30 degrees of motion. Abduction movement is limited by gracilis muscle and adduction by tensor fascia latae and the iliotibial band.

Internal rotation of the hip occurs in a transverse plane around a longitudinal axis with a range of 0 to 30 degrees to 70 degrees. External rotation occurs in a range from 0 to 45 degrees to 90 degrees. (Differences in normative values are due to differences in measurement procedures.)

While the ROM values reflect norms for each motion, daily activities involving the lower extremities require much less ROM. For example, while the normal value for hip abduction is 0 to 30 degrees to 50 degrees, tying a shoe with the foot on the floor requires only about 19 degrees of ROM in the frontal plane. This illustrates that while a client may not have full or normal ROM, the client may be able to perform daily tasks successfully.

The head of the femur is convex while the acetabulum is concave, so most motions of the femoral head will be in a direction opposite to the motion of the distal end of the femur (Norkin & Levangie, 1992) (Table 9-1). The motions of flexion and extension are almost purely spin, with spinning occurring in a posterior direction for flexion and anteriorly for extension. Abduction and adduction are combined spin and glide, but again in a direction opposite to the motion of the distal end of the femur when the femur is the moving segment. However, when the hip is weight bearing, the femur is fixed. The motion of the hip is produced by the movement of the pelvis on the femur. While this motion is more common, the acetabulum now moves in the same direction as the opposite side of the pelvis (Norkin & Levangie, 1992) (Table 9-2).

Hip flexors are those muscles on the anterior or anteromedial surface of the hip region. The rectus femoris and iliopsoas muscles both cross the hip anterior to the frontal axis and act as hip flexors (Figure 9-6). The iliopsoas muscle (sometimes referred to as two separate muscles, the iliacus and psoas muscles) is a powerful muscle especially useful in the initial part of hip flexion. As flexion progresses, the iliopsoas muscle becomes shorter and less effective. This mechanism has led to the development of the "crunch" to exercise the abdominal muscles as they flex the spine. By bending the knees while in a supine position, the iliopsoas is rendered ineffective so that the "crunch" involves the abdominals and not synergistic muscles (Gench et al., 1995). The rectus femoris exerts little power in flexion until other muscles have initiated the flexion action and its action is complementary to the iliopsoas muscle. Pectineus, with a relatively long force arm and advantageous angle of insertion, is a powerful flexor as well as adductor muscle. Sartorius, the longest muscle in the body, is an effective hip flexor because its force arm is longest to the frontal axis and tensor fascia latae also participates with this movement. Anterior fibers of gluteus medius and gluteus minimus contribute to hip flexion, as do adductor magnus, adductor longus, and adductor brevis. The gracilis muscle, depending upon the location of the femur, can assist with flexion and extension, in addition to the adductor action at the hip (Gench et al., 1995).

The muscles that extend the thigh lie on the posterior aspect of the thigh (Figure 9-7). Gluteus maximus, while a large muscle on the posterior buttocks, is a strong extensor. However, Gench et al. (1995) state that this muscle is "notoriously lazy during actions associated with daily living", which may account for the ease with which this muscle loses its firmness and attracts fat deposits (p. 197). The posterior portions of gluteus medius also contribute to hip extension, as do the lower portions of the adductor magnus muscle. Posterior hamstring muscles (semimembranosus, semitendinosus, and biceps femoris) lie posterior to the joint axis and can act as extensors. All three muscles have essentially the same mechanical advantage in moving the femur. Since the posterior hamstrings extend the thigh and flex the leg, they are not strong

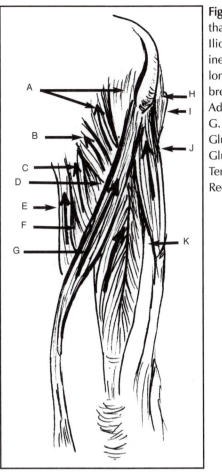

Figure 9-6. Muscles that flex the hip. A. Iliopsoas; B. Pectineus; C. Adductor longus; D. Adductor brevis; E. Gracilis; F. Adductor magnus; G. Sartorius; H. Gluteus minimus; I. Gluteus medius; J. Tensor fascia lata; K. Rectus femoris.

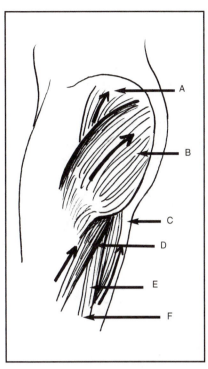

Figure 9-7. Muscles that extend the thigh. A. Gluteus medius; B. Gluteus maximus; C. Adductor magnus; D. Biceps; E. Semitendinosus; F. Semimembranosus.

contributors to extension unless the knee is kept in extension. When the leg is kept extended and the thigh is flexed (as in touching one's toes or high-kicking activities), pain may be felt behind the knee due to the posterior hamstrings. The posterior hamstrings are active in any forward bending at the hips and act as antigravity postural muscles (Jenkins, 1998).

The function of the muscles that abduct the thigh is to keep the pelvis in a horizontal placement when weight is put on the limb (Jenkins, 1998) (Figure 9-8). Two muscles are particularly strong in supporting the pelvis: gluteus medius and gluteus minimus. Both of these muscles pass the sagittal axis of the hip joint to the lateral side, so they are strong abductors and both have similar angles of attachment, which give these muscles superior mechanical advantages at the hip (Gench et al., 1995). Since the gluteus minimus is a smaller muscle, it is less powerful than the medius. Tensor fascia latae also contributes to the movement of the limb in abduction, but only when the limb is weight bearing (Jenkins, 1998). Sartorius, and to a lesser degree the piriformis, obturator internus, and the upper fibers of the gluteus maximus, assists with abduction. When the thigh is flexed to 90 degrees, the gluteus maximus then becomes an abductor; in other positions, this muscle is an adductor (Jenkins, 1998).

Adductor muscles are anteriorly placed on the thigh and include pectineus, adductor longus and brevis, and the obturator

portion of the adductor magnus (Figure 9-9). The adductor magnus is well-placed to adduct, but is recruited only when resistance is met (Gench et al., 1995). Adductor longus and brevis are active in all stages of adduction whether there is resistance or not (Gench et al., 1995), and pectineus has both a long force arm and advantageous angle of insertion, so it is a strong adductor. Crossing the hip joint on the medial side of the sagittal axis, gracilis is well placed for adduction action. Muscles that also contribute to adduction include gluteus maximus, quadratus femoris, obturator externus, the hamstrings, gracilis, and iliopsoas (when the thigh is flexed), although not all sources indicate that these muscles function in adduction (Gench et al., 1995; Goss, 1976; Jacobs & Bettencourt, 1995; Sine et al., 2000).

The muscle actions of medial and lateral rotation are often the secondary result of other movements and there is some variability in the categorization of muscles that rotate the thigh. Muscles that laterally rotate the thigh are numerous. Gluteus maximus is a powerful lateral rotator. Piriformis, obturator internus, obturator externus, quadratus femoris, and superior and inferior gemelli are small muscles that lie deep in the pelvis with the primary action of external rotation. These six muscles are often grouped together and called the *outward rotators* (Gench et al., 1995). These six small rotator muscles hold the femur in acetabulum just like the rotator cuff muscles of glenohumeral joint and they either laterally rotate the femur or balance the pelvis and trunk. Biceps femoris, posterior fibers of the gluteus medius, and sartorius also produce weak lateral rotation.

Medial rotation is produced by gluteus minimus, tensor fascia latae, and anterior fibers of gluteus medius. Semimembranosus and semitendinosus are credited with weak internal rotation (Figure 9-10).

Figure 9-8. Muscles that abduct the thigh. A. Tensor fascia latae; B. Sartorius; C. Gluteus medius; D. Gluteus minimus; E. Piriformis.

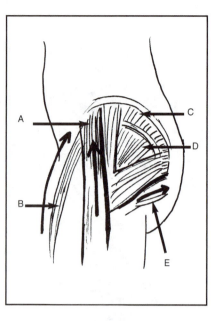

Figure 9-9. Muscles that adduct the thigh. A. Pectineus; B. Adductor brevis; C. Adductor longus; D. Adductor magnus; E. Gracilis.

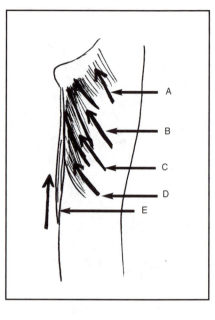

Due to the gluteals and hamstrings, the hip is very strong in extension. Perhaps extension of the hip is even more critical than hip flexion because extension is needed for an upright posture as well as sitting and standing. The hip extensors are active when gravity pulls the upper body into flexion and they prevent this forward motion of the trunk (Hinkle, 1997). The hip extensors and flexors also maintain lumbar curve, with iliopsoas seen as a key postural muscle as it pulls anteriorly on lumbar vertebras and ilium to reinforce lumbar curve and anterior pelvic tilt (Hinkle, 1997, p. 121) and the flexors help to maintain the anterior and posterior trunk balance.

The two joint function of rectus femoris and hamstrings (semitendinosus, semimembranosus, and biceps femoris) requires further discussion. When the hip is flexed, the rectus femoris acts as the agonist and hamstrings work antagonistically. In hip extension, the hamstrings are acting as agonists, while the rectus femoris is the antagonist. In knee flexion, the hamstrings have an agonist function and rectus is antagonist, and in knee extension, the muscle roles reverse. If hip and knee actions are performed simultaneously, the relationships are more complex. For example, a place kick in soccer requires hip flexion and knee extension so the rectus femoris contracts to flex the hip and extend the knee, whereas the hamstrings must relax to allow the leg to move. The hamstrings are capable of generating more force than the rectus femoris at the hip due to a longer force arm, just as the rectus femoris is more forceful at the knee. Simultaneous hip and knee flexion or hip and knee extension requires both hamstrings and rectus femoris be agonists at one joint and antagonists at the other. This is contradictory to muscle action in the upper extremity, where a muscle will act as an agonist at all of the joints it crosses. For example, the extensor digitorum longus crosses five joints, causing extension at each; flexor digitorum profundus crosses four joints, causing flexion at each joint. Due to this, these upper extremity muscles can be easily overstretched or overshortened.

Figure 9-10. Medial rotators of the thigh. A. Semimembranosus; B. Semitendinosus; C. Gluteus medius; D. Gluteus minimus; E. Tensor fascia latae.

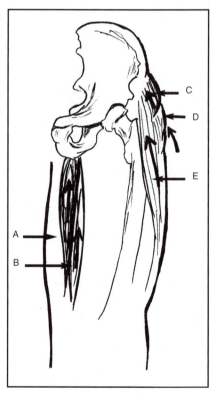

In walking, the abductors control the pelvis and the hamstrings control the amount of hip flexion and some propulsion. Abduction of the femur separates the feet, providing a wider base of support. Without adequate abductor strength, the hip of a swinging leg would drop (Trendelenburg sign) and ambulation would be more cumbersome and less energy efficient (Hinkle, 1997). Lateral rotation accompanies abduction and extension of hip and provides stability by allowing the feet and lower leg to be positioned before striking the ground or in balancing on one leg as we walk and run.

When lateral rotation is diminished, the foot points toward the midline, which adds stress to the knees (Hinkle, 1997). Muscles controlling hip abduction and adduction are also important in maintenance of dynamic sitting balance, as are medial rotators, which control diagonal balance and weight shifts.

Gench et al. (1995) state that "the muscles of spine and pelvic girdle are at the mercy of the demands of upright posture" (p. 184), which constantly needs to overcome the forces of gravity and sustain loads. If the muscles are unable to overcome these forces, the forces and movements tend to be transmitted to the spine rather than the pelvis, creating pain, decreased movement, and structural damage. Tight hip extensors can cause an increase in lumbar flexion when the thigh is flexed and tight hip flexors will cause increased lumbar extension as the thigh extends. If the adductor muscles are tight, this can cause lateral pelvic tilt on the opposite side and side bending of the trunk toward side of tightness. The opposite result occurs with tight abductors (Gench et al., 1995; Hinkle, 1997).

POSTURE

Posture is influenced by many factors, including general health status, body build, gender, strength and endurance, visual and kinesthetic awareness, and personal habits (Galley & Forster, 1987). Being in an upright stance has definite advantages for using one's hands in complex tasks, but also creates a position that is inherently unstable because the center of gravity of the body is over a relatively small base of support (Galley & Forster, 1987).

The anatomic factors that affect posture are:
1. Bony contours.
2. Laxity of ligamentous structures.
3. Fascial and musculotendinous tightness (e.g., hamstrings, tensor fascae latae, pectorals, hip flexors).
4. Muscle tone (gluteus maximus, abdominals, erector spinae).
5. Pelvic angle (normal is 30 degrees).
6. Joint position and mobility.
7. Neurogenic outflow and inflow (Magee, 1992, p. 581).

Posture is the position of the head, limbs, and trunk and their relationships to each other. Changes in posture occur when any part is moved—adjusting the position of the head and limbs in relation to trunk, adjusting the trunk in relation to the head or limbs when these are fixed, and making finely adjusted vertebral movements. Posture also communicates nonverbal body language to observers, reflecting self-esteem and attitude.

Standing upright depends on the weight distribution on each foot, between the two feet and the balance of the pelvis over the feet, the trunk over the pelvis and the head over the trunk (Kisner & Colby, 1990). Posture and balance has been compared to stacking movable blocks, where balance is achieved between each block and the weight is distributed between two sides of the body. Changes in position of the pelvis results in automatic realignment of the spine, especially in the lumbar region. If the head is too far forward or too far back, tension, strain and pain in neck muscles, headache, and eye strain may result. Ideal erect standing posture is

when the line of gravity passes through the mastoid process of the jaw, a point just in front of the shoulder, a point just behind the center of the hip joint, a point just in front of the center of knee joints and approximately 5 to 6 centimeters in front of the ankle. The pelvis is neutral and there is a natural lordosis of the lumbar spine (Cook & Hussey, 1995, p. 254) (Table 9-3).

A balanced posture reduces work done by muscles and not all muscles are active in standing posture. The intrinsic muscles of feet are quiescent as are the quadriceps and hamstrings. There is slight activity in the gluteus maximus and the abdominal muscles are quiescent except for the lower fibers of internal obliques, which are active to protect the inguinal canal. The soleus is continuously active (as is iliopsoas) in all cases because gravity tends to pull the body forward over feet. Erector spinae are active, counteracting gravity's effect to pull the body forward. Gastrocnemius and the posterior tibial muscles are less frequently active and tibialis anterior is quiescent, but this changes if high heels are worn. Lateral postural sway is counteracted by gluteus medius and tensor fascia latae.

Various postures can be assumed in a standing position. Several types of faulty posture are shown in Tables 9-3 and 9-4, and also in Appendix K.

One cannot maintain a symmetrical stance for long and standing is not a static activity. There is a continuous slight sway and the magnitude of the sway tends to be larger in those who are very old or very young. The alternating activity enables muscle spindles to be activated irregularly so fatigue in any one motor unit is prevented and venous return is assisted. Sitting provides a more stable posture because the supporting surface area of the buttocks, back of thighs, and feet is greater. The center of gravity is lowered and this posture allows relaxation of lower extremity muscles and less energy use. Pelvic stability, though, is greater in standing than sitting due to the passive locking mechanism at the hip by ligaments when the hips are fully extended during standing. When seated, the hips are flexed and the locking mechanism is lost. The pelvis rotates backwards causing lumbar lordosis to convert to a kyphotic or flexed position due to tension of hip extensors, especially hamstrings (Cook & Hussey, 1995).

Optimal sitting posture is described as:
- Pelvis: no pelvic obliquity, slight anterior pelvic tilt, no pelvic rotation.
- Trunk: slight lumbar lordosis, slight thoracic kyphosis, slight cervical extension.
- LE: neutral IR/ER, slight abduction at the hips, flexion of hips, knees and ankles to 90 degrees.
- UE: elbows slightly forward of shoulders, forearms supported, hands toward midline.
- Head: midline, eyes facing forward (Perr, 1998).

Various sitting postures are possible. One can be sitting supported or in a relaxed unsupported or erect unsupported position, or in a forward sitting posture. This has been called the *functional task position* or the *posture of readiness* (Cook & Hussey, 1995), in which the person's center of gravity shifts in the direction of the activity. In unsupported sitting, the muscles of the spine are activated to overcome the backward rotation of the pelvis and lumbar

Table 9-3.

FAULTY POSTURES

Name	Description	Potential Sources	Muscle Imbalances	Causes of Pain
Lordotic posture two types: 1. exaggerated 2. swayback	Military	Increase in lumbosacral angle, in lumbar lordosis, in anterior pelvic tilt and hip flexion	Stress to anterior long-itudinal ligament; narrow-ing of the intervertebral foramen, which may compress the dura and blood vessels of nerve roots; may cause approx-imation of the articular facets that makes them weight bear and may cause synovial irritation and joint inflammation.	Tight hip flexors (iliopsoas, tensor fascia latae, rectus femoris) and lumbar extensors (erector spinae); may be stretched and weak abdominal muscles (rectus abdominis, in-ternal and external obliques), faulty posture, pregnancy, obesity, weak abdominal muscles.
Relaxed, slouch-ed or swayback posture (lordosis)	Sway back	Excessive shifting of the pelvic segment anteriorly. This results in hip extension and a shift of the thoracic region posteriorly. Increased thoracic kyphosis and forward head placement also occurs.	Stress to iliofemoral ligament, anterior longi-tudinal ligament and posterior longitudinal ligament; if asymmetrical posture, also stress to iliotibial band on side of elevated hip; narrowing of intervertebral foramen in lower lumbar spine may compress blood vessels, dura, nerve roots.	Muscle imbalance in tight upper abdominal muscle (rectus abdom-inis and obliques), in-ternal intercostal, hip extensor, lower lumbar extensor muscle and fascia; stretched and weak lower abdominals (rectus abdominis and obliques), extensor muscles of lower thor-acic and hip flexors.
Kyphosis-lordosis posture		Head is forward; cervical spine, lumbar spine (lordosis) are hyperextended and knees are extended with increased flexion of thoracic spine (kyphosis).	See both lordosis and kyphosis.	Weakness in anterior neck and upper back muscles and muscles of lower abdomen. Shortness occurs in hip flexors and possibly the low back.
Kyphosis: Flat low-back posture Kyphosis: 4 types: 1. flat back 2. hump back 3. round back 4. dowagers hump		Decreased lumbosacral angle, decreased lumbar lordosis, hip extension and posterior tilt of pelvis.	Lack of normal physio-logic lumbar curve that reduces shock absorbing and predisposed to injury; stress to posterior longi-tudinal ligament; increase in posterior disc space so nucleus produces more fluid and may protrude posteriorly.	Tight trunk flexors (rectus abdominis and intercostals) and hip extensors; stretched and weak lumbar extensor and possibly hip flexor muscles, continued slouching or flexing in sitting or standing; over-emphasis on flexion exercises.

Table 9-3, continued.

Name	Description	Potential Sources	Muscle Imbalances	Causes of Pain
Flat upper back		Decrease thoracic curve, depresses scapulae, depressed clavicle, flat neck; associated with exaggerated military posture but not common.	Fatigue of muscles, compression of neurovascular bundle in thoracic outlet between clavicle and ribs.	Tight thoracic erector spinae, scapular protractors and potentially restricted scapular movement; weak scapular protractors and intercostals; common cause: exaggerating the upright posture.
Round back or increased kyphosis		Increased pelvic angle; increased thoracic curve, protracted scapulae and forward head.	Stress to posterior longitudinal ligament; fatigue in thoracic erector spinae and rhomboid muscles; thoracic outlet syndrome; cervical posture syndromes	Tight anterior thorax (intercostal), UE originating on thorax (pectoralis major and minor, latissimus dorsi, serratus anterior), muscles of cervical spine (levator scapulae, upper trapezius) and muscles of cervical region, stretched and weak thoracic erector spinae and scapular retractors (rhomboids and upper and lower trapezius).
Scoliosis		Usually thoracic and lumbar; in right handed, mild right thoracic, left lumbar S-shaped curve or mild left thoracic-lumbar C-curve; may be asymmetry in hips, pelvis, and LE.	Muscle fatigue and ligamentous strain on side of convexity; nerve root irritation on side of concavity.	Tight on concave side; stretched on convex; long-term asymmetrical postural and functional activities, handedness, and developmental patterns.
Forward head posture muscles		Increased flexion of lower cervical and upper thoracic, increased extension of occiput on first cervical vertebra, increased extension of upper cervical; may be TMJ too.	Stress to anterior longitudinal ligament and posterior; muscle tension and fatigue, irritation of facet joints in cervical spine; narrowing of intervertebral foramina, which may impinge on blood vessels and nerve roots; impingement on neurovascular bundle from anterior scalene muscle tightness; impingement on	Tight levator scapulae, sternocleidomastoid, scalene, suboccipital and maybe upper trapezius and muscles of mastication; stretched and weakened anterior throat and lower cervical and upper thoracic erector spinae; occupational or functional postures requiring leaning forward long periods

Table 9-3, continued.

Name	Description	Potential Sources	Muscle Imbalances	Causes of Pain
Forward head posture muscles			cervical plexis from impingement on occipital nerves from tight upper trapezius leading to tension headaches; lower cervical disk lesions; muscle levator scapulae muscle; suboccipital headaches by pinching of the greater occipital nerve; TMJ by altering occlusal relationship of teeth; loss of upper thoracic mobility with resultant degenerative changes in intervertebral discs; diminished respiratory capacity due to less able to use diaphragm.	or result of faulty pelvic or lumbar spine posture.
Flat neck posture	Decreased cervical lordosis, increased flexion of occipit on atlas; may be seen with exaggerated military posture (flat upper back); may be TMJ dysfunction	TMJ and occlusive changes; decrease in shock absorbing function of lordotic curve may predispose neck to injury; stress to ligamentum nuchae.	Imbalances to short anterior neck muscles, stretched or weakened levator scapulae, sternocleidomastoid and scalene; uncommon but could be due to exaggerated use of this posture for prolonged periods.

Adapted from Kisner, C. & Colby, L. A. (1990). *Therapeutic exercise: Foundations and techniques* (2nd ed.). Philadelphia: F.A. Davis; and Kendall, F. P. & McCreary, E. K. (1983). *Muscles: Testing and function* (3rd ed.). Baltimore: Williams & Wilkins.

kyphosis and achieve erect or lordotic sitting posture. The pelvis rotates forward and line of gravity through ischial tuberosities (Cook & Hussey, 1995).

Use of correct sitting posture has the following health benefits:
1. Decrease in ligamentous strain to prevent overstretching.
2. A decrease in muscular strain and overstretching of the back muscles, which causes muscle imbalances.
3. A decrease in intradiskal pressure.
4. A healthy spine along the whole kinetic chain because of a reduction in stress on the thoracic and cervical spine and shoulder girdle.
5. More efficient muscle work and reduction in fatigue because the postural muscles are used to support the spine and rib cage while the extremities are used to conduct work.
6. A greater ROM of the upper extremities when the worker reaches to shoulder level and overhead because the upper body is not flexed, which limits this range.
7. Efficient diaphragmatic breathing because there is a greater distance between the sternum and pelvis.
8. More air entering the lungs because breathing increases, providing more oxygenated blood to vital organs, including the brain. Efficient breathing diminishes fatigue, resulting in increased productivity and accurate work.
9. Improved lower extremity circulation with proper seat tilt and depth.
10. Good posture that promotes a positive self-image (Jacobs & Bettencourt, 1995).

Prolonged sitting can have deleterious effects on the lumbar spine. Unsupported sitting requires higher muscle activity in the thoracic region and more of a load on the lumbar spine because of the backward tilt and flattening of the low back and the forward shifting of the center of gravity, which adds an additional load on the disks. Jacobs & Bettencourt (1995) indicate that "research has provided a dichotomy: disk pressures are reduced when a person sits in an erect posture and maintains the three natural spinal curves but the trunk muscles exert less energy when a person sits in a

Table 9-4.

EFFECTS ON BODY STRUCTURES

Deviation	Compression	Distraction	Stretching	Shortening
Excessive anterior tilt of pelvis	Posterior vertebral bodies Interdiskal pressure L-5-S-1 increased	Lumbosacral angle increased Shearing forces at L-5-S-1 Likelihood of forward slippage of L-5 on S-1 increased	Abdominals	Iliopsoas
Excessive lumbar lordosis	Posterior vertebral bodies and facet joints Interdiskal pressures increased Intervertebral foramina narrowed	Anterior annulus fibers	Anterior longitudinal ligament	Posterior longitudinal ligament Interspinous ligaments Ligamentum flavum Lumbar extensors Lumbar extensors
Excessive dorsal kyphosis	Anterior vertebral bodies Intradiskal pressures	Facet joint capsules and posterior annulus fibers increased	Dorsal back extensors Posterior ligaments Scapular muscles	Anterior longitudinal ligament Upper abdominals Anterior shoulder girdle musculature
Excessive cervical lordosis	Posterior vertebral bodies and facet joints Interdiskal pressure increased Intervertebral foramina narrowed	Anterior annulus fibers	Anterior longitudinal ligament	Posterior ligaments Neck extensors

Reprinted with permission from Norkin, C. & Levangie, P. (1992). *Joint structure and function: A comprehensive analysis*. Philadelphia: F. A. Davis Co.

slightly flexed or slouched position" (p. 140). For this reason, periodic changes in position and properly designed chairs are essential to the maintenance of good posture. Positions of least pressure are sidelying and lying supine.

The height of a properly fitted chair should be equal to length of the leg from the back of the knee to the base of the heel with knee bent to 90 degrees and feet flat on the floor. If the seat is too long, there is pressure behind the knee. If too short, there will be pressure on the posterior surface of the thigh and more pressure on the feet. The chair back should be inclined back slightly and with a lumbar support.

An ergonomically well-designed chair would include:
- Seat height that is easily adjustable, as in a pneumatic chair.
- Backrest that is easily adjustable to support the lumbar spine vertically (height) and horizontally (forward and backward) and is narrow enough so that the operator's arm or torso do not strike it if rotation is required.
- The seat tilts forward and backward independently of the backrest. This feature is useful with fine detail work and office work.
- The seat edge is curved to reduce pressure under the legs.
- There is enough space between the back of the chair and the seat to accommodate the buttocks.

- The adjustable armrests (optional) are small and low enough to fit under the work surface and to support the back when the worker works close to the work surface.
- The base has five points (safety).
- The worker can make adjustments easily with one hand while seated.
- The upholstery fabric is comfortable, reduces heat transfer in warm climates and static electricity in cold weather, and is stain resistant and easily cleaned.
- Training is provided to ensure that workers are familiar with the features and adjustments of an optimally fitting chair.

Sitting in a wheelchair presents several challenges that this text will only briefly discuss. Many wheelchairs have a sling seat, which is good for transport of the chair since it can be easily folded and placed in a trunk or backseat. However, the position of the person in the wheelchair is one where the hips slide forward and rotate inward, which brings the knees together. This position in the wheelchair is not particularly comfortable for long periods of time and makes it more difficult to effectively use one's hands in activities. There are ramifications related to pressure distribution as well as to posture and comfort. With the posterior pelvic tilt, there is additional weight on the ischial tuberosities, coccyx, and possibly lower sacrum, which may precipitate scoliosis or promote pelvic obliquity. Cook and Hussey (1995) add that a "sling seat conforms to the forces generated by the individual instead of providing forces that resist and stabilize. This is an application of Newton's Third Law: Each action (force) has an equal but opposite reaction. The internal forces of the body are not balanced by external forces from the sling seat" (p. 257). These present challenges for the comfort, safety, and function of our clients in wheelchairs.

SUMMARY

- The spine is formed by 33 bones, including the cervical, thoracic, lumbar, sacral, and coccygeal vertebral bones. There are distinct differences in each of the spinal segments dependent upon the purpose and function of these segments.
- The spine has four naturally occurring curves. If there is more or less of a curve than what naturally occurs, the balance of the spine, pelvis, and body is disturbed. This can result in pain, deformity, and loss of function.
- The lower extremities absorb high forces and support the body weight as well as providing a mechanism for movement.
- The hip, a ball and socket joint, is capable of a wide variety of movement. The hip generally serves to provide stability, weight bearing, and balance.
- Movements of the pelvis include pelvic tilt, pelvic shift, rotation, and lumbar-pelvic rhythm. These movements enable flexion/extension, abduction/adduction, and internal/external rotation of the hip.
- The two-joint function of rectus femoris and the hamstrings (semitendinosus, semimembranosus, and biceps femoris) can act as an agonist at one joint and as an antagonist at another. This action is contradictory to the muscle action in the upper extremity, where a two-joint muscle acts as an agonist at all of the joints it crosses.

- Correct posture in sitting, standing, or lying maintains forces in the body and expends the least amount of energy. Postural control is maintained by automatic postural adjustments and is affected by body build, natural movement ability, central nervous system functioning, vision, vestibular system function, perception, muscle tone, and other factors.
- Faulty sitting or standing postures limit function and expend excess energy. Good posture is achieved when the body weight is borne evenly on various surfaces and natural spinal curves are maintained. Careful attention to posture, whether seated or standing, is essential to functional performance.

REFERENCES

Cook, A. M., & Hussey, S. M. (1995). *Assistive technologies: Principles and practice.* St. Louis, MO: C. V. Mosby.

Esch, D. L. (1989). *Musculoskeletal function: An anatomy and kinesiology laboratory manual.* Minneapolis: University of Minnesota.

Galley, P. M., & Forster, A. L. (1987). *Human movement: An introductory text for physiotherapy students* (2nd ed.). New York: Churchill-Livingstone.

Gench, B. E., Hinson, M. M., & Harvey, P. T. (1995). Anatomical kinesiology. Dubuque, IA: Eddie Bowers Publishing, Inc.

Goss, C. M. (Ed.) (1976). *Gray's anatomy of the human body* (29th ed.). Philadelphia: Lea and Febiger.

Hamil, J., & Knutzen, K. M. (1995). *Biomechanical basis of human movement.* Baltimore: Williams & Wilkins.

Hinkle, C. Z. (1997). *Fundamentals of anatomy and movement: A workbook and guide.* St. Louis, MO: C. V. Mosby.

Jacobs, K., & Bettencourt, C. M. (1995). *Ergonomics for therapists.* Boston: Butterworth-Heinemann.

Jenkins, D. B. (1998). *Hollingshead's functional anatomy of the limbs and back* (7th ed.). Philadelphia: W. B. Saunders Co.

Kendall, F. P., & McCreary, E. K. (1983). *Muscles: Testing and function* (3rd ed.). Baltimore: Williams & Wilkins.

Kisner, C., & Colby, L. A. (1990). *Therapeutic exercise: Foundations and techniques* (2nd ed.). Philadelphia: F. A. Davis Co.

Magee, D. J. (1992). *Orthopedic physical assessment.* Philadelphia: W. B. Saunders Co.

Norkin, C. C., & Levangie, P. K. (1992). *Joint structure and function: A comprehensive analysis* (2nd ed.). Philadelphia: F. A. Davis Co.

Perr, A. (1998). Elements of seating and wheeled mobility intervention. *OT Practice,* 16-24.

Sine, R., Liss, S. E., Rousch, R. E., Holcomb, J. D., & Wilson, G. (2000). *Basic rehabilitation techniques: A self instructional guide* (4th ed.). Gaithersburg, MD: Aspen Publishers.

Smith, L. K., Weiss, E. L., & Lehmkuhl, L. D. (1996). *Brunnstrom's clinical kinesiology* (5th ed.). Philadelphia: F. A. Davis Co.

BIBLIOGRAPHY

Basmajian, J. V., & DeLuca, C. J. (1985). *Muscles alive* (5th ed.). Baltimore: Williams & Wilkins.

Baxter, R. (1998). *Pocket guide to musculoskeletal assessment.* Philadelphia: W. B. Saunders Co.

Burstein, A. H., & Wright, T. M. (1994). *Fundamentals of orthopaedic biomechanics*. Baltimore: Williams & Wilkins.

Daniels, L., & Worthingham, C. (1977). *Therapeutic exercise for body alignment and function* (2nd ed.). Philadelphia: W. B. Saunders Co.

Demeter, S. L., Andersson, G. B. J., & Smith, G. M. (1996). *Disability evaluation*. St. Louis, MO: C. V. Mosby.

Durward, B. R., Baer, G. D., & Rowe, P. J. (1999). *Functional human movement: Measurement and analysis*. Oxford: Butterworth Heineman.

Greene, D. P., & Roberts, S. L. (1999). *Kinesiology: Movement in the context of activity*. St. Louis, MO: C. V. Mosby.

Hartley, A. (1995). *Practical joint assessment: Lower quadrant* (2nd ed.). St. Louis, MO: C. V. Mosby.

Konin, J. G. (1999). *Practical kinesiology for the physical therapist assistant*. Thorofare, NJ: SLACK Incorporated.

Loth, T., & Wadsworth, C. T. (1998). *Orthopedic review for physical therapists*. St. Louis, MO: C. V. Mosby.

Lumley, J. S. P. (1990). *Surface anatomy: The anatomical basis of clinical examination*. New York: Churchill Livingstone.

MacKenna, B. R., & Callender, R. (1990). *Illustrated physiology* (5th ed.). New York: Churchill Livingstone.

Nordin, M., & Frankel, V. H. (1989). *Basic biomechanics of the musculoskeletal system* (2nd ed.). Philadelphia: Lea and Febiger

Palastanga, N., Field, D., & Soames, R. (1989). *Anatomy and human movement: Structure and function*. Philadelphia: Lippincott Williams & Wilkins.

Palmer, M. L., & Epler, M. E. (1998). *Fundamentals of musculoskeletal assessment techniques* (2nd ed.). Philadelphia: J. B. Lippincott.

Perry, J. F., Rohe, D. A., & Garcia, A. O. (1996). *Kinesiology workbook*. Philadelphia: F. A. Davis Co.

Swedberg, L. (1998). Low-tech adaptations for seating and positioning. *OT Practice*, pp 26-31.

The Knee, Ankle, and Foot

Chapter 10

THE KNEE

The knee, with the hip and ankle, supports the body. In addition, the knee "functionally lengthens and shortens the lower extremity to raise and lower the body or move the foot in space" (Kendall & McCreary, 1983, p. 345). While occupational therapists rarely remediate the knee, ankle, or foot by either stretch or strengthening, this chapter will serve as an overview of the contributions that these structures add to functional performance and skills in occupations.

While the knee is often considered a simple hinge or ginglymus joint, it is actually made up of three articulations. Two articulations are between each condyle of the femur and condyle of the tibia and are called the *inferior and superior tibiofibular joints*. These are condyloid joints and only the superior tibiofibular articulation is contained within the knee. A partly arthrodial joint, formed by the articulation between the patella and femur, forms the third articulation or the *patellofemoral joint* (Goss, 1976; Nordin & Frankel, 1989). The tibia and fibula have been seen as corresponding to the ulna and radius of the upper extremity while the anterior surface of the leg is seen to correspond to the extensor surface of the forearm (Jenkins, 1998).

Of the two bones in the leg, the tibia is larger, more medially located, and articulates with both the knee and ankle. The fibula is smaller, more lateral in location, articulates only with the ankle but not the knee. The knee joint is actually the articulation of the lower femur and upper tibia and acts as a double condyloid joint, producing the movements of knee flexion and extension in a sagittal plane around a coronal axis and medial and lateral rotation, which occurs in the transverse plane around a vertical axis. The joint capsule does not form a complete covering around the joint but contributes to knee stability. Stability of the knee is provided primarily by the ligaments, muscles, menisci, joint capsule, and cartilage, while the bones provide mobility (Smith, Weiss, & Lehmkuhl, 1996) (Figure 10-1A, B).

The ligaments of the knee are important especially because there are no bony restraints to knee movements. The ligaments resist or control:

1. Excessive knee extension.
2. Varus and valgus stresses of the knee (attempted adduction or abduction of tibia).
3. Anterior or posterior displacements of the tibia beneath the femur.
4. Medial or lateral rotation of the tibia beneath the femur.
5. Combinations of anterior-posterior displacement and rotation of tibia (Norkin & Levangie, 1992, p. 347).

There are two collateral and two cruciate ligaments that function as passive load carrying structures and as a back up for the muscles. The *medial collateral ligament* (MCL), or medial tibial ligament, attaches to the medial aspect of the medial femoral epicondyle and supports the knee against valgus forces and offers some resistance to rotational stresses. This ligament is taut with knee extension. The thinner *lateral collateral ligament* (LCL) provides the main resistance to varus forces and lateral rotation, and is also taut in knee extension. In full extension, the collateral ligaments are assisted by the tightening of the posteromedial and posterolateral joint capsules, making extension the most stable position of the knee joint. When the knee is flexed, the ligaments are lax so that the tibia can rotate around the long axis. When the knee is extended, the tight ligaments and bony structures are more congruent, which prevents tibial rotation. Since the knee often is in a flexed position (as in dressing, bathing, etc.), effort should be made to ensure that the muscles of the knee, which are the last line of defense against injury, be maintained at peak strength to avoid injurious twisting of the tibia (Gench, Hinson, & Harvey, 1995).

The *iliotibial band* (ITB) is formed from the fascia from tensor fascia latae, gluteus maximus, and gluteus medius muscles. It reinforces the anterolateral aspect of the knee joint and assists with preventing posterior displacement of the femur when the tibia is fixed and knee is in extension (Norkin & Levangie, 1992).

The two cruciate ligaments are important in controlling anterior-posterior and rotational movements. The *anterior cruciate ligament* (ACL) is the primary restraint for anterior movement of the tibia relative to the femur. Different parts of the ACL are tight in different positions—the anterior portions are tight in extension, the middle portions are tight in internal rotation, and the posterior portions are tight in flexion. Like the collateral ligaments, the ACL as a whole is taut in extension. The ACL has secondary functions of limiting internal and external rotation.

The *posterior cruciate ligament* (PCL) is the primary restraint to posterior movement of the tibia on the femur. The posterior fibers

Figure 10-1A. Bones of the knee. A. Patellofemoral joint; B. Lateral femoral condyle; C. Fibula; D. Patella; E. Medial femoral condyle; F. Tibiofemoral joint; G. Tibial tuberosity.

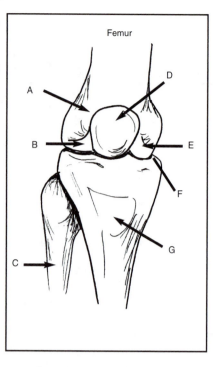

Figure 10-1B. Bones of the knee. A. Lateral femoral condyle; B. Medial femoral condyle; C. Intercondylar notch; D. Lateral condyle facet; E. Intercondylar eminence; F. Medial condyle facet.

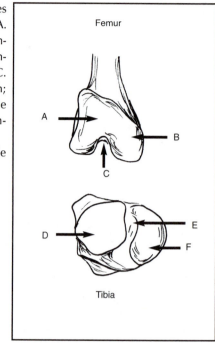

of the PCL are taut in extension, while the anterior portion is taut in midflexion and posterior in full flexion (Hamil & Knutzen, 1995). In spite of the numerous ligaments that support the knee, it is the most frequently injured joint in the body (Hamil & Knutzen, 1995). The palpable structures in the knee are listed below.

Femur

Medial and Lateral Condyles

With the knee flexed, these distal enlargements or rounded projections of femur or condyles can be easily felt anteriorly on both sides of the patella (Esch, 1989; Sine, Liss, Rousch, Holcomb, & Wilson, 2000) and are easily palpated.

Medial and Lateral Epicondyles

These are two roughened prominences proximal to the condyles.

Patella

This flat, rounded, triangular sesamoid bone is easily seen and palpated on the front of the knee. When the knee is extended, the patella is freely movable because the quadriceps are relaxed (Esch, 1989; Goss, 1976).

Tibia

Tuberosity of the Tibia

Located anteriorly on the tibia and below the tibial condyles, this roughened area is easily palpated 2 inches below the inferior border of patella with the knee flexed.

Anterior Crest (or Border) of the Tibia

This is sharp and can be followed distally to the ankle (Smith et al., 1996).

Fibula

The head is irregular and flat in shape and is located on the posterior and lateral aspect of lateral condyle of the tibia at the level of the tibial tuberosity (Esch, 1989).

Tibiofemoral Joint

This biaxial modified hinge joint (Kisner & Colby, 1990), which some consider to be a double condyloid (Norkin & Levangie, 1992), is made up of two large condyles on the distal femur and two asymmetrical concave tibial plateaus or condyles on the proximal tibia. The medial condyle is longer than lateral and contributes to locking of the knee. There are two fibrocartilaginous joint disks called *menisci* that enhance joint stability by deepening the contact surface on the tibia. The menisci also aid in shock absorption, help to protect underlying articular cartilage and subchondral bone, serve to reduce the load per unit area on tibiofemoral contact sites, enhance lubrication, and limit the motion between the tibia and femur (Hamil & Knutzen, 1995). The medial menisci are subject to injury if there is a lateral blow to the knee joint.

Stability is provided by ligaments. Tibial and fibular (or medial and lateral) collateral ligaments prevent passive movements of the knee in the frontal plane (Smith et al., 1996). These ligaments prevent abduction and adduction of the tibia on the femur, which would produce *genu valgum* (knock knee) and *genu varum* (bowleg), respectively. Anterior-posterior stability is provided via the poste-

Table 10-1. PHYSIOLOGIC MOTION OF THE KNEE	
Physiologic Motion of the Tibia if Moveable	*Direction of Slide*
Flexion	Posterior
Extension	Anterior
Physiologic Motion of the Tibia if Fixed	*Direction of Slide*
Flexion	Anterior
Extension	Posterior

rior and anterior cruciate ligaments. Coronary ligaments attach the menisci to the joint capsule.

Patellofemoral Joint

The patella is a sesamoid bone in the quadriceps tendon that articulates with the anterior aspect of the distal femur. The patella is embedded in the anterior portion of joint capsule and is connected to the tibia by the ligamentum patellae (Kisner & Colby, 1990). Many bursae surround the patella. The patella slides caudally with flexion of knee and slides cranially with extension. Patellofemoral surface motion simultaneously occurs in two planes, the frontal and transverse, but the greatest motion occurs in the frontal plane. Support for this joint is by the quadriceps tendon and the patellar ligament.

The angle formed between the femur and in relation to the position of the patella is known as the Q angle. The Q angle is greater in females due to wider pelvic girdles and increases in this angle will increase the valgus stress on the knees (Hamil & Knutzen, 1995).

The patella is helpful in knee extension because it serves to extend the lever arm of the quadriceps muscle throughout the entire range of motion (ROM) and allows a wide distribution of compressive stress on the femur (Magee, 1992).

Joint action between the patella and femur is important. Vastus medialis and vastus lateralis exert opposite forces on the patella and if there are muscular imbalances, contraction of the quadriceps will pull the patella off center. The patella can be kept in balance by exercising the knee joint through full range of extension.

Movements of the Knee

Movements that take place at the knee joint occur due to the motion at the tibiofemoral joint. These motions (primarily flexion and extension but also rotation of the tibia on the femur in nonweight bearing positions) occur in three planes simultaneously, with the greatest amount of motion occurring in the sagittal plane. The movements of flexion and extension differ from the move-

ments at the elbow in that: 1) the axis of motion is not a fixed axis but shifts anteriorly during extension and posteriorly during flexion, and 2) the beginning of flexion and ending of extension are accompanied by rotary movements associated with fixation of the limb (Goss, 1976). This mechanical movement of extension with external rotation and flexion with internal rotation has been called the "screw-home mechanism" and provides mechanical stability that is energy efficient to withstand forces occurring in the sagittal plane.

The axis for flexion is a few centimeters above the joint line transversely through femoral condyles. Clinically, the joint axis can be located approximately through the center of lateral and medial condyles of the femur. The shifting of the joint axis creates problems when fitting for orthoses (such as long leg braces or below the knee prosthetic devices), or when using goniometers or isokinetic dynamometers. When one moves from extension to flexion, the anatomic axis moves 2 centimeters, while the mechanical axis remains fixed. It is important to carefully align the devices to prevent discomfort and abrasions. The muscles that cross anterior to this axis are extensors and those crossing posterior to the axis are flexors. Internal and external rotation occur around the long axis and muscles that insert medial to the axis will internally rotate the leg, whereas those inserting laterally will externally rotate (Gench et al., 1995).

Arthrokinematically, if the motion of the tibia is in an open chain, the concave tibial plateaus slide in the same direction as the bone motion (Kisner & Colby, 1990). However, if the motions of the femur occur on a fixed tibia (or closed kinetic chain), the convex condyles slide in the direction opposite to bone motion (Table 10-1).

The large articular surface of the femur and relatively small tibial condyle create problems as the femur initiates flexion on the tibia. If there was only rolling of the fibial condyle on the tibial condyle, the femur would roll off of the tibia. For this reason, there must be simultaneous rolling and sliding during flexion and extension. The femoral condyle rolls posteriorly while simultaneously sliding anteriorly during flexion. The opposite motions occur during extension with anterior rolling of the femoral condyle while there is simultaneous sliding in a posterior direction.

Internal Kinetics

Knee flexion occurs in a range from 0 to 120 degrees to 145. The motion is due to the three hamstring muscles (biceps femoris, semimembranosus, and semitendinosus muscles) and is accompanied by internal rotation of the tibia, which is produced by sartorius, popliteus, and gracilis (as well as semimembranosus and semitendinosus). The semitendinosus and semimembranosus are particularly well-suited to flex and internally rotate the leg because they are located posteriorly to the frontal axis as it crosses the knee and medially to the long axis. For example, biceps femoris, while active in flexion, does not assist with internal rotation because its location lateral to the long axis makes this muscle responsible for external rotation of the tibia. It is an important muscle for knee stability because it will neutralize the internal rotation of the other knee flexors (Gench et al., 1995). Sartorius courses diagonally and medially in the front of the thigh and acts both as a flexor and internal rotator, although it should be noted that in some individuals, the muscle crosses anterior to the knee joint rather than posteriorly, which would make this muscle an extensor of the knee (Gench et al., 1995). There are several calf muscles that extend across the knee and have a flexor action there, including gastrocnemius, plantaris, and popliteus.

The quadriceps femoris group is made up of the vastus lateralis, vastus medialis, vastus intermedius, and rectus femoris muscles and these participate in extension of the leg. The iliotibial band, with its origins from the tensor fascia latae, gluteus maximus, and gluteus medius, has been reported to have an effect on the knee through this band (Jenkins, 1998). Some sources also cite gastrocnemius and soleus as contributors to knee extension (Jenkins, 1998).

The *medial rotators* are essentially the same muscles indicated as flexors. Sartorius, gracilis, semimembranosus, and semitendinosus all cross the joint medial to the axis and act as internal rotators. Popliteus also crosses the knee joint distally and medially and acts as a medial rotator. *Lateral rotation* is achieved by the biceps femoris muscle, which passes on the lateral side of the joint axis (Jenkins, 1998).

Knee stabilization can be categorized on the basis of function, structure, or location of supporting structures. Categorization based on location refers to embryonic joint compartments (Norkin & Levangie, 1992). Functional stabilizers can be static (joint capsule and ligaments) or dynamic (muscles and aponeurosis). The joint capsule and coronary, meniscopatellar, patellofemoral, middle and lateral collateral and anterior and posterior cruciate ligaments, as well as the oblique popliteal, arcuate, and transverse ligaments are all static stabilizers. Muscles providing dynamic stabilization are the quadriceps femoris, extensor retinaculum, popliteus, biceps femoris, semimembranosus, and the pes anserinus (made up of the semitendinosus, sartorius, and gracilis muscles) (Norkin & Levangie, 1992).

Supporting structures can be categorized according to location. Medial compartment structures include: medial patellar retinaculum, medial collateral ligament, oblique popliteal ligament, and posterior cruciate ligament, as well as the medial head of the gastrocnemius, pes anserinus, and semimembranosus muscles. The lateral compartment structures are the iliotibial band, biceps femoris, popliteus muscles, lateral cruciate ligament, meniscofemoral ligament, arcuate ligament and anterior cruciate ligament with the lateral patellar retinaculum (Norkin & Levangie, 1992).

Anterioposterior stabilization is achieved by the extensor retinaculum, which is comprised of fibers from quadriceps femoris and fuses with fibers from the joint capsule. This supports the anteromedial and anterolateral aspects of the knee. The medial and lateral head of gastrocnemius reinforce medial and lateral aspects of the posterior capsule, with popliteus being an important posterolateral stabilizer with posterior cruciate ligament. The anterior cruciate ligament and the hamstrings (especially semimembranosus) work together to resist anterior displacement of tibia and shear forces on the femur posteriorly. The patella helps with posterior knee stability by preventing the femur from sliding forward and off the tibia (Norkin & Levangie, 1992).

Contributors to medial-lateral stabilization are the soft tissue and tibial tubercles and menisci when the knee is extended. The knee is reinforced medially and laterally by the medial and lateral collateral ligaments. Laterally, the iliotibial tract, lateral collateral ligament, popliteus tendon, and biceps tendon contribute to stability and the posteriolateral capsule is important for varus stability in extension (Norkin & Levangie, 1992).

Passive mechanisms seem to contribute to rotational stabilization. The cruciate ligaments seem especially important, especially in the extended knee. Rotational stability is also credited to the medial and lateral collateral ligaments, the posteromedial and posterolateral capsule, and the popliteus tendon. The menisci are important in medial-lateral stability (Norkin & Levangie, 1992).

ANKLE/FOOT COMPLEX

The foot and ankle together have 26 bones, 30 synovial joints, 100 ligaments, and 30 muscles, so it a very stable complex. In fact, Norkin and Levangie (1992) state that the ankle joint is the most congruent joint in the body (p. 384). Structurally, the ankle/foot complex is comparable to the wrist/hand, although the hand is more critical to daily life tasks. The ankle/foot complex needs to balance conflicting demands for stability and mobility. On one hand, the ankle and foot meet stability demands of providing a stable base of support for the body without undue muscular or energy demands and acts as a rigid lever for propulsive weight bearing. On the other hand, mobility demands of dampening the rotations imposed by the more proximal joints of the lower extremity, having the flexibility to absorb shock of body weight, and permitting the foot to adjust to varied terrains, are also met by this section of the lower extremity (Norkin & Levangie, 1992). The flexible-rigid characteristics of the ankle/foot complex provide these functions:

- Support of superincumbent weight.
- Control and stabilization of the leg on planted foot.
- Adjustments to irregular surfaces.
- Elevation of body, as in standing on toes, climbing, or jumping.
- Shock absorption.
- Operation of machine tools.
- Substitution for hand function in persons with upper extremity amputations or muscle paralysis (Smith et al., 1996).

The ankle joint is actually composed of the talocrural articulation (tibiotarsal or talotibial/tibiotalar) and the tibiofibular joints, although when discussing the ankle, reference is made to the talocrural joint because anatomically the inferior and superior tibiofibular articulations are separate from the ankle. The forces acting on the ankle can be as much as five times the body weight and the talocrural joint transmits approximately 1/6th of the force exerted through the foot (Norkin & Levangie, 1992). The talocrural articulation is the articulation of the tibia and fibula with the talus of the foot. This is a ginglymus joint, which is supported by strong ligaments, including the medial (deltoid) and lateral collateral ligaments (posterior and anterior talofibular and calcaneofibular ligaments) (Kisner & Colby, 1990).

Since this is a hinge joint, there is 1 degree of freedom permitting flexion and extension of the foot, which is known as plantarflexion, and dorsiflexion is the motion that occurs in the sagittal plane around a transverse axis. Plantarflexion occurs in a range of 0 to 50 degrees and ankle flexion is due to the gastrocnemius, soleus, flexor digitorum longus, peroneus longus and brevis, flexor hallucis longus, and tibialis posterior (Jenkins, 1998). The large size of the gastrocnemius and the long force arm enable this muscle to be a strong plantarflexor of the ankle, but only when ankle motion is needed, not when standing at ease (Gench et al., 1995). Gastrocnemius and soleus (together known as the triceps surae) work powerfully on the calcaneus to push the foot down and the soleus is more involved in static standing. The tendons of these two muscles form the large, easily palpated tendon on the posterior distal leg known as the *Achilles' tendon*. Since tibialis posterior, flexor digitorum longus, and flexor hallucis longus cross the joint posterior to the joint axis, these muscles act to plantarflex the ankle in addition to other actions. These three muscles are fondly referred to as: *Tom* for tibialis posterior, *Dick* for flexor digitorum longus, and *Harry* for flexor hallucis longus. Peroneus longus changes direction twice before insertion and is close but posterior to the axis, so it acts only as a weak plantarflexor, as does peroneus brevis. The plantarflexion action is the strongest movement of the foot and important in propulsion force.

Dorsiflexion of the foot occurs in a range of 0 to 20 degrees to 30 degrees and the muscles producing the movement cross anterior the joint axis. One of the most important muscles in this action is tibialis anterior; this is the muscle that gives our legs the roundness of the shank portion. Extensor digitorum longus crosses the joint anterior to the axis with a long force arm and is effective as a dorsiflexor. Peroneus tertius, which appears to be a part of the extensor digitorum longus, and is, incidentally, often missing in individuals, crosses the ankle in the same manner as the extensor digitorum longus and has similar action on the joint. Similarly, extensor hallucis longus, with primary action involving the big toe, also crosses the joint anterior to the axis and is contributory to dorsiflexion. Generally, these muscles are weak and not capable of generating high forces (Hamil & Knutzen, 1995).

The ankle/foot complex is capable of moving the foot up and down as well as in and out. Much variability exists in the literature about how to define these motions. The movement of the foot and ankle toward and away from the midline in the transverse plane around a vertical axis is referred to as adduction and abduction and there is minimal ROM in these movements of adduction and abduction at the ankle/foot complex. Frontal plane motion of the foot turning inward (*inversion*) or outward (*eversion*) occurs in the anterior-posterior axis, although some authors use the terms *supination* (to turn up or medial tilt or varus) and *pronation* (to turn down or lateral tilt or valgus) to describe this motion. Often the terms eversion-inversion will be used to describe motion in open kinetic chains and pronation-supination to describe a closed chain motion (Kendall & McCreary, 1983; Sine et al., 2000). Other authors use the term pronation to describe a combination of dorsiflexion, eversion, and abduction, while supination is a combination of plantarflexion, inversion, and adduction. For simplicity, the terms inversion and eversion will be used in this text to describe the motion at the ankle, although the definition based on the combined movements more aptly describes the actual motion that occurs. Inversion and eversion occur primarily around the subtalar and transverse tarsal joints with very little movement at the talocrural joint. Due to these motions, the foot can be positioned to travel uneven ground, and the ability to invert/evert one's foot is helpful in bathing and dressing of the lower extremity.

The superior (or proximal) tibiofibular is a plane synovial joint formed by the articulation of the head to fibula with the posterior and lateral surfaces of the tibia. Motions are variable and limited and have been described as superior and inferior sliding of the fibula and as fibular rotation (Norkin & Levangie, 1992). The distal tibiofibular joint is a syndesmosis or fibrous joint between the tibia and the fibula. The tibia and fibula do not actually come into contact because they are separated by fibroadipose tissue. The tibiofibular joints are essential to dorsiflexion and plantarflexion due to the mortise-like arrangement of the bones that allows the tibia and fibula to grasp and hold onto the distal joint segments (Norkin & Levangie, 1992).

The foot is divided into the forefoot, midfoot, and hindfoot. The anterior segment of the foot is made up of the five metatarsals, and 14 phalanges which make up the five toes. The midfoot is the middle section of the foot and is made up of five bones—the navicular, the cuboid, and the three cuneiforms. The most posterior segment, the hindfoot, is formed by the talus and calcaneus bones (Figure 10-2).

As with the hand, there are arches in the foot—two longitudinal and one transverse (Figure 10-3). These arches create an elastic shock-absorbing system and the flexibility of these arches is critical in walking and running. The lateral longitudinal arch is a relatively flat arch that plays a support role in weight bearing and has limited function in mobility. The medial longitudinal arch is more flexible and mobile and plays a greater role in shock absorption. When one takes a step, the force is absorbed by a fat pad on the inferior surface of calcaneus. This force then causes an elongation of the medial arch that continues to maximum elongation at toe contact with the ground. This portion of the foot rarely touches the ground unless the person has flat feet. The medial longitudinal arch helps to diminish the impact by transmitting vertical loads through the deflection of the arch (Hamil & Knutzen, 1995). The transverse arch supports a significant portion of weight during weight bearing (Hamil & Knutzen, p. 253).

The subtalar (or talocalcaneal) joint is the area where the talus articulates with the calcaneus. This is a synovial gliding joint and the talus presents with three facets that correspond to three facets on the calcaneus. With the three articulations, the convex-concave facets limit mobility of the joint. When the talus moves on posterior facet of calcaneus, the articular surface of the talus should slide in the same direction as the bones move. However, at middle and anterior joints, the talar surfaces should glide in a direction opposite to the movement of bone. What actually occurs is a screw-like or twisting motion around a triplanar axis (Smith et al., 1996). When inversion (supination) occurs, the posterior articulation slides in a lateral direction and with inversion (pronation),

Figure 10-2. Parts of the foot.

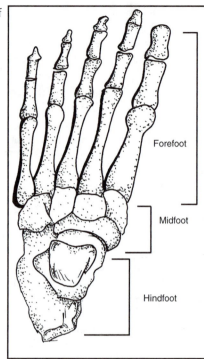

Forefoot

Midfoot

Hindfoot

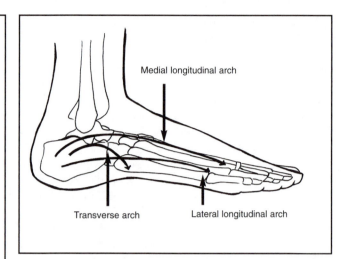

Figure 10-3. Arches of the foot.

Medial longitudinal arch

Transverse arch

Lateral longitudinal arch

there is a medial slide of the posterior articulating surfaces (Kisner & Colby, 1990).

The transverse tarsal joint, also called the midtarsal joint, forms an S-shaped joint line between the talonavicular and calcaneocuboid joints. The midtarsal joint participates in movement of the forefoot on the hindfoot to lower the longitudinal arch in pronation and raise it in supination. The midtarsal joint also contributes to eversion (pronation) and inversion (supination) and in absorbing forces of contact.

Inversion occurs when the muscles pass around the medial border of the foot. This includes tibialis posterior, flexor digitorum longus, flexor hallucis longus, tibialis anterior, and extensor hallucis longus. Of these, tibialis anterior is the strongest inverter of the foot, while extensor hallucis longus is the weakest. By pulling the feet inward (inversion or supination), the arches are maintained and the body weight distributed to the lateral sides of the feet.

Eversion of the foot is produced by peroneus longus, brevis and tertius and by extensor digitorum longus. Extensor digitorum longus, while primarily involved in extension of the interphalangeal joints, does cross the joint anterior and lateral to the joint axis, so it has a long force arm for producing dorsiflexion and eversion of the ankle. By pulling the sole of the foot outward into eversion, body weight is distributed to the medial side of the foot.

Additional articulations of the foot that contribute to movements are:
- The articulation of the talus with the navicular or the talocalcaneonavicular joint.

- Calcaneus with fourth tarsal, cuboid to form the calcaneocuboid articulation.
- Intertarsal joints are the articulations between the tarsal bones.
- Tarsometatarsal joints where the three cuneiforms and cuboid articulate with base of 5 metatarsals; the tarsometatarsal joints in the midfoot function to stabilize the second metatarsal making it rigid forefoot bone and carry most of the load while walking.
- Metatarsophalangeal where metatarsals articulate with phalanges.
- Interphalangeal joints between the phalanges, which aid in keeping the toes in contact with the ground.

Essentially, the tarsals transmit the weight of the body to the heel and the ball of the foot. Tarsals are seen to correspond structurally to the carpals of the hand. The metatarsals and phalanges, then, correspond to the metacarpals of the hand and these form the instep of the foot (Smith et al., 1996).

Summary

- While not the direct focus for intervention by occupational therapists, an overview of the structures of the knee, ankle, and foot is provided to understand the contribution these structures make to function.
- The knee, with the hip and ankle, supports the body and also serves to help in foot placement in space.
- The ligaments of the knee are especially important because there are no bony restraints to knee movement.
- The ankle and foot are seen as very stable due to the large number of bones, ligaments, and muscle that comprise these joints.
- These joints balance the conflicting demands of providing a stable base of support while also permitting the foot to adjust to different terrains and to movement.

REFERENCES

Baxter, R. (1998). *Pocket guide to musculoskeletal assessment*. Philadelphia: W. B. Saunders Co.

Esch, D. L. (1989). *Musculoskeletal function: An anatomy and kinesiology laboratory manual*. Minneapolis: University of Minnesota.

Gench, B. E., Hinson, M. M., & Harvey, P. T. (1995). Anatomical kinesiology. Dubuque, IA: Eddie Bowers Publishing, Inc.

Goss, C. M. (Ed.) (1976). *Gray's anatomy of the human body* (29th ed.). Philadelphia: Lea and Febiger.

Hamil, J., & Knutzen, K. M. (1995). *Biomechanical basis of human movement*. Baltimore: Williams & Wilkins.

Jenkins, D. B. (1998). *Hollingshead's functional anatomy of the limbs and back* (7th ed.). Philadelphia: W. B. Saunders Co.

Kendall, F. P., & McCreary, E. K. (1983). *Muscles: Testing and function* (3rd ed.). Baltimore: Williams & Wilkins.

Kisner, C., & Colby, L. A. (1990). *Therapeutic exercise: Foundations and techniques* (2nd ed.). Philadelphia: F. A. Davis.

Magee, D. J. (1992). *Orthopedic physical assessment*. Philadelphia: W. B. Saunders Co.

Nordin, M., & Frankel, V. H. (1989). *Basic biomechanics of the musculoskeletal system* (2nd ed.). Philadelphia: Lea and Febiger.

Norkin, C. C., & Levangie, P. K. (1992). *Joint structure and function: A comprehensive analysis* (2nd ed.). Philadelphia: F. A. Davis Co.

Sine, R., Liss, S. E., Rousch, R. E., Holcomb, J. D., & Wilson, G. (2000). *Basic rehabilitation techniques: A self instructional guide* (4th ed.). Gaithersburg, MD: Aspen Publishers.

Smith, L. K., Weiss, E. L., & Lehmkuhl, L. D. (1996). *Brunnstrom's clinical kinesiology* (5th ed.). Philadelphia: F. A. Davis Co.

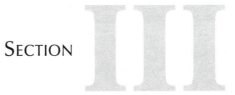

Occupational Therapy Intervention

Biomechanical Remediation Intervention Approach

Chapter 11

SELECTION CRITERIA

In selecting an intervention approach, remediation or restorative approaches are selected when there is an expectation for:

1. Significant reduction in impairment that leads to:

    a) prevention of further activity limitations and participation restrictions

    b) resolution of activity limitations or increased participation in areas of occupations

2. Learning of new performance skills.
3. Slowing declines in impairments and task abilities.
4. Maintaining or improving quality of life.
5. Consistency of approach with performance context (McGinnis, 1999).

Remediation is "an intervention approach designed to change client variables to establish a skill or ability that has not yet developed or to restore a skill or ability that has been impaired" (McGinnis, 1999, p. 47). In particular, the focus is performance skills, performance patterns, and client factors with the underlying belief that by establishing or restoring these factors, resumption of valued roles and successful participation in areas of occupation will be possible (Table 11-1).

The biomechanical approach is used to explain function utilizing anatomical and physiological concepts with exercise physiology, kinetics, anatomy, and kinematics as the theoretical base (Trombly, 1995). Occupational therapists use their knowledge of activity analysis and apply it to understanding movement created by muscles, joints, and soft tissues and those circumstances that prevent or permit motion to occur (Pedretti, 1996). The biomechanical approach is a study of the relationship between musculoskeletal function and how the body is designed for and used in the performance of daily occupations. The effect, purpose, and meaning of engagement in these activities influence the client's compliance, effort, fatigue, and improvement in movement capacity (Kielhofner, 1992).

ASSUMPTIONS

There are several assumptions underlying the biomechanical approach. These are listed in Table 11-2.

This approach assumes that the client has the capacity for voluntary control of body (muscle control) and mind (motivation) (Trombly, 1995). It is anatomy and physiology that determine normal function and that humans are biomechanical beings whose range of motion (ROM), strength, and endurance have physiological and kinetic potential as well as role-relevant behaviors (Smith, Weiss, & Lehmkuhl, 1996). Humans are able to perform role-relevant behaviors most efficiently when they assume and maintain positions that are biomechanically advantageous. Further, the environment can be specifically designed to facilitate the development or recovery of voluntary control of skeletal musculature (Trombly, 1995).

The biomechanical approach involves the musculoskeletal system, peripheral nerves, integumentary and/or cardiopulmonary systems and requires an intact brain and central nervous system to produce isolated, voluntary, coordinated movements (Table 11-3). Intervention is aimed at improving strength, ROM, endurance, and coordination of these systems. This approach is most effective for clients with orthopedic disorders (fractures, rheumatoid arthritis) and lower motor neuron disorders resulting in weakness and flaccidity (peripheral nerve injuries and diseases, Guillian Barré Syndrome, polio, spinal cord injuries and diseases) as well as clients with hand injuries, burns, cardiopulmonary disease and those with amputations. For the intervention techniques to be effective, the client must have motor pathways available with the potential for recovery in strength, ROM, endurance, and/or coordination. Some sensory feedback must be available in order to provide information about movement to the muscles and nervous system. Since the focus of intervention is on strength, endurance, and ROM, muscles and tendons must be free to move and relatively free of pain. In addition, the client must be able to understand the directions and purpose of the intervention and be interested and motivated to perform the activities and exercises.

FOCUS ON MUSCULOSKELETAL SYSTEM

The focus on musculoskeletal systems defines biomechanical intervention and also focuses on the issue of physical fitness and health. While not the only frame of reference to accentuate the value of health promotion, many of the physical fitness goals are biomechanical in nature. In *The Guide to Occupational Therapy*

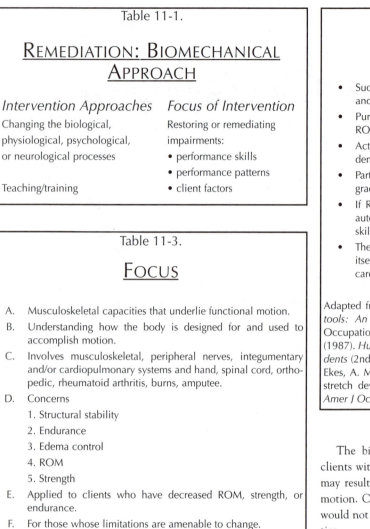

Table 11-1.

REMEDIATION: BIOMECHANICAL APPROACH

Intervention Approaches	Focus of Intervention
Changing the biological, physiological, psychological, or neurological processes	Restoring or remediating impairments:
	• performance skills
	• performance patterns
Teaching/training	• client factors

Table 11-3.

FOCUS

A. Musculoskeletal capacities that underlie functional motion.

B. Understanding how the body is designed for and used to accomplish motion.

C. Involves musculoskeletal, peripheral nerves, integumentary and/or cardiopulmonary systems and hand, spinal cord, orthopedic, rheumatoid arthritis, burns, amputee.

D. Concerns
  1. Structural stability
  2. Endurance
  3. Edema control
  4. ROM
  5. Strength

E. Applied to clients who have decreased ROM, strength, or endurance.

F. For those whose limitations are amenable to change.

Table 11-2.

ASSUMPTIONS

• Successful human motor activity is based on physical mobility and strength.

• Purposeful activities can be prescribed to remediate loss of ROM, strength, and endurance.

• Activities can be graded progressively to meet particular demands within an intervention program.

• Participation in activities involving repeated, specific, and graded movements maintains and improves function.

• If ROM, strength, and endurance are regained, a client will automatically use these prerequisite skills to regain functional skills.

• The principle of rest and stress; the body needs time to heal itself and then gradually add stress to the musculoskeletal and cardiovascular systems to regain normal function.

Adapted from Asher, I. E. (1996). *Occupational therapy assessment tools: An annotated index* (2nd ed.). Bethesda, MD: American Occupational Therapy Association; Galley, P. M., & Forster, A. L. (1987). *Human movement: An introductory text for physiotherapy students* (2nd ed.). New York: Churchill-Livingstone; and Nuismer, B. A., Ekes, A. M., & Holm, M. B. (1997). The use of low load prolonged stretch devices in rehabilitation program in the pacific northwest. *Amer J Occup Ther, 51*(37), 538-545.

Practice, health promotion and wellness involve a "lifestyle redesign" (AOTA, 2002) and it is stated that occupational therapists believe that occupation is an important component to staying healthy. Health involves the body, the self, and the environment and may include:

• Body: physical fitness; adapted fitness programs; nutrition; avoidance of alcohol, drugs and tobacco; safe sex practices.

• Self: balance of work, play, and self-care; engagement in purposeful and meaningful occupations; building habits that support social interaction.

• Environment: match the context with the interests and values of the person; family planning; avoidance of violent and abusive behavior; positive value of peer groups (Moyers, 1999).

Other aspects of health and physical fitness are also intricately linked to these areas of intervention and cannot be separated from them. These include:

• Cardiovascular function
• Age
• Fitness levels prior to injury/illness–levels of deconditioning
• Hereditary factors (Christiansen & Baum, 1997).

The biomechanical approach would not be appropriate for clients with impairments in central nervous system function that may result in spasticity and lack of voluntary control of isolated motion. Clients with inflamed joints or those just out of surgery would not be appropriate for vigorous exercise regimes and activities.

Function, according to the biomechanical approach, is the capacity for movement in bones, joints, muscles, tendons, peripheral nerves, heart, lungs, and skin as demonstrated by adequate ROM, strength, and endurance for physical abilities and performance skills needed in role-relevant behavior. The functioning person is able to assume and maintain positions that are biomechanically advantageous and promote efficiency of motion. Performance depends on simultaneous actions of muscles across joints to produce the movement and the stability that is required of the task (Trombly, 1995).

Dysfunction is characterized by the inability to demonstrate adequate ROM, strength, and endurance for physical subskills and independent lift skills in role-relevant behaviors. The person is unable to assume and maintain positions that are biomechanically advantageous and promote efficiency of motion due to alterations or decreased capacity for movement in joints and bones, muscles, and tendons resulting in impairments in strength, ROM, coordination, or endurance that interfere with occupational performance.

Assessment in this approach involves identification of ROM, strength, and endurance subskills needed to perform role-relevant behaviors (Pedretti, 1996). Activity analyses will enable an understanding of the most biomechanically advantageous and efficient positions to assume when participating in desired activities and will help ascertain discrepancies between the physical requirements of the activity and the client's baseline performance. Specific assessments usually include ROM, strength testing (manual muscle testing and grasp/pinch via dynamometer and pinchmeter), as well as assessment of edema and endurance.

Moyers (1999) identified two main techniques used in remediation approaches. The first is that of teaching new skills, behaviors, or habits where outdated or maladaptive skills, behaviors, or habits are replaced. This is done by modifying the existing performance skills and performance patterns.

The second technique used in remediation approaches is to change the biological, physiological, psychological, or neurological processes. The focus is on decreasing the client's pain and reducing the impact of impairments on occupational performance.

While sensorimotor techniques, graded exercise and activities, physical agent modalities, and manual techniques are used as intervention strategies in this approach, Moyers adds that "...simply expecting improvements in impairments to automatically produce changes in the level of disablement without addressing performance in occupations within the intervention plan is inappropriate. The relationship between the impairment and the level of disablement is complex and is affected by many factors in addition to changes in the impairment" (Moyers, 1999, p. 276).

This typifies a cited limitation of this therapeutic approach in which it cannot be assumed that increases in ROM, strength, and endurance will automatically be used by the client in functional activities. Dutton cites several studies that show a low correlation of dexterity with activities of daily living (ADL) and asks the question, "How can skills such as manual dexterity and strength have such a low correlation with ADLs?" (1995, p. 31). If dexterity is not a needed client physical ability for successful performance in areas of occupation, should this be an area of intervention? This is an area needing further research to substantiate this assumption or to refute it.

Another cited limitation of this approach is that the focus of the intervention on the client abilities and performance skills seems reductionistic. Pedretti (1996) describes a variety of activities that are used in intervention that are, in fact, considered non-purposeful and without an inherent goal of engaging both the physical and mental attributes of the individual. These intermediate activities are called *enabling activities* and are done to:

1. Practice specific motor patterns.
2. Train in perceptual and cognitive skills.
3. Practice sensorimotor skills.

Examples are having clients work on inclined sanding boards, cone stacking, puzzles, fastener boards, work simulators, and some computer programs as used in cognitive remediation programs. Pedretti adds that while these activities are seen as the intermediate means to achieve long-term goals, enabling activities "should be used judiciously and are often used with adjunctive modalities and purposeful activities as part of a comprehensive treatment program" (Pedretti, 1996, p. 300). These activities may be analogous to Fisher's continua classification of "contrived occupation" (1998).

Adjunctive modalities are defined as "preliminary to the use of purposeful activities and that prepare the client for occupational performance" (Pedretti, 1996, p. 300). These modalities include exercise, orthotics, sensory stimulation, and physical agent modalities. These adjunctive modalities are necessary to provide structural stability, to position parts to prevent deformities, to provide rest for a part, and to increase function in components for use in occupations. These are roughly analogous to Fisher's (1998) "exercise" where there is little meaning to the client with the focus on remediation of impairments. The *Occupational Therapy Practice Framework Domain and Process* would classify adjunctive modalities as preparatory methods in anticipation of future purposeful and occupation-based activities.

The use of enabling and adjunctive modalities seems inherently at odds with the core values of occupational therapy and would be true if the ultimate intervention goal is simply remediation of an impairment and not one of functional improvement in meaningful tasks. Occupational therapists see clients earlier in the recovery phase, see clients who are more acutely ill, and often have shorter lengths of stays that necessitate these preliminary interventions. Again, it must be reiterated that without the ultimate focus of a functional outcome, using adjunctive or enabling activities should not be considered occupational therapy practice. Activities used in this intervention can also be purposeful, i.e., goal directed within a designed context, or engagement in actual occupations in activities that are client directed and important to that person (Table 11-4).

Other limitations of this approach are that it focuses only on the physical performance of occupations and does not include aspects of volition, context, role, or environment (Pedretti, 1996) and little reference is made to motivation or to the psychological, emotional, or social aspects of rehabilitation. There is no attention to the holistic values held by occupational therapists that address the need for balance in daily life and higher levels of self-esteem and self-actualization (Pedretti, 1996). This approach is seen as reductionistic, with the client being a passive recipient in a program that does not reflect the client's interests, needs, or improved occupational performance (Pedretti, 1996, p. 51). Again, this would be true if exercise is the focus of intervention at the expense of improved occupational performance.

However, it must be seen that clinically the biomechanical approach is used to restore those variables than can be improved to enhance client participation in work, play, and self-care. Thoughtful clinical reasoning is used to determine what aspects of performance can be improved and which need compensatory strategies based on an in-depth understanding of the client as a person (interactive reasoning). Intervention occurs not only because there are impairments in biological, physiological, psychological, or neurological processes, but because these impairments interfere with the successful living of this person's life. The remediation of strength or ROM is only one small part of the total intervention strategies used, and the biomechanical approach is often used with other approaches to address these other areas simultaneously. While the biomechanical approach relies heavily on procedural reasoning to incorporate disease and prognostic information into intervention planning, that is not to say that other aspects of reasoning are not also occurring concurrently.

Table 11-4.

COMPARISON OF OT REMEDIATION INTERVENTION CONTINUA

OT Framework	*Pedretti*	*Fisher*
Preparatory Methods Prepares client for occupational performance. Includes sensory input, physical agent modalities, orthotics/splinting, exercise.	**Adjunctive Methods** "Preliminary to the use of purposeful activities and that prepare the client for occupational performance." Include exercise, orthotics, sensory stimulation, physical agent modalities, ROM, inhibition/facilitation techniques. Necessary to provide structural stability, prevent deformities, provide rest for a part, to increase function in client factors (body structure/function).	**Exercise** Rote exercise and practice activities. A purpose but no goal. Little meaning.
Purposeful Activity Goal directed behaviors or activities within therapeutically designed context that leads to occupation. Examples: practice slicing vegetables, role play to manage anger.	**Enabling Methods** Intermediate activities. Practice specific motor patterns. Train in perceptual and cognitive skills. Practice sensorimotor skills. Examples: inclined sanding boards, cone stacking, puzzles, fastening boards, work simulators, pegboards, computer programs. Lack client-centered goals.	**Contrived Occupation** Exercise with added purpose or occupation with contrived component. Little meaning. Examples: exercise embedded in an activity; pounding nails into a board to pretend to build a birdhouse.
	Purposeful Activities Identifiable goal and frequently areas of occupation are addressed. Skill generalization greater than for adjunctive or enabling methods.	**Therapeutic Occupation** Client actively participates in areas of occupation. Client sees task as purposeful and meaningful. Real objects used in context. Still focused on remediation.
Occupation-Based Activity Actual occupation part of their own context and meeting their goals. Examples: grocery shopping, dressing without assistance.	**Occupation-Based Intervention** Includes information about client needs, wants, goals, expectations. Most beneficial to client and most challenging. Activities in appropriate context and match client goals. Goal directed, meaningful.	**Adaptive or Compensatory Occupation** Active participant in areas of occupation that they choose. Focus on improved performance in areas of occupation. May include assistive devices, teaching alternative or compensatory strategies, modification of environment.

Adapted from Fisher, A. G. (1998). Uniting practice and theory in an occupational framework: 1998 Eleanor Clarke Slagle lecture. *Amer J Occup Ther*, 52(7), 509-521; Pedretti, L. W. (1996). *Occupational therapy: Practice skills for physical dysfunction* (4th ed.). St Louis, MO: C.V. Mosby; and American Occupational Therapy Association (2002). Occupational therapy practice framework: Domain and process. *Amer J Occup Ther*, 56(6), 609-639.

The biomechanical approach makes good use of media and equipment to promote physical function and the techniques can be applied to a variety of creative and constructive activities. Knowledge of activity analysis is applied to understanding movements needed and to planning appropriate activities and exercises. The utilization of anatomical, physiological, and mechanical knowledge has led to the development of specific techniques for measuring movement, strength, and endurance (Dutton, 1995). There is a direct cause and effect relationship that can be seen in the treatment process and prevention of deformities that can be clearly seen and demonstrated.

To ensure that the activities used in intervention will achieve goals that are of value to the client, these activities must:

- Correlate the physical demands of the graded activities to subskills and role-relevant behaviors.
- Provide activities that are motivating; the activities must have meaning to the person in meeting individual needs and interests in relation to social roles.
- Short-term goals may relate to performance of subskills in clinic or school environment.
- Long-term goals must relate to role-relevant behaviors and performance in the community environment in which they are ultimately expected to occur.
- Be designed to prevent or reverse dysfunction and/or to develop new skills to enhance performance in life roles.
- Provide graded activities that simulate the physical requirements of the tasks and demand increasing levels of ROM, strength, and endurance (Demeter, Andersson, & Smith, 1996; Norkin & Levangie, 1992; Smith et al., 1996; Steinbeck, 1986).

STRUCTURAL STABILITY

Occupational therapists are involved in intervention programs for the entire spectrum of clients—from wellness programs to those who are critically ill. In hospital settings, occupational therapists previously would be consulted to work with clients who were medically stable. Now, our clients are more severely disabled and acutely ill so there is the need to balance early mobilization with rest. Clients do not always come to occupational therapy with stable cardiovascular and respiratory function. In addition, shorter lengths of stay greatly influence intervention. Intervention is based on where the client currently is in the continuum of care and what further services are needed and expected.

Structural stability is necessary to regain prior to implementation of other intervention goals. Splints or devices that are worn temporarily to enforce rest to enable healing are enabling changes in the biological, physiological, or neurological processes by temporarily immobilizing the part. Positioning devices can also serve to temporarily enforce rest to promote healing. By changing the damaged structures, this would be considered a remediation goal of the biomechanical approach.

Devices and orthoses can be used to remediate, compensate, or to prevent further disability. If the orthosis or device was used in joints too weak to resist the force of gravity to maintain functional alignment with the goal of preventing development of contractures and deformities, then this would be more a goal of prevention

of disability. The use of a lapboard for a dependent hemiplegic arm, used to prevent further injury to the extremity, might also be an example of prevention of disability. Neither of these devices is used to remediate the lack of function of that extremity. The use of a universal cuff with utensils inserted is a means of compensating for lost function, not to prevent disability or promote healing. However, if a foam wedge was used by a client with a hip replacement, this object will be used temporarily until the structures relative to the hip surgery are healed. The wedge does not serve to compensate for lost function (compensation) nor to prevent disability; rather, the function of the wedge is to promote healing and enforce positioning. While the distinction between the use of these devices seems academic, why one is using a particular device or positioning technique has much to do with clinical reasoning, responsible use of adaptive equipment, and client outcomes.

While goal statements seem awkward and wordy, the focus of biomechanical intervention is actually the short-term improvement of performance components and physical client abilities that will result in the long-term outcomes of improvements in the areas of occupation of work, play, leisure, self-care/ADL, instrumental activities of daily living (IADL), and social participation. Biomechanical goals are actually short-term goals. By writing one goal that includes the short-term objectives of intervention (e.g., increasing ROM, an aspect of motor skills and client factors) and the reason the goal is being attempted (e.g., the functional outcome of the ability to put on a shirt, or area of occupation), the focus on function is clear. This answers the question "so what"; so what is so great about an increase of 50 degrees of additional ROM? It can mean the difference between being independent in dressing and being dependent upon others and this needs to be clear in the goal statement (Table 11-5).

TISSUE INTEGRITY

Issues relative to the maintenance of soft tissue integrity involve remolding of scar tissue as well as reduction in edema. Intervention can be viewed as both a biomechanical change in structures as well as prevention of further disability due to the damage that edema and scarring can do to adjacent structures and in resultant function.

Edema is a barrier to function because ROM is limited and there is decreased coordination and pain. Untreated edema may result in permanent losses of ROM if fluids become fibrotic. Nerve compression can cause losses in sensation. Loss of active movement combined with compromised nutrition of distal parts can ultimately lead to amputation (Dutton, 1995). Maintenance and remediation of the anatomical and physiological condition of interstitial tissue and skin are important aspects of intervention.

Compression is often used in the control of edema. Retrograde massage is an effective method of applying compression. Teaching self-massage to the client is helpful in desensitizing painful parts and in giving the client a sense of control and responsibility in the management of the edema. Compression can be applied by pressure garments, gloves, elastic wraps, or even string. When performing massage or in wrapping parts for compression, it is important that

Table 11-5.

REGAINING STRUCTURAL STABILITY

Goal	Method	Principle/Rationale	Example
Client will be (independent/ modified independent/ require maximal/moderate/ or minimal assistance) in performance of _____ tasks (specify) by regaining structural stability in damaged structures by using...	Orthoses Positioning	Which are worn/used to temporarily enforce rest until the damaged structures are healed.	Dorsal rubber band splint for flexor tendon repair Body jacket/body case Stryker frame Wedge for hip replacement No resistive exercise during an arthritic flare-up Non-weight bearing for hip replacement
	Procedures	Which gradually stress structures that are healed.	Stump toughening and shaping LE weight bearing for fracture

Adapted from Dutton, R. (1995). *Clinical reasoning in physical disabilities*. Baltimore: Williams & Wilkins; and Marrelli, T. M., & Krulish, L. H. (1999). *Home care therapy: Quality, documentation and reimbursement*. Boca Grande, FL: Marrelli and Associates, Inc.

the application of the compressive force be distal to proximal. The idea is to push the fluid from the part toward the heart. For example, if the dorsum of the hand is swollen, begin at the fingertips and massage toward the wrist, from the wrist to the elbow, etc. In addition, the choice of material for application of compression needs to be considered with regards to the skin surface to which it will be applied. Coban would be contraindicated for open wounds and skin grafts as it leaves a ribbed, uncosmetic imprint. While pressure garments are smooth and would leave fewer marks on the skin, they also are expensive and take time to receive from vendors. Use of a fitted pressure garment may be more applicable to maintaining edema reduction than for actually reducing edema (Dutton, 1995).

Normal muscle contraction serves to increase circulation so active movement and use of weight bearing positions stimulate these normal muscle actions and can be useful in decreasing edema. However, active motion that is too forceful in early stages of recovery may aggravate edema instead of reducing it, so parameters of movement need to be controlled.

Modalities used in the treatment of edema may include ice baths or contrast baths. Ice baths or ice dips are used by having the client immerse an edematous hand for 3 seconds in water at a temperature of 12° C (48° F). The client would then squeeze the hand or wiggle it while in water and this would be repeated two to three times. Contrast baths are used if the client cannot tolerate ice or is experiencing hypersensitivity. The client alternately places an edematous hand in cold water (66° F) for 30 seconds and then warm water (96° F) for 3 minutes, ending with cool water. The client does active movements while immersed in the warm water.

Adaptive equipment is also used to decrease edema, such as an arm trough placed on the wheelchair of a client with hemiplegia.

The arm trough positions the arm safely and elevates to facilitate circulation of the fluid from the hand toward the heart. Continuous passive motion (CPM) devices are also used to prevent and decrease edema. The use of elevation is practical when the client is at rest or is not able to use the extremity. However, once the extremity can be used in activities, some adaptive equipment can actually prevent active use of the arm and should be discontinued. For example, a sling may enable a dependent extremity to be placed in an elevated position but may prevent active motion. In this case, other positioning devices would be better for the extremity that is capable of active motion, such as using a trough or pillow for optimal positioning (Dutton, 1995).

Scar prevention and management begins as soon as tissues are damaged and can continue for as long as 18 months after the injury. Hypertrophic scar formation prevention begins about 3 weeks after burns, starting with the use of pressure dressings as soon as grafts have taken or epithelialization begins. The sequence of dressings may start with Ace wraps initially, followed by tubular/coban next, and then pressure garments. Pressure garments are worn nearly all day for as long as 6 months to 2 years. Elastomer molds may also be worn for the chest, palms of the hand, and the face. Pressure garments and elastomer molds use compression to decrease blood flow, which may slow collagen synthesis (Dutton, 1995). These garments may also produce friction and shear forces, putting the part at risk for ischemia, so wear schedules and skin monitoring should be done periodically. Since scar management can take such an extended period of time, patient compliance is an important issue in intervention (Table 11-6).

Table 11-6.

TISSUE INTEGRITY

Goal	Method	Principle/Rationale	Example
Client will be (independent/ modified independent/require maximal/moderate/minimal assistance) in reducing peripheral edema by using...	Elevation	Which allows gravity to remove excess accumulation of peripheral fluids.	Arm sling Wheelchair arm trough
	Pressure	Which prevents filtration of fluids from capillaries into interstitial tissues.	Coban wrap Retrograde massage
	Temperature control	Which stimulates localized vascular responses.	Icing Contrast baths
	Active range of motion	Which pumps fluids out of interstitial and joint structures.	Gentle active range of motion Active assistive range of motion

Adapted from Dutton, R. (1995). *Clinical reasoning in physical disabilities*. Baltimore: Williams & Wilkins; and Marrelli, T. M., & Krulish, L. H. (1999). *Home care therapy: Quality, documentation and reimbursement*. Boca Grande, FL: Marrelli and Associates, Inc.

RANGE OF MOTION/FLEXIBILITY

ROM may be limited for a variety of reasons, including disease, injury, edema, pain, skin tightness, muscle spasticity, muscle and tendon shortening (tightness/contractures), and prolonged immobilization. *Flexibility* is the ROM of a joint and is determined by:
- The elasticity of soft tissues.
- Conditions within the joint.
- Excessive body fat or muscle mass.
- Pain (Hamil & Knutzen, 1995).

Flexibility is further defined as *static* or *dynamic*. Static flexibility is measured with a goniometer, whereas dynamic flexibility is seen to be the ease of movement or "amount of resistance to a joint to movement or the ability of a joint to make rapid and repeated flexing movement". Other definitions are that flexibility is the amount of resistance to passive motion of a joint or tone. Kisner and Colby define flexibility as "the ability of muscle to relax and yield to a stretch force" (Kisner & Colby, 1990, p. 110).

In interpreting ROM values made via goniometric measurements, it is important to remember that the available range varies with age, occupation, gender, specific joint, and activity levels. Earlier discussions described problems with reliability and validity, especially since normative values rarely describe how the measurement was made, from what population the values were taken, and the standard deviation for the mean values.

Limitations in ROM are the focus of intervention only if the limitation prevents successful engagement in areas of occupation that are of value to the client. Full ROM is not needed to achieve many tasks, and functional range is sufficient for many occupations. This illustrates that the clinical collaboration between the therapist and the client is vital and use of this approach must go beyond the procedural reasoning about the knowledge of musculoskeletal function and prognosis. It is only by assessing contextual variables and knowing the patient, using interactive reasoning, that meaningful interventions take place. For example, if a client lacks 90 degrees of shoulder flexion but is still able to dress himself and this is of value to him, then increasing ROM is not indicated. If the client lacks 120 degrees of shoulder flexion, is unable to put on a shirt but the spouse will dress the client, then increasing ROM for the shoulder may not be indicated. Intervention directed at remediation of ROM itself is not a valid intervention goal unless directed toward a functional outcome related to work, play, or self-care.

The main principle regarding ROM is that there must be movement through full ROM. There are many different ways to assure that the movement produced is through the complete range.

Exercise and activities can occur in anatomical planes of motion. For example, passive range of motion (PROM) for flexion of the shoulder would need to occur in a sagittal plane and in a frontal axis. By grasping the client's arm under the elbow, and with the other hand grasping the wrist, the client's arm would be lifted straight up parallel to the trunk. Similarly, abduction would occur in a frontal plane and a sagittal axis and the arm would be moved in a direction perpendicular to the trunk. The therapist could perform this motion or the client or caregiver could be instructed in the procedure through the available ROM.

Another method of providing ROM would be to move or have the client move the part in the direction of the muscle range of elongation. Knowledge of muscle fiber composition and line of pull would be necessary since ROM exercise would be antagonistic to the line of pull of the muscle (Kisner & Colby, 1990, p. 23).

Combined patterns (as in proprioceptive neuromuscular facilitation [PNF] patterns) are seen as a very functional way of incorporating ROM actions with movement in several planes of motion. An example might be to have the client sitting or lying supine. The starting position is: shoulder hyperextended, slightly abducted, internally rotated with the forearm pronated. Next, move the client to: shoulder flexion, horizontal adduction, external rotation with forearm supination. Several motions and planes are combined in one smooth movement. The disadvantage with these patterned movements is the complexity of the movement planning involved and in the ability to follow multistep directions. Again, these combined patterns can be performed actively by the client as exercise or as part of an activity, and can be taught to caregivers.

Functional patterns of movement associated with functional tasks can also be encouraged. This would be an appropriate screening strategy or could be considered an aspect of the top-down approach where occupational performance areas of work, play, and ADL are assessed rather than an initial focus on performance component. Observation of functional patterns of movement is actually a constant ongoing assessment occupational therapists make and is part of what comprises conditional clinical reasoning.

A continuous passive motion (CPM) device is often used to provide constant movement through specified ranges for a predetermined duration for clients following orthopedic surgery. Muscle fatigue is not a factor because the motion is passive.

If a client experiences unilateral deficits in ROM, then self ROM exercises can be taught for independence in maintenance of ROM. These can be exercises that use the unaffected hand and arm to move the affected side or can use a variety of tools such as those used in wand, cane, or dowel exercises (Figures 11-1 through 11-3).

Other tools and devices used in ROM exercises include:
- Finger ladder
- Shoulder wheel
- Overhead pulleys
- Suspension (e.g., Swedish suspension sling)
- Skate or powder board

INCREASING RANGE OF MOTION

When soft tissues around a joint are shortened and there is a loss of ROM, elongating these soft tissues will result in increased range. The shortening of soft issues may be due to prolonged immobilization, restricted mobility, connective tissue or neuromuscular disease, tissue pathology secondary to trauma, or due to congenital and acquired bony deformities (Kisner & Colby, 1990, p. 109).

Shortening of muscle or other tissues that cross a joint produces a *contracture*. Note that this is not synonymous with *contraction*, which is the process by which tension develops in a muscle during shortening or lengthening. Contractures can be defined and classified by the soft tissues affected. A myostatic contracture has no specific tissue pathology and yet there is loss of range that is usually mild and transient. Myostatic contractures often are resolved quickly with gentle stretching. *Tightness* is a term often used to describe loss of ROM at the outer limits of ROM that occurs in otherwise healthy tissues (Jacobs & Bettencourt, 1995, p. 111).

Scar tissue adhesions occur when scar tissue adheres to healthy tissue and limits motion. Contractures due to scar tissue adhesions can occur in muscles, tendons, joint capsules, or skin. Knowledge of the healing process and subsequent intervention can prevent scar tissue adhesions and exercise is helpful once scar tissue develops.

Once scars have formed, these need to be remodeled by making the tissue more pliable. This is achieved via deep friction massage, tendon gliding exercises, and by pressure garments that help to separate deep structures (tendons, nerves, blood vessels) that are stuck by the collagen bundles so that these deep structures can move separately (Demeter et al., 1996). Once the structures move separately, slow stretch forces can be applied. Rapid stretching causes scar tissue to tear while slow stretching produces small gains and is more effective than aggressive, rapid overstretching (Demeter et al., 1996, p. 52).

Chronic inflammation and fibrotic changes in soft tissues can lead to fibrotic adhesions that are difficult to reduce. *Irreversible contractures* are those in which there is a permanent loss of extensibility of soft tissues (Kielhofner, 1992). Irreversible contractures often are released surgically and occur when normal tissue is replaced by bone or fibrotic tissue. Hypertonicity can also cause a limitation of joint ROM as a result of central nervous system lesions. The muscle is in a state of high tone and constant contraction resulting in a *pseudomyostatic contracture* (Kisner & Colby, 1990).

To elongate the tissues, a stretch force is applied. The force, velocity, speed, and extent of the stretch force must be controlled and the joint movement needs to exceed the currently available range.

> Principle: Stretch that is done beyond the current ROM elongates collagen fibers in soft tissue.

When a tissue is stretched, this causes stress inside of the tissue. *Stress* is a force per unit area and is an internal reaction force within the material. Stress is not visible.

When stress is applied to a tissue, as when a muscle is elongated beyond the current range, the size and shape of the tissue changes or deforms. The amount of deformation depends upon the amount of the load and the ability of the material to resist the load. The percentage of deformation that occurs is known as *strain*. These two ideas, stress and strain, are reflected in Hook's Law, which states: "deformation increases proportionally to the applied force or strain increases proportionally to the stress of resisting the applied load" (Irion, 2000).

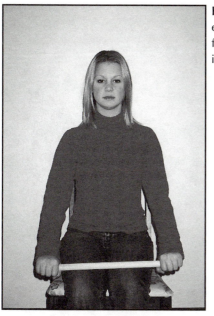

Figure 11-1A. Cane exercise for shoulder flexion, starting position.

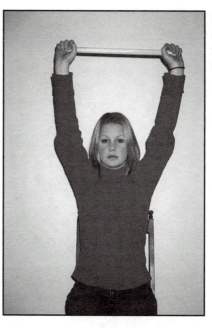

Figure 11-1B. Cane exercise for shoulder flexion, end position.

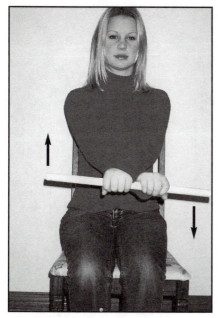

Figure 11-2A. Cane exercise for pronation and supination, starting position.

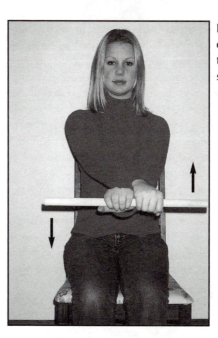

Figure 11-2B. Cane exercise for pronation and supination, starting position.

Both the contractile and noncontractile elements of muscle fibers influence stretching of soft tissues and both contribute to the temporary (elasticity) and permanent (plastic) changes in tissue length. Noncontractile tissue, comprised of collagen, elastin, reticulin fibers, and ground substance (mostly a gel containing water), can develop tightness and contractures, and limit joint motion and function. Since collagen is the element that absorbs most of the tensile stresses, tissues with a greater proportion of collagen fibers will provide greater stability, while soft tissue with a greater proportion of elastin fibers will have greater extensibility and flexibility.

When stress is applied to a muscle, the reaction of the muscle follows a predictable pattern shown in the stress-strain curve

(Figure 11-4). When a muscle is passively stretched, there is an initial lengthening of the series elastic components due to a mechanical disruption of the cross bridges as the actin and myosin proteins slide apart. This causes the sarcomere to lengthen until the stretch force is released. This is the toe region where most functional activity normally occurs (Kisner & Colby, 1990, p. 118). Once the force is stopped, the muscle returns to its original resting length, illustrating the elastic nature of the short-term stretch.

If, however, the muscle is immobilized in a lengthened position for a prolonged period of time, the changes in the muscle will be more permanent and a plastic change has occurred. This is due to the greater number of sarcomeres in series allowing the greatest functional overlap of actin and myosin proteins (Kisner & Colby,

Figure 11-3A. Cane exercise for shoulder hyperextension, starting position.

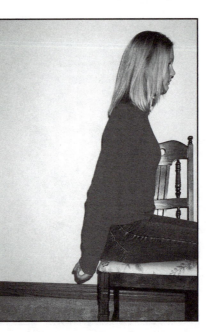

Figure 11-3B. Cane exercise for shoulder hyperextension, end position.

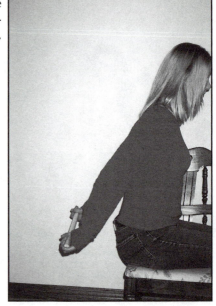

1990, p. 113). This more permanent change is the result of sequential failure of the collagen bonds, which respond to forces by remodeling and rebonding over time in the lines of stress (p. 118).

The muscle may also be immobilized for prolonged periods of time in a shortened position. In this case, the muscle produces increased amounts of connective tissue to protect the muscle against stretch. There are fewer sarcomeres due to sarcomere absorption. The changes in sarcomere length are transient and they will resume the original position if the muscle is allowed to return to normal length after immobilization.

If stress continues to be applied to a muscle in the plastic range, plastic changes can only continue up to a point, known as *necking*. This is the point of ultimate strength of the muscle. Past this point, there may be increased strain without an increase in stress so that even with less loads applied, the tissue is under increased strain. After this point, the tissue fails rapidly either due to a single maximal force applied or repeated submaximal stresses.

It is important for the therapist to be aware of the way that the tissue feels when stretching because when the strain is increased but the resistance felt in the muscle decreases and when less force is needed for deformation to occur, necking may be occurring with tissue failure imminent even with smaller loads (Fisher, 1998).

Creeping is the application of "low magnitude loads over prolonged periods of time [that] increases the plastic deformation of noncontractile tissue, which allows a gradual rearrangement of collagen fibers" (Kisner & Colby, 1990, p. 119). The remodeling and rebonding of the collagen fibers require time for healing. Intensive stretching is usually done every other day to allow this time for healing. This is especially true in tissues of elderly clients because a normal age-related change is a reduction in collagen and there is decreased capillary supply that reduces the healing abilities in the elderly (Kisner & Colby, 1990). In addition, there is a decrease in tensile strength and rate of adaptation to stress in the elderly.

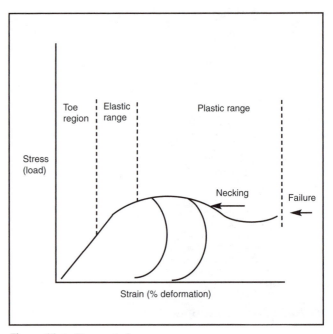

Figure 11-4. Stress-strain curve.

Heat increases creep and therefore the elasticity of collagen fibers, making tissues more amenable to stretch (Demeter, Andersson & Smith, 1996; Kisner & Colby, 1990) and making the stretching of tissues more comfortable for the client. For this reason, both superficial and deep heat modalities increase the extensibility of tissue and are often used prior to stretch. Other techniques used to relax the tissues prior to stretch force application might include active inhibition techniques, local relaxation, progressive relaxation techniques (which may include controlled breathing techniques or progressive muscle relaxation), and biofeedback. Low intensity exercise or activity can also be used to warm the tissues prior to stretch. Massage done before stretching serves to increase circulation and decrease muscle spasms and stiffness. Cognitive relaxation techniques, such as disassociative visualization (pleasant memory or image), autogenic relaxation (similar to self hypnosis), use of videotapes, audiotapes, music or meditation, also serves to relax the client prior to stretch. Several nontraditional techniques such as the Feldenkrais Method, Alexander technique, or hatha yoga can also be used.

Two sensory receptors are directly involved in muscle function and to application of stretch forces. The *muscle spindle* is a major sensory organ of the muscle and consists of microscopic intrafusal fibers that lie parallel to the extrafusal (skeletal) muscle fibers. These fibers are sensitive to the length and velocity of the lengthening of extrafusal muscle fibers and the muscle spindle initiates muscle contraction. Once a muscle shortens, the spindles are no longer activated because they are no longer stretched. Since the muscle spindle lies parallel to the extrafusal muscle fibers, when the muscle is lengthened, the muscle spindle is also lengthened and responds by initiating a muscle contraction. The muscle spindle has been called a "comparator" because the spindle compares the length of the spindle with the length of the skeletal muscle fiber. If the length of the extrafusal muscle fiber is less than the spindle, the spindle is less active. Conversely, when the spindle is stretched, more nerve impulses are sent to activate the extrafusal fibers (Pedretti, 1996, p. 102). When the patella is tapped by a small hammer, this illustrates the activation of the muscle spindle in a brief contraction called the stretch reflex, muscle spindle reflex (MSR), myostatic or monosynaptic stretch reflex, or deep tendon reflex (DTR).

The *golgi tendon organ* (GTO) wraps around the extrafusal fibers of the muscle in neuromuscular junctions between the muscles and tendons. This sensory receptor is sensitive to the tension in muscles, either due to passive stretch or active muscle contraction. It serves a protective function to inhibit the contraction of a muscle in which it lies and has a low threshold (fires easily) after active muscle contraction. The GTO has a high threshold (fires less easily) to passive stretch. Due to the GTO, the force that can be developed in a muscle is limited.

The implications of the action of these two receptors on the stretching of extrafusal skeletal muscles is that if a muscle is stretched too quickly (too great a velocity) or too far, the muscle spindle will be stretched. This in turn will produce increased tension in the skeletal muscle. This is counterproductive to efforts to lengthen this muscle. Stretching done at too high a velocity may actually increase the tension in a muscle that you are trying to lengthen. When a muscle is stretched slowly, the GTO fires, which inhibits increased tension development in that muscle and allows lengthening to occur by permitting the sarcomeres to lengthen.

Stretch can be applied actively or passively, statically and dynamically. Situations for passive stretch would be in cases when the client is unable to stretch the part actively due to muscle weakness; when the client cannot learn how to prevent substitu-

tion movements; or when the goal is to increase ROM at the end of range.

Some general concepts related to stretch are:
- Static stretching is preferable to ballistic.
- Increased flexibility and ROM is produced by overstretching but the motion should not exceed normal muscle length by more than 10%.
- More repetitions are needed to increase flexibility than to maintain it.
- Stretching should be done before and after strengthening activities.

Passive stretch can be applied by means of *joint mobilization*, which involves passive rocking, and oscillatory movements aimed at increasing joint play. Joint play is not under the patient's voluntary control and is used when there is joint stiffness, pain, or reversible joint hypomobility (Trombly, 1995). Another technique, called *myofascial release*, is the stretching and breaking up of adhesions of the fascia. Joint manipulation is done to break up massive adhesions and is usually done under anesthesia. These three techniques require extensive training beyond entry level competence and the scope of this text.

Manual passive stretch is a short duration stretch where the tissue is elongated beyond resting length by a therapist applying external force. The therapist controls the direction, speed, intensity, and duration of the stretch. It is important to point out that manual passive stretch is not the same as PROM. PROM moves the part through unrestricted, available range while manual passive stretch is done to the point of maximal stretch or a few degrees past the point of discomfort (Thompson & Floyd, 1994). Excessive overstretching occurs when the movement overcomes the natural supportive function of the joint and tissues resulting in hypermobility, joint instability, and increased risk of strain and injury. Signs of excessive overstretching are pain, redness, and swelling that persist for several hours. Nonverbal danger signals that may be observed might include a sudden increase in sweat, visual signs of stretching on the skin, gradual loss of slack, the client looks away suddenly, or there is a sudden constriction of the pupils (Table 11-7).

Gains in muscle elongation due to manual passive stretch are transient and are attributed to temporary sarcomere give (Kisner & Colby, 1990). The stretch force applied is dependent upon the client's tolerance and the therapist's strength and endurance. Low intensity stretches applied for prolonged periods of time are more comfortable for the client (Kisner & Colby, 1990).

Prolonged mechanical stretch is a low intensity external load (5 to 15 pounds) that is applied to a part for a prolonged period of time by means of positioning, traction, braces, splints (static), or serial casting. The force is applied from 20 to 30 minutes to several hours. The longer duration of low intensity force application permits the sarcomeres to be added and for remodeling and rebonding of collagen fibers to occur so more plastic changes occur. Prolonged mechanical passive stretching is seen to be more effective and more comfortable for the client than manual passive stretch. This static

Table 11-7.

PRECAUTIONS RELATED TO STRETCH

1. Do not force the tissue beyond normal limits of ROM.
2. Newly united fractures should be protected and stabilized.
3. Osteoporosis.
4. Avoid vigorous stretching in tissues that have been immobilized for a long period of time because connective tissue can lose strength.
5. If soreness or pain occurs 24 hours after a stretch, too much force was used.
6. Allow time for healing/remodeling to occur so you do not need to stretch daily.
7. Avoid stretching edematous tissues because these are more susceptible to injury and stretching can actually increase the pain and edema.

Figure 11-5. Pendulum exercises.

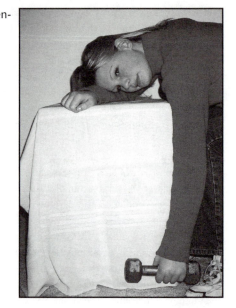

stretching technique is seen as less labor intensive because the body part or object is providing the stretch force.

Active stretching is done in cases where the client is afraid of passive stretch due to loss of control, fear of reinjury, or low tolerance for discomfort. When passive stretch is harmful (for example, in newly sutured tendons or grafted skin), active stretching can be done. Since the client is providing or controlling the stretch force, there is less chance of overstretching. This can mean that injury and discomfort will be minimized or it could also prevent sufficient lengthening of the soft tissues and for a long enough duration to enable permanent elongation. In active stretching, the resistance force is minimal. Active stretching can be done by self stretching one's own muscles, by means of the shoulder wheel or finger boards, or by using PNF diagonal patterns of movement. Self stretching is done by the client using weight of a body part or gravity as the stretch force (Figures 11-5 and 11-6).

Active stretch done during occupational activities and tasks that are meaningful to the client serves to distract the patient who has pain, can be a motivational factor, and can reduce psychological dependence on the therapist (Dutton, 1995). Whether passive or active stretching is done, it is vital to incorporate tasks and activities that the client actually needs to be able to successfully perform as a major focus of intervention. The goal of occupational therapy is to enable clients to return to the daily activities that are important to them and it cannot be assumed that increases in ROM will automatically be assimilated into these meaningful tasks.

Active inhibition techniques are used in collaboration with the patient to actively stretch shortened tissues. The patient must have normally innervated muscles capable of volitional control and the stretch affects contractile elements by stretching the elastic tissues. Kisner and Colby indicate that the assumption is that the sarcomere will give more easily when the muscle is relaxed and there is less active resistance in the muscle as it is elongated (Kisner & Colby, 1990, p. 123). While active inhibition is generally more

comfortable for the client than other types of stretches, the gains are usually temporary. Whether contract-relax (hold relax), contract-relax-contract (hold-relax-contract), or agonist-contraction methods are used, the client is asked to first relax and then elongate tight muscles. These relaxation and inhibition techniques have been used to relieve pain, muscle tension, tension headaches, high blood pressure, and respiratory distress (Kisner & Colby, 1990).

Studies to determine the optimal type of load and duration of force application have used a variety of stretch mechanisms and methods. Low load prolonged stretch (LLPS) is used to reduce contractures, often by means of an orthotic device. High load brief stretch (HLBS) and exercise in PNF diagonal patterns was compared with LLPS. In this case, LLPS was found to be superior in the results while a study comparing the use of a Dynasplint (Severna Park, MD) with PROM and manual stretching found no difference between this regime and LLPS (provided by the Dynasplint). Serial casting often is used as a means of providing a LLPS and this has been found to result in significant increases in PROM as compared with other methods (Nuismer, Ekes, & Holm, 1997).

Stretching soft tissues would be contraindicated immediately following surgery or if the joint lacks structural stability as in unhealed fractures (Dutton, 1995). Kisner and Colby state that "the only true contraindications to stretching techniques are hypermobility, joint effusion (swelling) and inflammation" (Kisner & Colby, 1990). If joint ROM is limited by bony blocks due to pathological ossification or bone fragments, stretching the soft tissue will not increase the ROM. If sharp, acute pain occurs with movement, stretching should be stopped. Extra caution should be used if there are hematomas.

In cases where shortened tissues are providing greater joint stability in lieu of normal stabilization or strength, stretching is contraindicated. This may occur in special cases such as cervical spinal cord injuries where intervention is aimed at the development of teneodesis action of the fingers and wrist. The development of

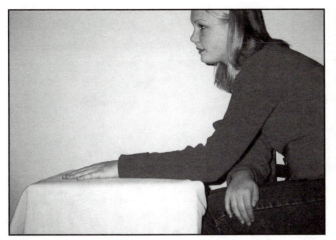

Figure 11-6A. Self stretch of shoulder flexors.

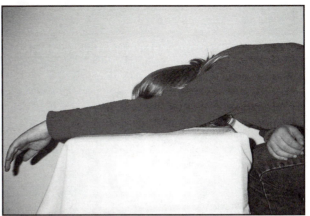

Figure 11-6B. Self stretch of shoulder flexors.

slight finger flexion tightness enables a better passive grasp of objects when the wrist is extended. To encourage this, the fingers are flexed while the wrist is extended or the fingers are extended while the wrist is flexed to avoid overstretching across all joints crossed.

Other special cases might include clients with rheumatoid arthritis. Stretching in acute, inflamed joints is avoided but gentle, prolonged stretch in postinflammatory phases prevents shortening of muscles and connective tissue into fixed deformities (Table 11-8).

STRENGTHENING

Muscle strength may be limited due to lower motor neuron diseases (e.g., polio, ALS), spinal cord injuries or disease, peripheral nerve damage, muscle diseases (e.g., muscular dystrophy), muscle overwork, trauma, disuse (due to muscle imbalance, pain, denervation of motor units), or immobilization (splints, casts, orthotic devices), which leads to shortened soft tissues, decreased circulation, atrophy, and smaller numbers of motor units.

Limitations in strength may be permanent or temporary and an understanding of the cause of the deficit will influence intervention strategies. Remediation intervention will be focused on those muscles in which improvement is possible.

Maintenance of strength might be an intervention focus if a client has been on bed rest for 6 to 10 days or more or a specific body part has been restricted (Dutton, 1995). Active movement and participation in grooming and hygiene activities can maintain muscle grades of F+ to good. In muscle grades of fair or greater, active movement is beneficial not only in maintaining strength but also in maintaining range (Dutton, 1995). Pedretti indicates that isometric activities and exercise without resistance can be used to maintain muscle strength when active motion is not possible or is contraindicated with muscle grades above trace. This type of activity is especially good for those in casts, after surgery, and with arthritis or burns (Pedretti, 1996). Since strength is maintained and not increased or changed, maintenance of strength may more

aptly be viewed as a rehabilitation goal or as one to prevent further structural limitations.

Increasing muscle strength would be the focus of intervention when muscle weakness interferes with occupational performance in work, play, and self-care. Muscle weakness is potentially deforming due to muscle imbalances and strengthening weak muscles will balance the forces of agonist and antagonist muscles.

Increasing strength occurs when more motor units are recruited due to the application of stress to a muscle to the point of fatigue. The stress to the muscle should be great enough to require a maximal motor unit response. A training effect occurs, which reflects the increased number of motor units involved in muscle contractions.

At the cellular level, increased strength of the muscle results in greater myofibril cross sectional area and size, which results in hypertrophy of the muscle as a whole. The increased fiber size results in more protein to the fibers and in greater capillary density. The actual number of myofibrils may also occur due to fiber splitting.

Strengthening programs are based on Hellebrandt's *overload principle*, which states that an increase in strength occurs only if the load is greater than that to which the tissue is accustomed and that the load is applied to the point of fatigue. The application of the appropriate stress will overload the system and cause adaptation. Without overload, there is no adaptation and no improvement in strength. *Adaptation* is defined as a fairly persistent change in the structure or function following repeated bouts of activity. Examples of adaptation include hypertrophy and increased strength, increased maximal oxygen consumption, or a change in body composition (Hamil & Knutzen, 1995). Overload is achieved by varying the parameters of intensity, duration, and frequency of the stress, with intensity being the most potent factor in yielding adaptation to stress.

Duration of exercise refers to the length or total time the client participates in the activity or exercise. When the duration increases, this causes fatigue, which leads to the recruitment of additional motor units. In addition, weak muscles activate more motor units than do strong muscles. If the client is engaged in activities that are

Table 11-8.

INCREASING JOINT RANGE OF MOTION

Goal	Method	Principle/Rationale	Example
Joint range of motion will be increased in (specify joint, R/L/B, and motion) by using...	Heat	Which increases the elasticity of collagen fibers in soft tissue.	Neutral warmth Warm water Paraffin Fluidotherapy Light activities or exercises
	Relaxation	Of soft tissues prior to stretch decreases tension.	Active inhibition techniques Progressive muscle relaxation Controlled breathing Low intensity activities or exercise Massage Cognitive relaxation strategies Nontraditional methods
	Scar remodeling procedures	Which provide stretch pressure to separate deeper structures, and compression, which slows collagen synthesis.	Deep friction massage Tendon-gliding exercises Transparent face mask Pressure garments
	Passive stretch	Beyond current range, which elongates collagen fibers in soft tissue.	Manual passive stretch Prolonged mechanical stretch Joint mobilization Joint manipulation Myofascial release
	Active stretch	Beyond current range against minimum resistance to elongate collagen.	Active activities and exercise Active inhibition techniques Finger boards Shoulder wheels PNF diagonal Active movement Self stretch Codman exercises
	Orthoses and positioning	Which maintains gains from stretching during cool-down and between treatment sessions. *or* Which provide gradually increasing amounts of prolonged static stretch.	Splints Serial casting

Table 11-8, continued.

Goal	Method	Principle/Rationale	Example
	Role-related activities	Through the increased range, which ensure that gains will be generalized to daily routines.	Reach for videotapes on third shelf of cabinet at work at TV station

Adapted from Dutton, R. (1995). *Clinical reasoning in physical disabilities.* Baltimore: Williams & Wilkins; and Marrelli, T. M., & Krulish, L. H. (1999). *Home care therapy: Quality, documentation and reimbursement.* Boca Grande, FL: Marrelli and Associates, Inc.

of high intensity and low duration, increases in strength are the objective. Usually programs that are of low intensity but high duration are aimed at increasing endurance. Activities that are of interest to the client will likely be done for longer periods of time, which increases the duration as well.

The *rate* or *velocity* is the speed of the activity or exercise. Generally it has been found that by using slower speeds, muscle strength can be increased more quickly and that slower, more constant rates tend to decrease the effects of momentum. Galley states that low speed, high load exercise produces greater increases in muscular force only at slow speed, whereas high power (high speed, low load) exercise produces increases in muscular force at all speeds as well as increases in endurance (Galley & Forster, 1987, p. 160). The velocity of the contraction should be based on the client's physical capacity at the time the exercise or activity is initiated.

It is critical to have knowledge of the rate of the activity for which the strengthening is directed. This reflects the SAID principle (specific adaptation to the imposed demand), which indicates that the choice of activity or exercise should be related to the activity in which you want a functional outcome. There is training specificity so an analysis of the motions required in daily tasks needs to be done in order to strengthen those muscles needed in those specific activities.

The type of muscle contraction is linked to velocity as well. In concentric muscle contractions, as the velocity of shortening increases, the force the muscle can generate decreases because the muscle does not have time to reach peak tension. Slow concentric contractions produce more torque than fast concentric. But, as Dutton points out, it is ironic that clients often prefer fast concentric activities and exercises because the speed recruits assistive, synergist muscles (Dutton, 1995). If using concentric contractions, the velocity should be slow.

In eccentric muscle contractions, as the velocity of lengthening increases against resistance, more tension can be generated because this serves as a protective measure when excessively loaded (Baxter, 1998; Berne & Levy, 1998; Galley & Forster, 1987). Fast eccentric contractions produce more torque than do slow eccentric muscle contractions but ballistic movements result, as when one slams a glass on a table. While more torque is produced in the fast contraction, this is not always the most desirable motion to produce, especially for those with fragile tissues such as clients with rheumatoid arthritis or burns (Dutton, 1995). Most activities and exercises use alternating concentric and eccentric contractions.

It is important to match the type of contraction used in intervention to that which is needed in the client's preferred and required occupational demands and interests. Analysis of the activities will help to determine the type of contraction needed to produce functional gains. Dutton (1995) cites three rules to determine the type of contraction based on three sources of movement that act together in activities:

- Rule 1: When the gravitational moment and what the object wants are the same as the desired motion, the contraction is eccentric.
- Rule 2: When either the gravitational moment or what the object wants is different from the desired motion, then the contraction is concentric.
- Rule 3: When no visible movement occurs, but muscle shortens, contraction is isometric.

Two examples of these rules follow.

Frequency is the number of times per day or number of days per week the activity or exercise is done. Frequency depends upon the types of fibers being strengthened, the type of activity for which the intervention is directed, the client's endurance and general health status, on the muscle grades, joint mobility, diagnosis, intervention goals, position of client, desirable plane of motion, and the level of fatigue.

Intensity is the level of exertion or energy expenditure and can be gauged by the client's heart rate, perceived exertion, and ability to speak normally. The amount of resistance needed to increase strength ranges from 50 to 67% of the maximum that the client can lift (repetition maximum [RM]). The number of repetitions varies from one to three sets of 10 repetitions with rest periods of 2 to 4 minutes between. The intensity and number of repetitions is based on the client's failure-to-lift in which all motor units in a muscle are strengthened. Optimally, one set of ten repetitions has been found to be adequate to increase strength if failure-to-lift occurs in the final repetitions. Signs that the client is approaching failure-to-lift include mild shaking, difficulty completing the full movement, grimacing, grunting, or sweating (Demeter et al., 1996). Watch for substitution movements since this would activate muscles other than the ones needing strengthening.

The type of fiber that predominates in the muscle (i.e., Type I, Type II) will also be a factor. For example, larger fast twitch muscle fibers have a greater capacity to develop tension and show a more pronounced hypertrophy in response to strength training than do smaller slow twitch muscle fibers.

Intensity can be graded by the type of exercise or activity that is performed, by the amount of resistance used, by changing the length of lever arm, by changing the point where the load is applied, or by changing plane of movement. Given the variety of ways intensity can be graded, increasing strength can be accomplished by many activities as well as by exercise regimes.

Whether activities or exercise are used to increase strength, *fatigue* is an important variable to be monitored. In order to increase strength, maximum stress is applied to the muscle to the point of fatigue. Excessive strengthening, however, may result in fatigue, pain, and temporary reduction of strength. If the muscle is *overworked*, it will be unable to contract.

Fatigue can be differentiated from overwork. Fatigue is the result of a maximal motor unit response, whereas overwork is an insidious loss of strength due to an overload on individual muscle strands. Overwork occurs in clients with spotty denervation, with or without sensory losses. These clients have fewer motor units and fewer contracting muscle fibers, so each fiber must work maximally. Since there is less waste product buildup, there is less sensation of fatigue and the client does not interpret the fatigue sensation properly. Overwork is frequently irreversible but fortunately occurs rarely.

Muscle fatigue levels vary from person to person. One's threshold for fatigue decreases in pathological states (Dutton, 1995) and clients may lack the sensation to be aware of their level of fatigue and others may push themselves beyond their tolerance. Local fatigue is normal and is characterized by a diminished response of muscles to repeated stimuli (Kisner & Colby, 1990).

Fatigue may be caused by synaptic fatigue, depletion of glycogen, build-up of lactic acid, shunt of blood to skin to control temperature, electrolyte imbalance, increased blood viscosity due to dehydration, or blood flow constriction by prolonged muscle action.

Signs of fatigue might include:
- Slowed performance
- Distraction
- Perspiration
- Increase in rate of respiration
- Performance of movement through decreased ROM
- Inability to complete prescribed number of repetitions
- Inability to maintain or repeat the production of a given force by muscular contraction resulting in decreased strength
- Decreased time of contraction
- Increased time for muscle lengthening
- Tremors with contraction
- Increased heart rate and respiration with no increase in load
- General sense of tiredness
- Attention wanders
- Incoordination
- Loss of concentration
- Substitution movements (Demeter et al., 1996; Kisner & Colby, 1990; Norkin & Levangie, 1992).

As the client performs activities, observe for signs of fatigue and distress. Distress may be evident in shortness of breath (dyspnea), confusion, profuse sweating in association with cold, clammy skin (diaphoresis), and straining while holding one's breath (Valsalva maneuver), which is especially dangerous in that it raises the blood pressure. More subtle signs of distress might be seen in escalating frustration, hurrying to finish the task, less ROM, chest pain, nausea, or lightheadedness (syncope) (Demeter et al., 1996). In the cases of chest pain or syncope, confusion, diaphoresis or level 2 dyspnea (defined as one who needs three breaths to count to 15), it is advisable to discontinue the activity and consult with the physician for further evaluation of these symptoms (Hamil & Knutzen, 1995).

Injuries to muscles can occur as a result of muscle strain or microtears in the muscle fibers. Client symptoms would be pain or muscle soreness, swelling, and possible deformity and dysfunction. Muscles at greatest risk are two-joint muscles, muscles used to terminate a ROM, and muscles used eccentrically. Two-joint muscles are especially prone to fatigue and strain since they can be stretched at two joints simultaneously. For example, to extend at the hip and flex at the knee, the rectus femoris muscle is vulnerable to injury because it is put on an extreme stretch (Hamil & Knutzen, 1995). Muscles that are used to terminate a motion are at risk because they are used to eccentrically slow a limb moving very rapidly, such as the hamstrings when slowing hip flexion or the posterior rotator cuff muscles when slowing the arm on the follow-through phase of a throw (Hamil & Knutzen, 1995).

While muscles may be the site of damage, soreness and strain is due to the connective tissues, especially at the muscle-tendon junction. Common injuries at this site are in the gastrocnemius, pectoralis major, rectus femoris, adductor longus, triceps brachii, semimembranosus, semitendinosus, and biceps femoris (Hamil & Knutzen, 1995).

Pain management is often a part of the intervention process because, without this, intervention will not yield successful outcomes. Often it is the complaint of pain that brings the client to the therapist for intervention and not the underlying component deficit. Pain presents both with sensory and emotional symptoms. Lack of comfort and often sleep, loss of activities, and loss of roles may cause withdrawal, introversion and depression, anger and aggression. Pain and lack of customary life roles may develop into learned helplessness where the client avoids strenuous activities and where secondary benefits are gained, such as excused participation in work activities or in less desired roles.

Acute pain is experienced immediately following a physical injury and is proportional to physical findings. Chronic pain lasts months or years and can change the client's personality, cause disassociation from physical problems, and can develop into a different clinical syndrome (Smith et al., 1996).

Assessment of pain can be done by means of a verbal rating scale (VBS), which is a list of adjectives that describe different levels of pain intensity (e.g., from no pain to extreme pain). Numerical rating scales (NRS) are used that can be from 1 to 10, 1 to 100 or any other predetermined scale so that the client can indicate the level of the pain intensity. A visual analogue scale (VAS) uses a line to visually define the level of pain.

No pain [----------------x----------------] Pain as bad as it could be

Table 11-9. SELECTED PAIN ASSESSMENTS			
Passive	*Active Assistive*	*Active*	*Resistive*
0	T, P-	P	P+
	F-	F	F+
			G-, G, G+

Twelve descriptor items with each centered over 21 horizontal dashes are used in a descriptor differential scale (DDS). The client would then rate the magnitude of pain on each descriptor. Pain discomfort scales (PDS) like the McGill Pain Questionnaire are often used, which uses words to describe sensory and affective dimensions of pain. Pain location, body diagrams, and mapping are other means of defining the location of pain (Trombly, 1995) (Table 11-9).

Pain management strategies draw upon the *gate control theory*. This theory indicates that impulses from large sensory nerve fibers at segmental levels of the spinal cord enable nonpainful sensory input to stimulate the same transmission cells that the pain receptors do. This would inhibit the transmission of the pain input. Every time you rub your knee after banging it against something, you are demonstrating this theory; mechanoreceptors are superseding the pain messages. The activation of the mechanoreceptors competes for transmission with the pain input, so by rubbing your knee, the sensation of pressure, not pain, is felt. One physiologic explanation for the gate theory mechanism is that the local stimulation of nonpain mediated sensory afferents closes the gate at the spinal cord level, thereby preventing further transmission of pain impulses. Another is that the body is stimulated to release endogenous opiate substances, which increases the circulation of neuropharmacologic agents (endorphins), which then decreases the pain. It has been found that the inhibition of pain input is enhanced by the client's concentration on competing activities that have important implications for occupational therapists and the use of meaningful occupation as the means of intervention.

Intervention for pain involves establishing functional goals. By working toward clear, functional goals, attention is directed away from the pain and toward an observable result of intervention. Clients may not become pain free but instead must be taught how to tolerate and manage their pain. Modalities are often used, such as localized heat (whirlpool, fluidotherapy, paraffin), deep heat (ultrasound, TENS, iontophoresis), massage, acupressure or acupuncture, and vibration (especially with amputees). Behavioral techniques might include hypnosis, relaxation techniques, biofeedback, behavioral modification programs, and counseling. Intractable pain may require medication or surgery.

Strengthening programs can use a variety of methods to increase strength that can include both activities and exercise. The use of therapeutic exercise is most beneficial to clients with muscle strength at the extremes of the manual muscle testing ratings (i.e., those muscles rated trace and poor or those with good muscle strength). Since occupational therapy intervention is developed based on client needs and interests, it is important to recognize that therapeutic exercise may be more acceptable to some clients than activities, while engaging in activities may be more meaningful to others.

Pedretti proposes eight purposes for the use of therapeutic exercise:
1. Develop awareness of normal movement patterns and improve voluntary, automatic movement responses.
2. Develop strength and endurance in patterns of movement that are acceptable and necessary and do not produce deformity.
3. Improve coordination, regardless of strength.
4. Increase power of specific isolated muscles or muscle groups.
5. Aid in overcoming ROM deficits.
6. Increase strength of muscles that will power hand splints, MAS, or other devices.
7. Increase work tolerance and physical endurance through increased strength.
8. Prevent or eliminate contractures developing as a result of imbalanced muscle power by strengthening antagonistic muscles (Pedretti, 1996, p. 300-301).

In developing strengthening intervention goals, the activity or exercise needs to match the client's muscle grades and endurance levels. The amount of stress applied to a muscle follows the continuum in progression from maximal assistance to maximal resistance.

Passive exercise would be the same as PROM. As such, no gains in strength are expected but rather the goal is for maintenance of the ROM.

Active assistive activities and exercises are those in which the client moves actively as far as possible and the therapist or a device completes the motion through the existing ROM. Because the patient moves actively as far as possible, there is stress to the muscle and recruitment and hypertrophy can occur. Exercise is graded so that the device/therapist gradually decreases the amount of support or assistance that is provided while the client provides more active (unassisted) movement.

Isotonic active assistive is appropriate for clients with T, P-, or F- muscle grades. For the trace muscle, the client contracts the muscle and the therapist completes the motion. Active assistive exercise in a gravity eliminated plane is used for P-, while with F- muscles, gravity is included as a factor. Bilateral activities are useful for active assistive exercise if only one extremity is affected and the assistance can be provided by the unaffected arm.

Progressive assistive exercise (PAE) is a type of assistive exercise where equipment (such as the Swedish suspension sling) provides the minimal amount of weight required to complete a motion. A skate with weights and pulley, dynamic orthoses, towel and dowel exercises are other examples of exercises that can be done assistively. Few activities provide assistive exercise without resistance, although some examples cited by Trombly include adapting floor looms or polishing a smooth surface (Trombly, 1995).

Active activities and exercise are those in which the client moves through the available ROM without resistance. Active activities

Figure 11-7A. Theraband exercises for shoulder abduction, end position.

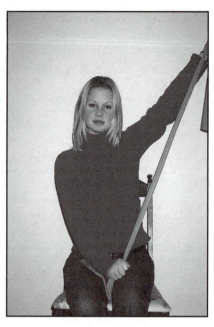

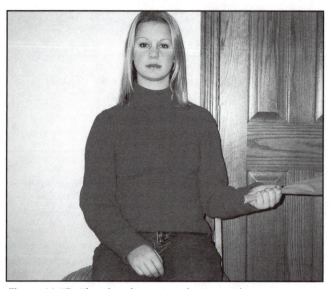

Figure 11-7B. Theraband exercises for external rotation.

and exercises increase muscle grades of P to F and higher. There are very few activities or exercises that are purely active exercise and even most ADL are resistive. Needlepoint completed in a gravity eliminated would be an active exercise for wrist extensors or elbow extensors. A fair muscle can move the wrist against gravity, as in a mosaic tile project (Pedretti, 1996). The goal of activities and exercises at this level is to progress to a point where some resistance other than gravity can be applied.

Resistive activities and exercise are done when an outside resistance is required to apply maximal stress to the muscle in order to promote adaptation. The resistance force may be applied manually (by the therapist) or by equipment, tools, or activity (Figure 11-7A-E). Use of resistance is necessary to increase the strength of P+, F+ to normal muscles by means of either isotonic or isometric muscle contractions. Isotonic resistive strengthening can also produce relaxation of antagonist to the contracting muscle and for stretching or relaxing hypertonic antagonists (Trombly, 1995).

In *manual resistive activities and exercise,* not only is the intensity of the resistance force controlled by the therapist, but also the site and direction of the force application. Force is usually applied at the distal end of the segment to which the muscle attaches, which provides a mechanical advantage for the therapist applying the force. The direction of force is directly opposite to the desired motion. Stabilization is important in order to avoid substitution or compensatory movements. The resistance is applied smoothly, steadily, slowly, and gradually so that the movement is pain free and through the maximal range. These criteria can be applied to either activities or to exercise regimes. For exercises, eight to ten repetitions are completed, one to two times per session, with rests of 2 to 4 minutes minimally between sets of application of resistance is recommended.

Mechanical resistive activities and exercise are any form of endeavor where the resistance is applied by mechanical equipment, tools or the placement of the task. Isotonic resistance equipment might

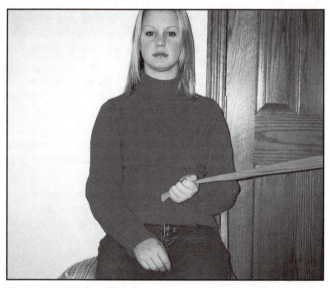

Figure 11-7C. Theraband exercises for internal rotation.

include free weights, elastic resistance devices (Theraband, tubing), pulley systems (using weights or springs) that may be free standing or wall mounted (e.g., Elgin exercise unit [Elgin Exercise Equipment, Lonbard, IL], Variable Resistance or Dynamic Variable Resistance [DVR]), systems (Nautilus [Louisville, CO], Cybex Eagle [Medway, MA], Keiser Cam II [Zurich]), or cycle ergometers (stationary bicycles) (Norkin & Levangie, 1992; Rantanen, Harris, Leveille, et al., 2000). Many of these devices are part of circuit weight training programs where the client exercises in short bouts, using light to moderate work loads with frequent repetitions with short rests. A specific sequence of exercise is followed.

Adding resistance can be done by changing the effect of gravity on the activity with a gravity eliminated plane, generally that which is parallel to the horizon. Additional resistance would be

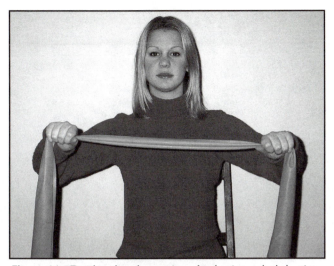

Figure 11-7D. Theraband exercises for horizontal abduction, starting position.

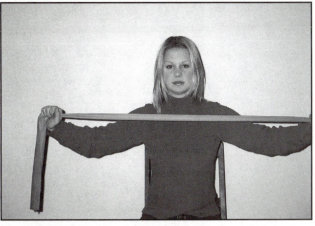

Figure 11-7E. Theraband exercises for horizontal abduction, end position.

achieved by using an inclined plane, additional resistance to the weight of the objects or tools used, or the duration of the activity. Activity analysis and adaptation are particular strengths of the occupational therapist and these skills are especially helpful in developing intervention aimed at increasing strength by means of activities of value and interest to the client. Occupations done daily can have a strengthening benefit without being contrived and have the added advantage of being a necessary part of one's life.

Isotonic strengthening activities and exercise require a dynamic effort with a constant load but uncontrolled speed of movement. The movement may require either eccentric or concentric contractions or both. A specific exercise regime was developed by DeLorme and is called *Progressive Resistive Exercise* (PRE). DeLorme based this exercise regime on the overload principle where several sets of repetitions are completed against a portion of the repetition maximum. The modified DeLorme PRE method first determines the RM, which is the greatest amount of weight that can be lifted, pulled, or pushed ten times through the full existing ROM. The RM is based on the muscle grades as a guide and is determined through trial and error. The client then performs 10 repetitions at 50% of the RM, 10 repetitions at 75% of the RM, then 10 repetitions at 100% of the RM with 2 to 4 minute rests in between exercise sets. These exercises should be performed once a day, 4 to 5 times per week for maximum strengthening benefit. An example might be that if a client is able to lift 12 pounds 10 times, this would be the 10 RM. The PRE program would be: 10 repetitions at 6 pounds, rest, 10 repetitions at 9 pounds, rest, 10 repetitions at 12 pounds.

Regressive resistive exercise (RRE) or Zinovieff's Oxford method, is essentially the opposite of the modified DeLorme PRE program. The client completes 10 repetitions at 100%, rests, 10 repetitions at 75%, rests, then 10 repetitions at 50%. The RRE program was designed to diminish the resistance as muscle fatigue develops, but this has been disproved as a theory of exercise.

Isometric activities and exercise are characterized by no visible joint movement nor appreciable change in muscle length but increased muscle tension. Because the joint does not move, isometric activities and exercise are well suited for clients with rheumatoid arthritis, those with pain or inflammation, and for clients with trace muscle strength. Isometric exercises have the advantage of being easy to perform with little setup or equipment needed and it takes minimal time since isometric contractions can be very fatiguing (Nuismer et al., 1997). Disadvantages of isometric exercise and activity are that the gains in strength do not necessarily transfer to dynamic activities, there is no effect on improving coordination, and it does not cause hypertrophy. The most serious disadvantage is that isometric contraction causes an increase in blood pressure, and so is contraindicated for patients with cardiovascular problems. Isometric activities with resistance are appropriate to use with muscle grades of F+ to normal. Using isometric contractions in activities is easily done when one considers that holding tools requires an isometric contraction (Figures 11-8 and 11-9).

Different isometric contraction exercises are:
- *Brief maximal isometric exercise regime*: a single isometric contraction is held against a fixed resistance for 5 to 6 seconds, once a day, 5 to 6 times per week. Longer duration contractions have been found to be more effective in increasing strength than one held for 5 to 6 seconds (Tan, 1998).
- *Brief repetitive isometric exercise (BRIME) regime*: the client completes 5 to 10 brief but maximum isometric contractions, each held 5 to 16 seconds and performed against resistance. This exercise regime is done daily (Tan, 1998).
- *Multiple angle isometric exercise regime*: resistance is applied at least every 20 degrees through ROM. For example, the client completes 10 sets of 10 repetitions with each contraction lasting 10 seconds in every 10 degrees of the ROM ("rule of tens") (Tan, 1998).
- *Prolonged method*: involves holding an isometric contraction as long as possible and then repeating this 10 times. The amount of time the client maintains the maximal effort for 10 repetitions is increased (Trombly, 1995).

Figure 11-8A. Self resistance for shoulder flexion.

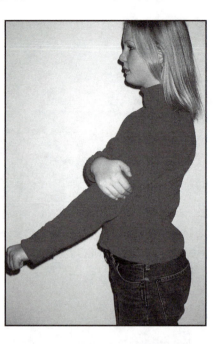

Figure 11-8B. Self resistance for shoulder abduction.

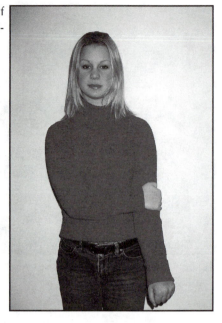

Figure 11-9A. Isometric shoulder flexion resistance.

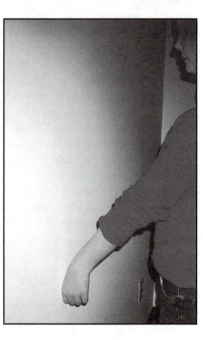

Figure 11-9B. Isometric resistance for shoulder abduction.

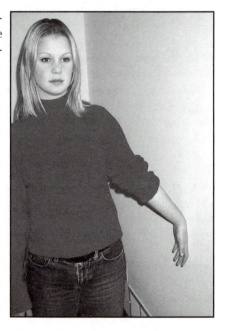

- *Weighted method:* when the client holds a contraction against resistance 30 to 45 seconds with a 15-second rest between each of the 10 repetitions (Trombly, 1995).

When using exercise machines such as Cybex (Medway, MA), Biodex (Shirley, NY), Kincom (Harrison, TN), Lido, Merac, and Orthotron II, isokinetic strengthening exercise is being done. This is a type of dynamic exercise performed with constant angular joint velocity (i.e., the muscle shortens/lengthens at a constant rate) and the load may be variable.

When clients are engaged in resistive, strengthening activities, it is important to caution them to avoid holding their breath while performing the task. By having them count, talk, or sing during the task, the Valsalva maneuver (holding the breath while exerting effort, which raises the blood pressure) will be avoided. This is especially important during isometric exercise and activities with heavy resistance.

Being aware of the level of fatigue will help prevent overwork of weak muscles and prevent substitution movements. Use care when developing strengthening programs for clients with osteoporosis, which may be suspected if the client has rheumatoid arthritis, if she is a postmenopausal woman, or has systemic steroidal use.

Be aware of the client's level of muscle soreness. Muscle soreness is usually delayed 24 to 48 hours after exercise and is caused by microtrauma to connective tissue and myofibrils. Muscle soreness

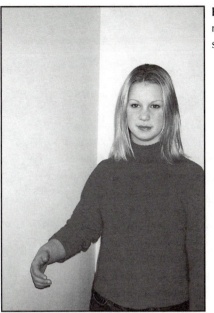

Figure 11-9C. Isometric resistance for shoulder rotation.

may be more severe and frequent with eccentric than concentric exercise against resistance. It can be minimized or prevented by ensuring a sufficient warm up and cool down prior to initiation of the activities, stretching prior to heavy resistance, and by gradually increasing the resistance as strength improves. Controlling the rate or velocity of the contraction also is a variable and contractions should be slow and controlled.

The benefits of warming up prior to strenuous activities are:
1. Cold muscles and tissues do not stretch very easily. Use of modalities will warm the tissues. Warming up the muscles and tissues tend to relax them, which make them more easily stretched.
2. With aerobic activities, the warm-up period prepares the heart, cardiovascular system, and muscles for activity. It has been shown that attempting to perform strenuous activities without adequate warm-up may precipitate cardiac arrhythmia even in those without heart disease.
3. Warming up causes the blood vessels that supply muscles involved in the activity to dilate and vessels supplying less involved parts to constrict. This provides additional oxygen to the muscles requiring the energy for the task.
4. Muscles not properly warmed up may work anaerobically without sufficient oxygen. As a result, the muscles may become prematurely fatigued and lactic acid will accumulate (Bird, 1992).

Warming up may involve gentle activities or exercises, followed by a few minutes of low intensity aerobic activities and then some gentle stretching. The warm-up period should be 5 to 10 minutes, which will prepare the body for more strenuous stress. Cooling down is similar to warming up but with decreasing physical demands placed on the body. Cooling down enables the body to eliminate metabolic wastes, bring in additional oxygen, and to gradually reduce the heart rate to resting level, which helps to reduce dizziness or fainting.

Developing intervention for clients is an individualized process. However, knowledge of different diagnostic categories not only provides information about the etiology and disease course but also prognostic information. By using this knowledge with procedural reasoning, intervention will be enhanced. Some special diagnosis-based cases relative to strengthening include:

- *Parkinson's disease.* In this case, strength is not the major presenting problem; rigidity is. Rigidity represents a problem in muscle tone that is more aptly treated using sensorimotor/neurodevelopmental approaches. Instead of focusing on increasing strength, activities and exercises should emphasize increasing mobility and rapid, rhythmical movements.
- *Cerebral vascular disease (CVA).* Many clients who have had a CVA have muscle tone problems ranging from flaccidity to spasticity. The generally accepted practice is to normalize tone and to strengthen only those muscles that are able to be controlled by the individual. Volitional control of muscles is required. Strengthening is not done with muscles moving in stereotypic, reflexive, or synergistic patterns. Much research is underway about tone and strengthening issues relative to clients who have had a CVA.
- *Cardiopulmonary diseases.* It is imperative to avoid isometric exercise because this type of muscle contraction increases heart rate and blood pressure. These individuals also fatigue more quickly due to decreased oxygen availability and they require a longer amount of time to recover from exercise.
- *Rheumatoid arthritis.* Strengthening may be done if the client is in remission and not in an acute, inflammatory phase. Isometric exercises and activities are preferred since no joint movement occurs.
- *Multiple sclerosis (MS).* Be aware that the client with MS will more likely be fatigued in the afternoon and more energetic early in the morning and in the evening, although this may vary based on the individual. In addition, the environment is important when working with the client with MS because heat is fatiguing to these individuals.
- *Guillian-Barré.* It is very important to avoid overfatiguing the recovering muscles (Table 11-10).

COORDINATION

Coordination can be defined as the ability to produce accurate, controlled movements characterized by smoothness, rhythm, appropriate speed, appropriate muscle tension, a minimal number of muscles involved to accomplish the movement, and adequate postural tone and equilibrium. A person is incoordinated when there are errors in rate, rhythm, range, direction and force of movement (Nuismer et al., 1997). Observation is important to identify irregular movements or sudden movements meant to compensate for incoordination. Factors that increase incoordination may include poor balance, fear, too much resistance, pain, fatigue, strong emotions, and prolonged inactivity.

Coordination involves smooth, rhythmical movement that is a function of the cerebellum. Also needed are intact proprioceptors and perceptual-motor systems, especially spatial orientation, vision and body scheme (closely associated with proprioceptors). Coordination is also influenced by the extrapyramidal system, and

Table 11-10.

INCREASING STRENGTH

Goal		Method	Principle/Rationale	Example
Strength will be increased (indicate where/which muscles, R/L/B) to ____ (what level of improvement) to perform (tasks) using...	[in a trace muscle]	Isometric exercise	Against no resistance, which recruits more motor units and increases proprioceptive awareness of individual muscles as they contract.	Electric stimulation Biofeedback machine Vibrators Manual contacts Isometric exercises: 　Brief maximal 　Brief repetitive 　Multiple angle 　Prolonged method 　Weighted methods
	[in a poor minus or fair minus muscle]	Active assistive exercise with assistance to complete the motion	Which recruits more motor units and causes hypertrophy of glycolytic fast twitch muscle fibers.	Therapeutic skate Deltoid aid Mobile arm support Manual assistance Bilateral activities: one side is affected
	[in a poor or fair and greater muscle]	Active exercise through full range of motion but against minimal resistance	Which recruits more motor units and causes hypertrophy of glycolytic fast-twitch muscle fibers.	Shoulder wheel Combing short hair Electric typewriter Clothespin races Needlepoint Mosaic tile project Computer work
	[in a poor plus, fair plus, or good minus and above muscle]	Progressive or regressive resistive exercise against the maximum resistance needed to produce failure-to-lift	Which recruits more motor units and causes hypertrophy of glycolytic fast-twitch muscle fibers.	Weight well Theraplast Theraputty Weighted weaving Overhead rug knotting ADL tasks like dressing Manual resistance via another person, activity Weighted exercises (isometric and isotonic)

Adapted from Dutton, R. (1995). *Clinical reasoning in physical disabilities*. Baltimore: Williams & Wilkins; and Marrelli, T. M., & Krulish, L. H. (1999). *Home care therapy: Quality, documentation and reimbursement*. Boca Grande, FL: Marrelli and Associates, Inc.

is also seen in the resting tremors (pill rolling) found in clients with Parkinson's disease. Note that coordination not only refers to the upper extremities but also to gait (ataxia), eyes (nystagmus), and facial muscles (dysarthria). *Dexterity* refers to coordination (smoothness, grace), especially skill and ease in using the hands.

The assessment and treatment of coordination does not seem to correspond with any one frame of reference. Coordination depends on accurate somatosensory feedback for normal reciprocal innervation and cocontraction, which is contrary to the biomechanical approach assumption that sensation is intact. In addition, biomechanical techniques, such as exercise, are often performed in linear patterns along anatomical planes with a constant rhythm. Normal movements are more diagonal with rotary components, irregular rhythms, and large numbers of muscles working together. Also, it is difficult to perform fine coordinated movements when maximum resistance is applied (Demeter et al., 1996). If you have strength and good endurance but are clumsy, you will not be able to resume satisfying life roles in the community. When coordination is an

Table 11-11.

PROBLEMS WITH COORDINATION AND LOCATION OF PROBLEM

Posterior Column Dysfunction: results in loss of proprioception, misjudgment of limb position and balance.
- Ataxia: reeling, wide based, unsteady gait.
- Romberg: inability to maintain balance with eyes closed.

Cerebellar Dysfunction: seen in regulation of loss of smooth voluntary movement and maintenance of upright posture.
- Adiadochokinesis or dysdiadochokinesis: inability or impairment in the ability to perform rapidly alternative movements.
- Dysmetria: inability to estimate the ROM necessary to reach the target of the movement (i.e., touches cheek instead of nose); "over-shooting".
- Tremor: intention tremor during voluntary movement intensified at the termination of the movement (often seen in multiple sclerosis); tremor is in proximal parts due to lack of stability.
- Nystagmus: involuntary movement of the eyeballs up and down and back and forth or in rotary motion.
- Hypotonia: decreased resistance to passive stretch.
- Dysarthria: explosive or slurred speech.
- Rebound Phenomenon of Holmes: lack of reflex to stop a strong, active motion (i.e., therapist applies pressure in the direction of elbow extension, releases pressure, and arm rebounds toward flexion).
- Asthenia: weak and easily tired muscles.

Basal Ganglia Dysfunction: functions in control of automatic, patterned movements of locomotion and initiation of rhythmical movements.
- Athetosis: slow, writhing motion primarily in distal parts, lack of stability in neck, trunk, and proximal joints; excessive mobility with increased speed but movement is involuntary and purposeless; not present during sleep.
- Dystonia: form of athetosis, characterized by postures (ex: lordosis); not present during sleep; bizarre writhing and twisting movements of trunk and proximal muscles of the extremities.

Extrapyramidal Dysfunction
- Tremors: resting tremors in pill rolling tremor in Parkinson's disease.
- Choreiform movements: irregular, purposeless, coarse, quick, jerky, and dysrhythmic movements; may occur during sleep.
- Spasms: involves contractions of large groups of muscles in arms, legs, and/or neck.
- Ballism: rare; produced by abrupt contractions of axial and proximal musculature of the extremities resulting in limb flying out suddenly; hemiballism = ballism on one side caused by subthalamic lesion on opposite side.

intervention goal, it is usually included after increased range and strength and may be the responsibility of the client, as an outpatient or as a home health goal, since length of stay is so reduced in inpatient facilities.

Neurodevelopmental or sensorimotor approaches (NDT, PNF, Rood) are often cited as treatment approaches to use for deficits in coordination. However, the focus of these interventions is not directly on the improvement of coordination. These approaches assume that good coordination will naturally follow if tone is remediated (Dutton, 1995). While neurodevelopmental approaches stress the sense of normal movement, these approaches are not designed to provide intervention directly for coordination training (Dutton, 1995).

Notice from the definition, a lack of coordination may be in the ability to move at the proper or appropriate *rate* (too fast or too slow). An example might be *dysdiadochokinesis*, or the inability to move within an appropriate range (e.g., Ballism when the limbs fly out suddenly), or to move in a planned, volitional direction (e.g., tremors), or in amount of force (e.g., Rebound Phenomenon of Holmes). Various types of incoordination have been identified along with the structural location of the problem (Table 11-11).

Many structural systems are involved in coordinated movement. Guidelines for evaluation suggested by Pedretti (1996) are varied and include:
- Assess tone and joint mobility.
- Observe client's sitting position and locate any hypertrophied muscles.
- Observe for ataxia proximally to distally.
- Stabilize joints proximally to distally and note differences in performance compared to performance without stabilization.
- Observe for resting or intention tremors. Are the eyes and speech involved?
- Does client's emotional status affect the incoordination?
- How does ataxia or incoordination affect function?

There are many tests of coordination and dexterity. Many are standardized and some are not (Table 11-12). As with any standardized test, it is important to administer the test exactly per protocols and to know with what population the test was standardized (e.g., norms for children ages 8 to 12 would not be applicable to adults). Some coordination and dexterity tests use functional tasks.

Table 11-12.

COORDINATION EVALUATIONS

Block and Box test
Minnesota Rate of Manipulation
Jensen-Taylor Hand Function test
Crawford Small Parts Dexterity Test
Hand Tool Dexterity Test, Bennett
O'Connor Tweezer Dexterity Test
Pennsylvania Bi-Manual Work sample
Purdue Pegboard
Stromberg Dexterity Test
Nine Hole Peg Test
Moberg's Pickup Test
Sister Kenny's Hand Function Test

Commercial Dexterity Tests, Work Samples, or Workstations

BTE Bolt Box and Assembly Tree
Easy Street Environments
Singer Work samples
Tower Work samples
Skills Assessment Module (SAM)
Coats Work samples
Bennett Hand Tool Dexterity Test
The Work System: work simulations for sustained productivity
Valpar Component Work samples
MESA Computerized Screening Tool
JEVS Work samples
BTE Work simulator
LIDO Work set
ERGOS Work simulator
Jacobs Prevocational Skills Assessment (JPSA)

For example, the Jensen Hand Function Test includes seven subtests (writing a short sentence, turning 3 x 5 inch cards over, placing small objects in container, stacking checkers, simulated eating, moving large cans that are light and those that are heavy). Other tools simulate ADL tasks and others have functional tasks plus grasp and pinch evaluations. Some coordination assessments evaluate unilateral function, some only bilateral use of the hands, and some test both. Some tools evaluate gross coordination, fine coordination, or both (Norkin & Levangie, 1992; Pedretti, 1996; Trombly, 1995). Knowing the performance skills required by the client in daily activities will aid in the appropriate tool to use in assessment of coordination.

Treatment of coordination deficits is difficult and may require several approaches. Lesions of the corticospinal system often use sensorimotor approaches to normalize tone and develop normal movement patterns. Normal motor learning to attain proximal stability then mobility and modulation of reflexes and synergies are also used, as are relearning of motor control mechanisms such as

righting and equilibrium reactions. Involuntary movements of cerebellar or extrapyramidal systems may be controlled pharmacologically to control tremors; weighting extremities with tremors is often suggested as a compensatory approach but is impractical in daily activities (Pedretti, 1996).

Exercises for training coordination have the general goal of achieving multimuscular motor patterns that are faster, more precise, and stronger. Repetition is used and the parts of the activity are broken down and attempted separately at first. Initially the tasks are simple and slow, requiring the conscious awareness of the client. Frequent rests are permitted and when the client can perform each step precisely and independently, the steps are made more difficult by grading for speed, force, and complexity (Pedretti, 1996).

ENDURANCE

Endurance is defined as "the ability to sustain cardiac, pulmonary, and musculoskeletal exertion over time" (AOTA, 1994). It would be reasonable to expect endurance limitations with clients who have deficits in local muscle metabolism (e.g., diabetes), cardiovascular system (e.g., congestive heart failure), respiratory system (e.g., emphysema), those on total bed rest 6 or more days, and in clients with paralysis (Dutton, 1995). Endurance may be limited due to activity restrictions, pathology of cardiac or pulmonary systems, or muscle diseases.

Endurance is influenced by three factors: muscle function, oxygen supply, and their combined effects. With cardiorespiratory dysfunction, breathing itself may be exhaustive.

Cardiovascular function is a factor of fitness. This is the ability of the body to take in, transport, and use oxygen (Christiansen & Baum, 1997). Ways to assess cardiorespiratory function are:

- Pulse
- Blood pressure
- Respiration
- Lung volume
- Vital capacity
- Breathing rate
- Pulmonary ventilation
- Cardiac output

Minor adds that "in the absence of pulmonary disease (COLD, COPD), most of the limitation to endurance performance depends not on our ability to inspire and diffuse oxygen, but on the ability of the heart and circulatory system to deliver oxygen and cellular mechanisms to use the oxygen for energy production" (Christiansen & Baum, 1997, p. 261). Cardiorespiratory decondition is seen in increased resting heart rate, decreased heart volume, loss of blood volume, decreased stroke volume, decreased cardiac output, decreased coronary blood flow, impaired orthostatic response, and diminished aerobic capacity. Clinical manifestations of cardiorespiratory deconditioning might include:

- Reduced exercise tolerance demonstrated by increased heart rate and respiration at low work loads.
- Early onset of fatigue.

- Exertional dyspnea.
- Perception of doing heavy or maximal work at low to moderate loads.
- Rise in heart rate and drop in blood pressure upon standing up (orthostatic hypotension), which produces syncope and fainting.

The Borg's rate of perceived exertion (RPE) scale is often used by the client to rate his or her perception of the level of intensity of the activity or exercise as well as the level of pain. While a subjective rating by the client, this scale is commonly used to rate angina, aches in muscles, levels of pain, and in exercise tolerance testing (Tan, 1998). Often the client is asked to rate the intensity or pain on a scale predetermined by the clinician or the client himself. Target heart rate range (THRR) is one way of monitoring aerobic activities. If the pulse rate exceeds the upper limit of the THRR, then the activity is too strenuous and similarly, if the heart rate is below the lower limits, then the intensity should be increased (Tan, 1998).

Another way of monitoring endurance aerobic activities is to use the Karvonen formula, which is:

Maximal HR - resting HR (40 to 85%) + resting HR = THRR.

Formulas have been developed to account for age differences as in the age-adjusted maximal heart rate (AAMHR) where the formula is:

(220-age) (65-85%) = THRR.

This formula is commonly used but is less accurate than the Karvonen formula.

It is the interaction of the cardiovascular and respiratory systems that influence endurance. A conditioned heart produces a greater cardiac output at a lower heart rate than the untrained heart. Less work results in lowered oxygen demand.

Diminished muscular endurance may be due to inactivity resulting in disuse atrophy. The deficits are most notable in the muscles of locomotion following bedrest and are associated with fast twitch/type II muscle fibers. The decreased maximal oxygen consumption is not only a consequence of diminished capacity of the heart to deliver oxygen but also the result of diminished capacity of muscle to use oxygen (Hamil & Knutzen, 1995). The rate of recovery of muscular endurance is much slower than the rate of loss of endurance (Berne & Levy, 1998).

To increase cardiorespiratory and muscular endurance there must be stress imposed on the systems to facilitate adaptation. The overload principle is applicable here but the systems need far less than maximal stress applied. The amount of resistance varies according to different authors from 15 to 40% (Pedretti, 1996) of the repetition maximum to less than 50% of the repetition maximum (Trombly, 1995), or 60 to 90% of the maximum heart rate or 50 to 85% of maximum oxygen uptake. Clients with very low endurance often resume activities based on metabolic equivalent (MET) levels. MET levels indicate endurance and activity tolerance and these levels are often used in cardiac rehabilitation programs. By referring to a table, one can determine the energy required to complete specific activities. Energy is measured by the amount of oxygen consumed while engaged in activities as well as the oxygen required to maintain metabolic functions (Trombly, 1995). The higher the MET level, the more vigorous the activity.

Usually endurance activities and exercises are designed to have less load for a longer duration (low load, high duration). These activities generally target the slow twitch/type I muscle fibers. While there is less than maximal load, there must be some resistance or adaptation will not occur. The probability that a client will engage in activities for a longer period of time is greatly enhanced if that activity is of interest and is meaningful because the client needs to sustain effort for increasingly longer periods of time (Smith et al., 1996). For example, the client may play 2 hours of wheelchair basketball but only do wheelchair laps on a track for 30 minutes (Dutton, 1995).

To facilitate cardiorespiratory and muscular endurance, an activity should require rhythmic, dynamic contractions of large muscle groups (Christiansen & Baum, 1997). As with exercises and activities to increase strength, the intensity, duration, and frequency are carefully controlled. Gradations are based on the client's current level of function with gradual progression. Warm-up and cool down activities are recommended to diminish muscle cramping, soreness, and syncope. Activities and exercises involving excessive use of the arms overhead or those requiring sustained isometric contractions should be avoided because these tend to elevate the blood pressure without cardiovascular (aerobic) benefits. A general guideline of 20 full range repetitions and sustaining the activity for at least 30 seconds done three to five times per week is recommended, but is variable based on individual client abilities (Bird, 1992). The intervention goal is to increase the client's ability to perform repeated motor tasks in daily living and to carry on sustained levels of activity.

Long-term effects of greater endurance and cardiorespiratory fitness include:
- ↓ HR at rest and submaximal effort.
- Submaximal effort with ↑ peak BP during maximal exercise.
- Small ↑ in cardiac output, ↑ coronary blood flow, ↓ exercise recovery time.

Low impact aerobic activities such as a stationary bicycle, cycling, race-walking, calisthenics, swimming, aquatic exercise, rowing, hiking, and cross country skiing can be used for less conditioned clients. High impact activities for more well conditioned clients might include jogging, running, volleyball, hopping, jumping, rope skipping, aerobic dance, and downhill skiing. These activities can be used to increase endurance and strength, and can be incorporated into discharge plans for the client's continued wellness.

The terms *tolerance* and *endurance* are often used interchangeably by therapists. For example, in documentation it may be stated that a client has "increased sitting tolerance from 10 to 20 minutes" where the client's ability to remain upright in the wheelchair has improved. Increases in the number of repetitions of an activity are indicators of increased endurance, such as increasing the num-

Table 11-13.

ENDURANCE

Goal	Method	Principle/Rationale	Example
Client will initially increase endurance (indicate level) to enable performance in (tasks) by using...	Increased duration Increased level in a cardiac step program Increased intensity Increased repetitions	Which gradually stresses cardio-pulmonary system while ensuring rest.	Sitting tolerance in minutes Tolerance for evaluation Graduate to eating while sitting up in a chair Stand instead of sitting to shave Cardiac target heart rate Dress in 10 fewer minutes Feed self 10 additional bites of food Walk 10 additional steps
Client will maximize endurance (indicate level) to enable performance in (tasks) using...	Increased duration Increased level in a cardiac step program Increased intensity Increased repetitions	Which gradually stresses the cardio-pulmonary system and local muscle metabolism of oxidative slow-twitch muscle fibers.	Increase the time involved in an activity (standing at table, completing a full meal) Increase levels on MET charts Perform activities at 50 to 70% maximum levels Dress 10 minutes faster than baseline Increase number of spoonfuls of food per meal Increase the number of wheelchair pushups

Adapted from Dutton, R. (1995). *Clinical reasoning in physical disabilities*. Baltimore: Williams & Wilkins; and Marrelli, T. M., & Krulish, L. H. (1999). *Home care therapy: Quality, documentation and reimbursement*. Boca Grande, FL: Marrelli and Associates, Inc.

ber of spoonfuls per meal (Pedretti, 1996). The client is increasing aspects of endurance where the activities or exercises are being performed at less than maximal levels of intensity for increased periods of time or number of repetitions.

Increased sitting tolerance is often an indication of improved postural control. This is the "ability to position and maintain head, neck and trunk with appropriate weight shift, midline orientation and righting reactions" (AOTA, 1994). Increasing postural control is seen in gradual increases in endurance by means of increased time or repetitions. Intervention that is aimed at remediation of righting reactions and weight bearing is usually a focus of neurodevelopmental/sensorimotor treatment approaches. Positioning and use of adapted seating devices could well be considered rehabilitation or compensatory strategies if used to compensate, not remediate, lost function (Table 11-13).

CASE STUDY

The following case study is provided to demonstrate how theory influences intervention. This case study has elements that are more appropriately considered within a remediation or biomechanical intervention approach, while other aspects are better served using a compensatory/adaptation or rehabilitation construct. This same case study is used in Chapter 12 so that the elements appropriate to each theory can be seen as they relate to this case. Other theories not covered in this text may also be appropriate and it is important to consider whether all of the approaches selected can be implemented concurrently with others, or if the design of the intervention needs to be sequential in nature.

Maggie

Maggie is a 61-year-old female referred to home health occupational therapy on October 29th with a diagnosis of right Colles fracture. Maggie fell while shopping at her neighborhood department store on October 27th. The physician has ordered occupational therapy to evaluate and treat.

On your first visit to see Maggie, you interview her and find out the following information. Maggie was in excellent health prior to this injury. Maggie's son, Fred, lives in the next town. She works part-time in her son's accounting office. A widow, she lives alone with her cat and her dog. Maggie is concerned that since she lives alone she needs to be able to do all of the cooking, cleaning, and care for her dog and cat. Her son is only able to come to her home every other day or every 3 days to assist with some of these activities.

Maggie is concerned about her present situation. She is right-handed and states that although she tries her best, she is not able to do very much for herself. Maggie has been very active in her local church organization. Maggie always heads up the Christmas crafts bazaar. Part of her responsibilities for the bazaar include organizing and teaching at craft nights. Maggie also has been one of the primary cooks for the annual fish dinner held just before Easter. She states that the church especially needs her this year as the other primary cook is moving to another state. She doesn't want to let the church organization down.

In the emergency room on October 27th, the emergency room physician performed a closed reduction and applied a plaster cast from mid-humeral level to the metacarpophalangeal (MCP) joints of the right hand. The elbow is casted in approximately 90 degrees of elbow flexion and the wrist is casted in approximately 30 degrees of wrist flexion. Maggie states that the physician has instructed her to stay home for the next 2 weeks and not to drive or do any housework. This is confirmed when you speak to the physician. A summary of information about Maggie as well as analysis of additional information that is needed and ideas about the next steps are as follows:

Facts

- 61-year-old female
- Enjoys shopping
- Right Colles fracture
- Fractures are immobilized, cause pain and edema
- Fractures may limit the use of the UE
- Lives alone
- Was independent in ADL, IADL
- Cares for dog and cat
- Active in church craft bazaar and fish dinner
- Anxious about present situation
- Immobilized in plaster cast
- Physician restricted activities for 2 weeks

Additional Information Needed

- How did Maggie fall?
- Precautions
- Medical management of Colles fracture
- Possible complications
- Prognosis to return to prior level of function
- Tasks that Maggie will need to do to resume roles

Action

- Continue dialogue with Maggie
- Review medical record
- Consult with physician
- Consult orthopedic textbooks and OT texts
- Perform OT assessments

From this information, an evaluation plan can be developed. Several assessments have been listed but these are not the only assessments that can be used to address the concerns about Maggie.

Evaluation Plan

Concerns

1. Maggie's perception of her strengths and weaknesses and her priorities for therapy.
2. Decreased ADL performance due to right (dominant) UE in cast.
3. Unable to carry out worker and volunteer roles.
4. Unable to participate in leisure pursuits.
5. Sensorimotor concerns (sensory): possible sensory loss or altered sensation due to pressure on nerves from swelling or tight cast.
6. Sensorimotor concerns (motor): potential for edema, stiffness and complex regional pain syndrome (CRPS) (previously known as reflex sympathetic dystrophy [RSD]) in right hand; potential for frozen right shoulder.
7. Psychological and cognitive concerns: potential for depression due to loss of role performance and feelings of helplessness.

Assessments

1. Canadian Occupational Therapy Performance Measure (COPM) or other client centered informal interview tool.
2. Observe Maggie attempting to perform ADL tasks; Klein-Bell ADL assessment; self report; Functional Independence Measure (FIM).
3. Interview Maggie to determine specific worker and volunteer tasks and activities.
4. Interest checklist; formal or informal interview.
5. Sensory evaluation to exposed areas; observe cast for fit, look for areas of redness where cast is pressing against the skin.
6. AROM and PROM of PIP and DIP joints of the right hand; circumferential edema measurements of the digits; pain assessment; AROM and PROM of right shoulder.
7. Formal and informal interview; observe Maggie during evaluation; speak with family members and other team members.

How Assessment Results Will be Used

1. Set client-centered goals for therapy; establish rapport; gain better understanding of Maggie's occupational context.
2. Assess potential for teaching compensatory techniques or use of adaptive equipment; determine components of ADL tasks causing difficulty; determine baseline for therapy.
3. Determine readiness for return to work and volunteer duties; assess potential for adapting tasks and activities.

4. Determine realistic leisure interest; assess potential for adapting leisure activities.

5. Set baseline for therapy; make suggestions for alterations of cast if necessary; determine need to teach compensatory techniques or sensory reeducation program if sensation is impaired or absent.

6. Set baseline for therapy; develop treatment plan that includes management of edema and home exercise program (HEP) to maintain ROM and prevent complications.

7. Determine Maggie's motivation for therapy; assess ability to follow directions and carry out HEP, set realistic goals appropriate for Maggie's cognitive and emotional status.

You evaluated Maggie and found the following:

Maggie is cognitively intact and motivated to be independent. Maggie is proud as she describes her success at figuring out how to open the foil packet of cat food with her left hand so that she could feed her cat. She is unable to don some types of blouses and dresses over the cast and is not able to don pants or skirts with closures. She requires minimal assistance to don a house dress, underpants and socks. She is unable to don her bra or panty hose, or tie her shoes/sneakers. Because of the inability to use her dominant right hand, Maggie is unable to manage buttons, has difficulty feeding herself with her nondominant left hand (spills food on herself frequently), requires minimal assist with personal hygiene after toileting, sponge bathing, and brushing her teeth. She requires maximal assistance in simple meal preparation. Maggie states she is able to get herself some simple food items, such as prepared foods (prepared by her son's wife) from plastic containers. She is dependent in household chores such as cleaning.

Through further interview, you learn that much of Maggie's work at her son's office involves working with Excel, a spreadsheet computer program. She has a computer at home and is an avid Internet user. She tells you that it is difficult to use the computer now because she cannot use her right hand.

Tasks associated with her responsibilities as chairperson of the Christmas craft bazaar include phoning church members to inform them of meeting times and craft supplies they will be required to bring, and delegation of other responsibilities such as making refreshments, teaching certain crafts, and clean-up duties. She is having difficulty using her rotary dial telephone to keep in touch with other church volunteers.

Maggie complains of (c/o) moderate pain in her right upper extremity, mainly the wrist and fingers. She rates her pain an 8 on a scale of 1 to 10. She describes it as a burning, throbbing type of pain. Severe edema is noted in all of the digits of the right hand (approximately two times the size of the left hand). She has a great deal of difficulty flexing her fingers to make a fist (the cast restricts the MP motion). She is unable to oppose her thumb to her index or any other finger. She is unable to hold any objects in her right hand because of the cast. She states that at times her hand feels numb and other times she has paresthesia. The fingers are discolored, a dusky reddish color.

In your conversation with the home health coordinator and the social worker, you find out that Maggie's insurance will cover home health occupational therapy for up to 3 months for the purpose of improving independence in ADL. The following would be an example of the intervention that would address biomechanical remediation concerns in this case. This is not a complete intervention plan in that many areas that can be addressed in treatment by an occupational therapist are not included. By combining the treatment plan for the compensation/adaptation/rehabilitation treatment plan with this, a more complete intervention for Maggie can be realized.

In Table 11-14, deficits as identified previously are related directed to long- and short-term outcomes. Specific principles or rationales are provided so that the reason for the specific intervention is clear.

SUMMARY

- The biomechanical frame of reference is a remediation intervention approach. In this approach, there is an expectation of an improvement in a performance component that will lead to improved occupational performance.

- The biomechanical frame of reference focuses on musculoskeletal system functions that include strength, endurance, range of motion, tissue integrity, and structural stability.

- Since this frame of reference focuses on the musculoskeletal system, physical fitness and health also are parts of this approach. Strategies to improve muscle function and range of motion in those with activity and participation limitations also apply to those without restrictions as part of an overall health promotion objective.

REFERENCES

American Occupational Therapy Association. (2002). Occupational therapy practice framework: Domain and process. *Am J Occup Ther*, 56, 609-639.

American Occupational Therapy Association. (1994). Uniform terminology for occupational therapy (3rd ed.). *Am J Occup Ther*, 48(11), 1047-1054.

Baxter, R. (1998). *Pocket guide to musculoskeletal assessment*. Philadelphia: W. B. Saunders Co.

Berne, R. M., & Levy, M. N. (1998). *Physiology* (4th ed.). St. Louis, MO: C. V. Mosby Co.

Bird, S. R. (1992). *Exercise physiology for health professionals*. San Diego, CA: Singular Publishing Group, Inc.

Christiansen, C., & Baum, C. (1997). *Occupational therapy: Enabling function and well being* (2nd ed.) Thorofare, NJ: SLACK Incorporated.

Demeter, S. L., Andersson, G. B. J., & Smith, G. M. (1996). *Disability evaluation*. St. Louis, MO: Mosby.

Dutton, R. (1995). *Clinical reasoning in physical disabilities*. Baltimore: Williams & Wilkins.

Table 11-14.

TREATMENT PLAN: BIOMECHANICAL REMEDIATION APPROACH

Deficits	Stage-Specific Cause	Short-Term Goals	Methods	Principle	Specific Activity/Modality
1. Potential for muscle wasting in right wrist extensors and flexors limiting functional use of right UE.	1. Immobilization in cast.	1. Client will perform HEP (home exercise program) of isometric exercises with minimal verbal cues.	1. Educate client in isometric exercises for right wrist muscles.	1. Active contraction of muscle fibers will maintain muscle bulk.	1. Client will learn techniques of performing isometric exercises for R wrist musculature using 10 repetitions of each exercise, 3 times a day.
2. Potential for active ROM and muscle strength to decrease in right shoulder, which will limit functional use of RUE.	2. Inability to use RUE for functional activities.	2. Client will perform home activity program with minimal assist to prevent decrease in AROM and muscle strength in right shoulder motions and muscle groups.	2. Client will be educated in activities/exercises to move UE through all shoulder motions.	2. Stretch of muscles on connective tissue through full ROM daily prevents shortening of these tissues. Stress provided by weight of cast will maintain or increase muscle bulk.	2. Therapist will provide written and videotaped guide to HEP to move UE through all shoulder motions. Client will learn a HEP.
3. Client has severe edema in right digits with potential for contractures, which limit functional use of RUE.	3. Immobilization in cast.	3. Client will independently perform self retrograde massage.	3. Application of pressure distally to proximally through massage of the hand.	3. Massage will prevent filtration of fluids from capillaries into the interstitial tissues and assist with blood and lymph flow.	3. Therapist will perform retrograde massage to R hand each treatment session. Client will be educated in self retrograde massage with instructions to perform 3 times a day.

Fisher, A. G. (1998). Uniting practice and theory in an occupational framework: 1998 Eleanor Clarke Slagle Lecture. *Amer J Occup Ther*, 52(7), 509-521.

Galley, P. M., & Forster, A. L. (1987). *Human movement: An introductory text for physiotherapy students* (2nd ed.). New York: Churchill-Livingstone.

Hamil, J., & Knutzen, K. M. (1995). *Biomechanical basis of human movement*. Baltimore: Williams & Wilkins,

Irion, G. (2000). *Physiology: The basis of clinical practice*. Thorofare, NJ: SLACK Incorporated.

Jacobs, K., & Bettencourt, C. M. (1995). *Ergonomics for therapists*. Boston: Butterworth-Heinemann.

Kielhofner, G. (1992). *Conceptual foundations of occupational therapy*. Philadelphia: F. A. Davis Co.

Kisner, C., & Colby, L. A. (1990). *Therapeutic exercise: Foundations and techniques* (2nd ed.). Philadelphia: F. A. Davis.

McGinnis, P. M. (1999). *Biomechanics of sport and exercise*. Champaign, IL: Human Kinetics.

Minor, A. D., Lippert, L. S., & Minor, S. D. (1998). *Kinesiology laboratory manual for physical therapy assistants*. Philadelphia: F.A. Davis Co.

Moyers, P. A. (1999). The guide to occupational therapy practice. *Amer J Occup Ther*, 53(3), 247-321.

Norkin, C. C., & Levangie, P. K. (1992). *Joint structure and function: A comprehensive analysis* (2nd ed.). Philadelphia: F. A. Davis Co.

Nuismer, B. A., Ekes, A. M., & Holm, M. B. (1997). The use of low load prolonged stretch devices in rehabilitation program in the pacific northwest. *Amer J Occup Ther*, 51(37), 538-545.

Pedretti, L. W. (1996). *Occupational therapy: Practice skills for physical dysfunction* (4th ed.). St Louis, MO: C.V. Mosby.

Rantanen, T., Harris, T., Leveille, S. G., Visser, M., Foley, D., Masaki, K., Guralnik, J. M.. (2000). Muscle strength and body mass index as long-term predictors of mortality in initially healthy men. *Journals of Gerontology. Series A, Biological Sciences and Medical*, 55(3), 168-73.

Smith, L. K., Weiss, E. L., & Lehmkuhl, L. D. (1996). *Brunnstrom's clinical kinesiology* (5th ed.). Philadelphia: F. A. Davis Co.

Steinbeck, T. (1986). Purposeful activity and performance. *Am J Occup Ther, 40*(8), 529-534.

Tan, J. C. (1998). *Practical manual of physical medicine and rehabilitation.* St. Louis, MO: C. V. Mosby

Thompson, C. W., & Floyd, R. T. (1994). *Manual of structural kinesiology* (12th ed.). St. Louis, MO: C. V. Mosby.

Trombly, C. A. (Ed.). (1995). *Occupational therapy for physical dysfunction* (4th ed.). Baltimore: Williams and Wilkins.

BIBLIOGRAPHY

American Occupational Therapy Association. (1995). Position paper: Occupational performance: Occupational therapy's definition of function. *Am J Occup Ther, 49*(10), 1019-1020.

American Occupational Therapy Association. (1997). Statement-Fundamental concepts of occupational therapy: Occupation, purposeful activity and function. *Am J Occup Ther, 51*(10), 864-866.

Andersen, L. T. (2001). *Adult physical disabilities: Case studies for learning.* SLACK Incorporated: Thorofare, NJ.

Asher, I. E. (1996). *Occupational therapy assessment tools: An annotated index* (2nd ed.). Bethesda, MD: American Occupational Therapy Association.

Caillet, R. (1996). *Soft tissue pain and disability* (3rd ed.). Philadelphia: F. A. Davis Co.

Daniels, L., & Worthingham, C. (1977). *Therapeutic exercise for body alignment and function* (2nd ed.). Philadelphia: W. B. Saunders Co.

Greene, D. P., & Roberts, S. L. (1999). *Kinesiology: Movement in the context of activity.* St. Louis, MO: Mosby.

Joe, B. E. (1996). Can you justify all those treatments? *OT Week, 10*(2), 15-16.

Konin, J. G. (1999). *Practical kinesiology for the physical therapist assistant.* Thorofare, NJ: SLACK Incorporated.

Marrelli, T. M., & Krulish, L. H. (1999). *Home care therapy: Quality, documentation and reimbursement.* Boca Grande, FL: Marrelli and Associates, Inc.

Neistadt, M. E., & Seymour, S. G. (1995). Treatment activity preferences of occupational therapists in adult physical dysfunction settings. *Amer J Occup Ther, 49*(5), 437-443.

Shankar, K. (1999). *Exercise prescription.* Philadelphia: Hanley & Belfus, Inc.

Turner, A., Foster, M., & Johnson, S. E. (1996). *Occupational therapy and physical dysfunction: Principles, skills and practice* (4th ed.). New York: Churchill Livingstone.

Van Deusen, J., & Brunt, D. (1997). *Assessment in occupational therapy and physical therapy.* Philadelphia: W. B. Saunders Co.

Zelenka, J. P., Floren, A. E., & Jordan, J. J. (1966). Minimal forces to move patients. *Am J Occup Ther, 50*(5), 354-361.

Rehabilitation

The rehabilitation frame of reference is a compensatory and adaptation approach. Often this approach is used when there is little or no expectation for change or improvement in the performance skills and abilities, leaving residual impairments and making remediation attempts futile or unproductive. When there is limited time for intervention or the client or family prefers a more immediate resolution to functional problems, rehabilitation approaches may also be used. Compensatory and adaptive strategies are valuable when activity limitations and participation restrictions interfere with occupational performance and when there are problems of safety during occupational performance (Moyers, 1999).

While some authors suggest that rehabilitation is a group of techniques rather than a theoretical approach (Dutton, 1995), this frame of reference has been used extensively in occupational therapy since the beginning of the practice of the profession.

ASSUMPTIONS

One assumption of this frame of reference is that the ability to function is essential to well-being and that there are secondary benefits to be gained by improving performance despite physical, cognitive, psychological, or social dysfunctions (Turner, Foster & Johnson, 1996). Humans are capable of adapting to their limitations by learning new methods of doing activities, by responding to new teaching processes, and by utilizing adapted objects and environments to their advantage. Clients are capable of capitalizing on their strengths as a healthy means of compensating for their limitations.

Through adaptation and compensation, clients can regain meaning and resumption of roles and a sense of purpose. Motivation for independence is based on the client's values, roles (volitional and habitual subsystems), and context (home environment, resources, financial status, family situation, age). The individual's involvement in choosing methods to improve daily life activities is also seen as an important part of the rehabilitation frame of reference. Use of compensatory strategies will facilitate integration of the client into the family, community, and previous life roles.

The reasoning used in this approach should reflect a top-down approach where successful accomplishment of activities of daily living (ADL), work tasks, and play and leisure pursuits are the focus of intervention rather than specific changes in anatomic, physiologic, or psychological attributes. In a top-down hierarchy, the intervention steps are to first identify the environmental demands and resources of the individual. What aspects of the context (including temporal aspects such as time and disability status) and environment (physical, social, and cultural aspects) are important variables to this person? It is imperative to ask the client and caregiver about the volitional and habitual subsystems. What does the client want to do? What does the client usually do? What does this person need to do to successfully engage in desired roles? How important are specific activities to this person? After gathering this information, an evaluation of the areas of occupation, including work, play, leisure, and self-care is completed to determine functional capabilities of the individual. Prerequisite skills that the patient lacks and task demands are compared with intervention aimed at matching the compensatory or adapted method with the prerequisite skill that the client lacks. Some authors indicate that in the rehabilitation approach, the client needs to acquire the ability to set his or her own life's direction, control it, and take responsibility for it with the acquisition of an attitude of independence as a basic part of the theoretical base (AOTA, 1995).

FUNCTION/DYSFUNCTION CRITERIA

The theoretical base of the rehabilitation frame of reference is in medicine and in the physical sciences. *Function* is the ability to maintain oneself, take care of others and the home; the ability to advance oneself through work, learning, and financial management; and to enhance the self through self-actualizing activities. This would necessitate certain levels of motor, sensory, cognitive, intrapersonal, and interpersonal subskills and role-relevant behaviors. Function is the ability to engage in constructive activity successfully along a continuum of independence.

Dysfunction is the loss of the ability to maintain and care for oneself and others and the home. It is the loss of the ability to advance oneself through work, learning, and the loss of financial management. While function occurs through normal development, dysfunction occurs through degenerative disorders, disease, or trauma (problems in structure or function).

Some merits to this intervention approach are that it is widely documented and extensively used. The foundational concepts are easy to explain to the client and caregiver with intervention often visual, concrete, and with rapid results. A range of options is available and can be easily matched to the needs of the individual. There is no rigid sequencing of intervention steps and the rehabilitation approach can be used to meet short-term needs as well as to compensate for permanent deficits.

Since the rehabilitation approach is associated with the medical model, there may be the tendency to be reductionistic and use recipe-like thinking rather than clinical reasoning to evaluate the range of intervention options. For example, one may be tempted to provide a long-handled sponge to all clients with total hip replacements without evaluating the actual need for the device. Often by providing adapted equipment or by teaching a modified technique, intervention can be relatively inexpensive and rapid. While this is a definite advantage to this approach, it is truly advantageous only if the intervention provided is what the client really needs, and not just done because it saved time and money or at the expense of a more in-depth evaluation of the client and his or her unique situation.

Some clients may refuse to participate in compensatory or adapted techniques or use of special equipment or tools because this acceptance forces a recognition of permanent loss of function. An understanding of the client's psychological adjustment to these losses is essential and depression has been found to be a strong predictor of rehabilitation failure. An attitude of assertiveness is helpful in adjustment, as is a high frustration tolerance and the ability to understand and learn new ways to do things.

Being able to understand abstract concepts, such as joint protection or safety precautions, is important in independent living. Using Allen cognitive levels, at Level 4, it is recommended that a caregiver be trained; at Level 5, clients are unable to implement abstract procedures; and at Level 6, it is important to stress problem solving rather than attempting to train the client in every possible means of compensation via rote learning (Dutton, 1995).

EVALUATION

Evaluation in the rehabilitation frame of reference focuses on those subskills and role-relevant behaviors that are necessary for independent functioning. The next step is to identify those subskills and role-relevant behaviors that cannot be performed independently, and/or those that will never be performed independently given the limitations imposed by the client's condition. Goals are established with the client based on the tasks the client is expected to perform, the expected environment, and factors such as time and cost. So while assessment starts with context and evaluation of areas of occupation as part of the occupational profile, a total analysis of client factors, performance skills, performance patterns, activity demands, and client factors is often necessary in this approach.

INTERVENTION

Intervention uses adaptive equipment and ways to adapt the environment to enable change. These adaptations replace normal function or compensate for abnormal function (AOTA, 1995).

These rehabilitation methods may include:

Changing the task via:
- Adapted task methods or procedures
- Adapting the task objects, adaptive devices, or orthotics

Changing the context via:
- Environmental modification
- Training the caregiver or family (see Appendix N)

The role of the therapist is to work with the client to determine the best method for performing a task and to determine the best teaching process for the client. The therapist will design, construct, recommend, and order the adaptive equipment. Adaptations to the home, work site, or school will be collaboratively decided upon by the therapist, client, family, and others. Identification of community resources is also an important part of the rehabilitation process in returning the client to his or her home environment and in enabling the client to assume the responsibility for his or her own health and well-being.

Changing the Task

This aspect of the rehabilitation approach is often referred to as *compensation* in that the aim is to match the task to the abilities of the client. Compensation may be made by altering the task method or procedures or by adapting the task objects.

Altering the Task Method

Altering the task method involves teaching the client new, more efficient and effective ways to complete a task using skills that closely correspond with the client's remaining capacities. Use of client skills and abilities in which there are no deficiencies is the aim in the altered task method. Because the client is altering a method and is doing a daily task in a new way, the client must have a sufficient capacity for new learning as well as adequate time for supervised practice of the new skill. Changing the way one puts on a shirt or the way one eats requires motivation by the client and/or caregiver to learn and apply the new methods to the task (Moyers, 1999).

Altering the task method may require modifications of techniques, learning new skills, or transferring existing skills to new situations. An example of a modifying technique is having a client with a paralyzed arm put the affected extremity into the shirt first and then dress the unaffected arm. A "trick" movement may be used by a client with C6 quadriplegia who extends and locks the elbow and externally rotates the shoulder as a compensatory movement for the loss of triceps function. Learning to use gravity as an assist rather than as a force to overcome is an adaptive technique, as is changing body mechanics or leverage used in activities so that they work to the client's advantage (e.g., letting gravity pull the forearm down to extend the elbow when there is paralysis of the triceps muscle).

Ways of altering task methods are numerous, flexible, and easily personalized. When the client is successful in performing the task, this enhances self-confidence and self-esteem. Modifying the procedure is usually cost-effective with long-term effectiveness.

Another advantage to altering the task method is that the changes made in how the task is done are rarely visible and so this may be more acceptable to clients (Dutton, 1995). While this is an advantage to some, to others the lack of external prompts as reminders is a disadvantage.

Disadvantages to changing the task by altering the procedure are that this requires new learning and a change of habit. The client and/or caregiver must be motivated and committed to making this change in daily activities. Dutton adds that some clients feel that an analysis of personal habits is seen as a form of criticism and that their privacy has been invaded (Dutton, 1995).

The specific examples presented are not meant to be an exhaustive list of all possible adaptations that can be made to the ways we do everyday activities. Whole texts are devoted to presenting numerous options for techniques if one has weakness on one side as occurs with a CVA or weakness or paralysis in all four extremities as may occur with a spinal cord injury. These examples are either commonly encountered or considered representative of adaptations that are encountered in practice.

Adapted Task Methods Used to Substitute for Lost or Decreased Range of Motion

Adapted task methods used to substitute for lost or decreased range of motion (ROM) will be addressed based on adaptations made for clients with specific diagnoses. The adaptations presented can be generalized from the specific categories to similar client factor and performance skill deficits that may not have the same diagnosis as those presented. For example, in clients with weakness in all four extremities due to multiple sclerosis, some of the adaptations for the spinal cord injured (SCI) client may also apply to the client with multiple sclerosis. Also, particular problems experienced by clients with loss of function on one side of the body (as in cerebral vascular accidents [CVA]) have been included in the adapted techniques for loss of ROM. Those clients experiencing weakness in all four extremities due to spinal cord injury are discussed in sections pertaining to loss of strength. This was an arbitrary decision and it is acknowledged that adapted techniques used by clients with CVA and SCI may be necessary due to limitations in both strength and ROM. However, the limitations experienced by a client with a CVA are likely to be due to loss of motion (whether due to abnormal tone or due to synergistic movements) and clients with SCI are most limited by decreased strength in remaining muscles.

Clients who have experienced a loss of ROM on one side of the body (e.g., CVA) can use the unaffected arm and leg to independently propel a wheelchair. Alternative ways of transferring, dressing, and moving from one place to another are necessary when the client is able to move only one side of the body.

Bed Mobility

Clients with loss on one side of the body will be able to roll toward the affected side but will have greater difficulty rolling toward the unaffected side. To roll to the unaffected side from supine, have the client place the unaffected foot under the affected leg. Slide the legs to the edge of the bed. Using the unaffected arm, carry the affected arm across body and then he or she pulls him- or herself over onto the unaffected side by holding the side of the bed. An alternative method advocated by Bobath is to have the client clasp both hands together with the thumb of the affected hand above the sound one, elbows extended, shoulder flexed above 90 degrees. The client then swings the clasped arms side to side to build momentum, which will carry him onto his side. Either method can be carried to the next step or that of coming to a sitting position. Once rolled onto the side, with the unaffected arm, push against the bed while swinging legs over the side of the bed to come to a sitting position. An alternative to crossing the affected leg over the unaffected is to bring the unaffected leg over the edge of the bed while simultaneously pushing against the bed with the unaffected arm. The affected leg will follow and the client will be in a sitting position. In either case, it is important to roll all of the way onto the side before pushing to sit up, as this will help to position the arm to push up and will create less strain on the back.

Transfers

A pivot transfer is a common transfer type for clients with loss of one side of the body. Since the patient can partially weight bear on one lower extremity, this transfer is a good choice and can be done independently or with assistance. If the client is unsafe with a pivot transfer or unable to perform the transfer even with assistance, sliding board transfers would be the next viable transfer option.

Pivot transfers generally are set up to move the person in a 90 degree angle, although some pivot transfers are in a 180 degree arc if in restricted spaces (like a bathroom) (Table 12-1). Initially, clients are taught to transfer to the uninvolved side and eventually teaching will involve transfers to the involved side, too, for greater independence. For the client to be considered independent in transfers, he or she should be able to:
- Demonstrate adequate safety awareness.
- Move in bed.
- Maintain a coactive trunk in sitting.
- Follow directions (simple verbal or written) (Palmer & Toms, 1992).

Dressing

Dressing for a client with loss of function on one side of the body generally follows the pattern that the affected extremity is dressed first and undressed last. In putting on a shirt, the overhead method is seen as less confusing for clients with sensory and perceptual impairments. This overhead method, however, is cumbersome for dresses and not possible for use with coats. Both methods are described below as are methods for donning trousers, shoes, and socks (Table 12-2).

Different ways of performing the everyday activities of cutting meat, opening packages, and brushing teeth can accomplish these tasks with little or no extra equipment or devices. Taping a nail file onto a table for filing nails or placing a jar inside a drawer to stabilize it are two alternative methods for everyday tasks.

Table 12-1.
PROCEDURE FOR PIVOT TRANSFER

- Position wheelchair.
- Lock wheelchair brakes.
- Move footrest/legrest out of the way on the side towards the destination surface.
- Have the patient come forward in the wheelchair; provide assistance so that both hips are even and that the person achieves an anterior pelvic tilt so that body weight is forward.
- Make sure the patient has a sufficiently wide base of support (shoulder distance).
- The therapist blocks the client's knees to provide stability.
- The client is encouraged to assist by pushing up with unaffected parts.
- The patient comes to a controlled stand; the therapist holds onto the client via gait or transfer belt.
- Client and therapist turn/pivot with therapist helping to move the client's affected foot.
- Client is encouraged to reach towards destination surface and ease self onto the surface by using unaffected parts; therapist assists by holding onto transfer belt and easing client onto surface while practicing good body mechanics.

Adapted Procedures and Methods that Substitute for Loss of Strength

Adapted procedures and methods that substitute for loss of strength reflect the principles of letting gravity assist, utilizing the mechanical principles of levers, using increased friction to decrease power requirements, and the use of two hands (Trombly, 1995).

Clients at the C5 spinal cord level can be taught to use their partially innervated deltoid and scapular muscles to perform the motions of shoulder external rotation and abduction. In doing these motions, the necessity to use supination (a lost function at this level) will be replaced and the client can use a mobile arm support for functional activities (Dutton, 1995).

A client at the C5 level of function and above can also be taught to hook the elbow around the wheelchair upright push handle. This positioning permits increased reach without loss of balance. Dutton adds that clients with C5 function also have selective tightening for a hook grasp if there is extrinsic tightness, which is useful in hooking fingers on the edge of a transfer board or wedging or "weaving" utensils or tools between tight fingers (Dutton, 1995).

Clients at the C6 spinal cord level lack triceps function and are unable to extend the elbow. The functional implications are that whenever the arm is brought to heights above the shoulder, the elbow will flex due to the pull of gravity. This use of gravity as an assist is very helpful when dressing and is a good principle of intervention.

Another functional ramification of loss of triceps is that the client will not be able to transfer using a sliding board without learning compensatory movements. Depression transfers can be successfully performed by clients at this level by having the client externally rotate the shoulder while locking the elbows as the weight of the body is shifted to that side. By depressing the scapula to shift the weight off the elbow, the client can inch forward on the sliding board. This same technique can be used in rolling onto the side and pushing up on the elbow during bed mobility activities and for push-ups in the wheelchair for pressure relief.

A very useful muscle action added at the C6 level is that of wrist extension due to the innervation of extensor carpi radialis longus and brevis muscles (radial wrist extensors). The addition of wrist extension is very helpful when trying to dress in that the client can use an extended wrist in sleeves and pant legs to assist with putting on the clothing. Two wrists extended and placed with palms together can hold clothing to pull it on or to straighten a shirt or blouse. These motions help to substitute or compensate for the lost ROM due to denervation caused by injury or disease.

Normally, when the wrist is actively extended, the fingers are passively flexed. If the fingers of a client with quadriplegia are allowed to develop some flexion tightness, then by using this tenodesis grasp, the client can pick up light objects and hook the wrist behind the wheelchair upright.

Even going through a door as a person with weakness in all four extremities requires a new method (Table 12-3).

Bed Mobility

Many activities require adaptation in the way that they are done if there is weakness in all four extremities. Some clients will require assistance with bed mobility where the caregiver will roll the client's body at one time with client assisting as possible (leg roll). Bed mobility will require altered methods in order to roll from side to side and to come to a sitting position. Clients with weakness of all four extremities may need to hold onto a bed rail, use a rope ladder, the side of the bed, a trapeze bar, or arm of a wheelchair in order to roll from side to side. They may need to grasp or hook their extended wrist or flexed elbow on these items if there is a decreased grasp. Momentum can be gained by rolling back and forth using proximal musculature and head when trunk muscles are affected. By hooking an extended wrist under the distal thigh, the leg can be pulled over or momentum can carry the legs. Rolling is made easier if the hands can be clasped together and the legs crossed prior to beginning the roll. To return to supine from sidelying, extend the wrist, lock the elbow in extension, and force the left shoulder back toward the bed (Pierson, 1994).

Coming to a sitting position when there is weakness of all four extremities can be achieved by:
1. Roll to one side, e.g., right.
2. Fling top arm (left) backward to rest the elbow on the bed.
3. Roll onto the left elbow and quickly fling the right arm back to rest the palm of the hand or fist on the bed.
4. Roll to the right and quickly move the left arm to rest the hand on the bed.

Table 12-2.

DRESSING ACTIVITIES

Putting on a Pullover Shirt

1. Begin sitting with shirt in lap, backside up, neck away from patient (label is facing down).
2. With left hand gather up the back of the shirt to expose the right armhole.
3. Using left hand, lift right hand and place it through the armhole and sleeve.
4. Place left arm through left armhole and sleeve up to the elbow.
5. Using left hand, push right sleeve above right elbow.
6. Gather back of shirt from collar to hemline.
7. Continue holding shirt and work shirt up both arms toward the shoulders.
8. Duck head and pull shirt over it.
9. Pull shirt down in back and front.

Putting on a Cardigan Garment

1. Begin sitting with shirt in lap, inside up, and collar away from body.
2. Using left arm, place right hand in right armhole (the armhole is diagonally opposite arm).
3. Pull sleeve over hand, grasp collar, and pull sleeve up onto the right shoulder.
4. Toss the rest of the garment behind body.
5. Reach left hand back and place it in armhole.
6. Work sleeve up arm and straighten shirt.
7. Button shirt (easier to start from bottom).

Putting on Trousers

1. Begin sitting on side of bed.
2. Using left hand, cross right leg over left.
3. Check to see that trousers are opened completely.
4. Grasp trousers at bottom of front opening and toss down toward right foot.
5. Pull right trouser leg up and over right foot.
6. Place right foot on floor and put left leg in other trouser leg.

7. Pull trousers up over knees.
8. Lie down, bend left hip and knee, push against bed, and raise buttocks.
9. Pull pants over hips; fasten. If patient can stand, omit step 8 and pull trousers on while standing; sit to fasten trousers.

Putting on Socks

1. Cross legs and pull on with left hand.

Putting on Shoes or Orthoses

1. Sew tongue to top of shoe at one side to prevent it from doubling over.
2. If brace is attached to shoe, be sure that the leg is in front of brace when putting shoe on.
3. Begin sitting on side of bed with right leg crossed over left.
4. Slip shoe on foot as far as possible.
5. Place a shoehorn in heel of shoe and place foot on floor.
6. Push down on knee, making sure shoehorn stays in place.
7. Fasten shoes (buckles, Velcro, or one-handed tie).

Tying a Shoe with One Hand

1. Knot one end of the shoe string and lace the shoe, leaving the knotted end at the lowest eyelet.
2. In the top eyelet, feed the end of the shoe string from outside to inside. Throw the end over the top of the laces.
3. Make a loop in the free end of the shoestring and pull it, loop within a loop.
4. Pull the lace tight, being careful not to pull the free end all the way through.
5. To untie, pull the free end.

Reprinted with permission from Palmer, M. L., & Toms, J. (1992). *Manual for functional training.* Philadelphia: F. A. Davis Co.

---

5. Having achieved a semi-sitting position resting on both hands, with the elbows extended or locked, the client "walks" his hand forward to come to a forward-leaning position of greater than 90 degrees of hip flexion to maintain balance.

An alternative way to come to a sitting position might be for the client to:
1. Place hands under hips or in pockets for stabilization.
2. Flex the neck and elbows until weight is on elbows.
3. Shift elbows backward, one at a time, until weight is on forearms.

4. Fling one arm backward, laterally rotating and extending the shoulder and elbow until the heel of the hand contacts the mattress (interphalangeal joints should be flexed).
5. Come to sitting by shifting weight onto extended arm and repeat this with the other arm.
6. Gain balance with weight on both extended arms.
7. Walk hands toward hips.

Using a rope ladder, overhead loops, or a trapeze can also assist with coming to a sitting position.

Table 12-3.

DOOR MANAGEMENT FROM A WHEELCHAIR

Through Doors (High Quadriplegic, C-4 or C-5, Pulling Door to Open)

1. Starting position: Back chair up to a double or a single door, the handrims just clearing the door that will be opened.
2. Motion:
   a. Place hand in door handle.
   b. Open the door slightly.
   c. Remove hand from door handle.
   d. Using hand against door, push door open until door is past the rim of the wheelchair.
   e. Using the rim to block the door open, turn chair toward the door, keeping the rim against the door.
   f. Propel chair forward with rim against the door until door is fully open.
   g. With the wheel continuing to block the door open, back chair with arm that is opposite the door.
   h. Push off from door and propel through doorway backward.
3. Teaching tip: Because of the tenodesis effect, it is important to place hand in door handle before turning the chair completely backward.

Through Doors (Low Quadriplegic, C-6 to C-7)

1. Starting position: Back chair up to a double or a single door, the handrims just clearing the door that will be opened.
2. Motion:
   a. Push door open far enough so that the door is blocked by the foot pedals.
   b. With the foot pedals against the door, turn wheelchair toward the open door.
   Caution: Feet will catch the door as the individual turns toward the door. To avoid injury to the feet let the chair roll back a little as the individual turns through the door.
   c. Hold elbow against the door to keep it open.
   d. Propel through.

Through Door (Pushing Forward)

1. Starting position: Approach the door to be opened at a slight angle (30 to 40 degrees).
2. Motion:
   a. Push the door open.
   b. Use toes and foot pedals to brace the door open.
   c. Turn wheelchair toward open door.
   Caution: Do not bang into the door with your toes.
3. Teaching tip: The weight of the door will straighten out the chair as it goes through.

Through Two Doors (Pushing Doors Open)

1. Starting position: Center wheelchair between the two doors with one foot pedal against each door.
2. Motion:
   a. Push doors with both feet until wheelchair is through the door past the handrims.
   b. With hands on the doors and elbows flexed, use trunk extension to push doors open.
   c. Propel through the doors.
   Caution: If you do not get far enough through the doors, the weight of the doors will push the chair backwards.

Reprinted with permission from Palmer, M. L., & Toms, J. (1992). *Manual for functional training.* Philadelphia: F. A. Davis Co.

Sliding Board Transfer

Getting from a bed into a wheelchair will require a transfer from one surface to another. The type of transfer and level of assistance or independence depends upon the degree of weakness. For clients who are very weak in all four extremities, they may need to be lift-ed or rolled over by another person or persons. These types of transfers are discussed in the section on caregiver education. Use of a transfer or sliding board is the most common transfer type for patients with loss of strength in all four extremities and for clients with C6 injuries and below.

Table 12-4.

PUTTING ON AND TAKING OFF A CARDIGAN GARMENT

1. Putting on a cardigan garment.
   The method may be adapted for jackets, blouses, sweaters, shirts, and top portion of dresses that open down the front.
   a. Patient is sitting in wheelchair. Position shirt on lap with back of shirt up and collar toward knees. The label of the shirt is facing down.
   b. Put arms under shirt back starting at shirt tail and into sleeve starting at armhole and working toward cuff. Push shirt past elbows.
   c. Using wrist extension, hook hands under shirt back and gather up material.
   d. Using shoulder abduction, scapular abduction and adduction, elbow flexion, and slight neck flexion, pass shirt over head.
   e. By relaxing wrist and shoulders, and with the aid of gravity, the hands may be removed from shirt back and the arms are now completely through the sleeves. Most of the material of the shirt is gathered up at back of patient's neck across shoulders and underarms.
   f. Shirt is worked into place over shoulders and trunk by alternately shrugging shoulders, leaning forward, with aid of wheelchair arms for balance if necessary, and using elbow flexion and wrist extension.
   g. Close shirt using buttons, snaps, or Velcro. If the shirt has not been buttoned previously, use a button hook, starting with bottom button, which is easier to see.

   Exceptions to this procedure would be as follows:
   a. Arrange shirt on table preparatory to putting on.
   b. When trunk stability is a problem, support elbows on table to assist in flipping shirt over head.

2. Removing a cardigan garment.
   a. Patient is in wheelchair. Unbutton only the necessary buttons. Use a hook, if necessary.
   b. Push one shoulder of cardigan at a time off shoulder. Elevate and depress shoulders, rotate trunk, and use gravity so cardigan will slip down arms as far as possible. Use thumbs alternately in armholes to slip sleeves farther down arms.
   c. Hold one cardigan cuff with opposite thumb and flex elbow to pull arm out of garment. Repeat for other arm. The thumb is used as a "hook" in this step.

Reprinted with permission from Palmer, M. L., & Toms, J. (1992). *Manual for functional training*. Philadelphia: F. A. Davis Co.

Dressing

Adapted techniques for clients with weakness in all four extremities require that certain levels of performance be met as prerequisites for dressing. Minimum criteria for upper extremity dressing are:

1. Neck stability is medically cleared.
2. Muscle strength fair to good in shoulder (deltoid, trapezius, serratus anterior, rotators) and elbow (biceps).
3. Shoulder flexion and abduction 0 to 90 degrees; medial and lateral rotation 0 to 30 degrees, and elbow extension and flexion 15 to 140 degrees.
4. Sitting tolerance and balance in bed and/or wheelchair achieved with assistance of bed siderails or wheelchair safety belts (Colenbrander & Fletcher, 1995).

Specific step-by-step directions for putting on and removing a cardigan appear in Table 12-4.

Putting on a bra is much the same procedure as putting on a cardigan as described above. It is easier to hook the bra in the front with the bra at waist level and then pull the straps up over the shoulder. Adaptations such as sewn loops or Velcro will enable independent fastening by the client.

An alternative method to putting on a cardigan would be to place the shirt on the lap, collar facing toward the legs. Place one hand into the sleeve, shaking the sleeve to help move it along the arm. Push the heel of the hand along the outside material of the sleeve to push the sleeve up to the elbows. Clients often use their teeth to assist with this and licking the heel of the hand helps, too, by providing a friction surface. At the axillary border of the sleeve (where the sleeve is sewn to the body of the shirt), have the client extend the wrist and pull the sleeve up over the shoulder. Putting the shirt material between the heels of each extended wrist also helps in pulling the shirt front down. Have the client hook the arm with the shirt sleeve pulled up to the shoulder over the upright of the wheelchair for balance. The client can then lean forward and insert the other arm into the remaining armhole. Pull the arm through the sleeve. Using both extended wrists, straighten the shirt by putting shirt material between the heels of both hands.

Minimum criteria for lower extremity dressing would be:
1. Muscle strength fair to good in pectorals, rhomboids, supinators, and radial wrist extensors.
2. ROM: knee flexion and extension 0 to 120 degrees to permit sitting with legs extended; hip flexion 0 to 110 degrees.
3. Body control, such as the ability to transfer from bed to wheelchair with minimum assistance; ability to roll from side to side, balance when sidelying (Pierson, 1994).

Step by step directions for putting on trousers can be found in Table 12-2.

Many people choose not to continue wearing undershorts for several reasons. One, this would be one more piece of clothing to put on in the morning. Dressing is very energy consuming and if it takes more than 1 hour to complete, it is not considered functional (AOTA, 1995). A second reason for not wearing undershorts or panties is that this is an additional potential source of skin breakdown. Clients should be cautioned to wear larger clothing that is loose-fitting and that does not bind or impinge the skin. Often blue jeans are a source of skin irritation due to the double seams and inflexible fabric. A final reason might be that the undershorts may interfere with the client's bowel and bladder programs.

There are some contraindications relative to UE and LE dressing, which might include:

1. Decreased breathing capacity; if vital capacity is below 50% (can often do UE dressing).
2. Pressure sores or an unusual tendency for skin breakdown when rolling or transferring.
3. Continued client resistance to dressing.
4. Pain in the neck or trunk that persists when attempting dressing training (Pierson, 1994).

Adapting the Task Method or Procedure to Provide Stability

Adapting the task method or procedure to provide stability due to ataxia or incoordination involves using stabilization to counteract the tremors or lack of controlled movement. Teaching the client to stabilize objects being used and to position the body in as stable a position as possible are compensatory ways of providing stability. Ways to position the body may include sitting when possible, bearing weight on the part, and holding the arms close to the body. It is helpful to stabilize proximal parts so the need to control body movement is reduced to just the distal body parts (AOTA, 1995). Using larger and less precise fasteners, tools, and objects also helps decrease frustration due to incoordination. For example, using roll-on deodorant is easier and safer for the person with decreased coordination and control. Increasing friction can add stability and can be as simple as placing an object on a wet cloth or towel, or using a nonskid mat. Dutton recommends using a two-handed proprioceptive neuromuscular facilitation (PNF) technique called "chop and lift" in daily activities such as getting a glass from a cupboard or washing one's face. Another PNF technique uses surface contact to increase friction and decrease instability. In this case, sliding the hand along the table toward the glass would be a more steady position for the arm. She suggests moving and stopping in the course of an action to improve controlled movement, such as resting on every shelf of a cabinet to lower one's hand (Dutton, 1995).

Adapting Methods to Inhibit Spasticity

While control or inhibition of spasticity is not a remediation goal of either the biomechanical or the rehabilitation frames of reference, some of the techniques advocated by theorists from the neurodevelopmental/sensorimotor frame of reference are useful in controlling spasticity or at least in minimizing the effect spasticity has on the performance of daily tasks. Using distal key points of control (NDT technique) was already discussed when it was recommended to put the unaffected leg under spastic leg during bed mobility and also when the hands were clasped in reaching activities and transfers. Another NDT technique, that of using proximal points of control, is seen if a client is instructed to lean forward to dangle a spastic arm to use the weight of that arm to protract the scapula and extend the elbow while putting on a shirt (Dutton, 1995). Dutton further recommends using placing, lowering, and weight bearing (NDT techniques) to control spasticity. An example of this might be seen when the client lowers a spastic arm to the table and uses the arm to hold down a piece of paper (Dutton, 1995).

Adapting Methods for Limited Vision

Clients with limited vision use organization as a method of compensating. If objects are organized in a specific way, in a particular place and routinely replaced after use, then the client with limited vision will always know where to find the object. Clothes can be organized by color in a closet. Pinning like items together after wearing them, but before laundering, will eliminate the need for visually sorting after washing and drying. By folding money differently for each denomination, the person with limited vision will be able to differentiate paper money. Food is cut by finding the edge of the food with the fork, moving the fork a bite-sized amount onto the meat, and then cutting, keeping the knife in contact with the food. Pouring liquid is based on the weight of the cup when it is full. Contrast is used to differentiate items for the low vision client, such as using a dark cutting board for cutting a potato and a light cutting board for cutting a tomato. Other contrast examples would be pouring coffee into a light-colored cup and using colored toothpaste, adding contrast to white brush bristles (Beaver & Mann, 1995; Cooper, 1985; Cristarella, 1977; Lempert & Lapolice, 1995).

Adapting Methods for Decreased Endurance

Many clients experience decreased endurance and they need to frequently schedule rests during the day. Energy conservation and work simplification principles are very applicable to those with cardiovascular and respiratory dysfunction, spinal cord injuries, and rheumatoid arthritis (Tables 12-5 & 12-6).

Adapting Task Objects, Adaptive Devices, and Orthotics

Adapting the task object involves changing or substituting the objects or tools used in activities. Adaptive equipment spans the continuum from low-tech buttonhooks to complex computer equipment. Adaptive equipment can be used to enable performance, to compensate for lost function, and to aid in efficient and safe performance of activities.

Recommendation of adaptive equipment seems deceptively simple but careful consideration of devices and client need is necessary to avoid costly errors in terms of equipment purchased and not used or used incorrectly. Some devices, used incorrectly, may

---

Table 12-5.

ENERGY CONSERVATION PRINCIPLES

1. Respect pain. Encourage clients to stop when pain occurs. To continue with an activity that is painful may restrict activities later in the day or even the next day.
2. Rest frequently. Plan regular rest periods throughout the day, alternating strenuous activities with rest.
3. Prioritize activities. Do the most important activities first while still rested and disregard less important activities if you are tired. Seek help with tasks and delegate some tasks to other family members.
4. Avoid isometric contractions or sustaining one static position for prolonged periods of time. For example, rest your elbow on the table while eating instead of holding it up in the air.
5. Avoid stressful positions such as raising your arms over shoulder height, crossing your legs (raises the blood pressure) and standing (which requires more energy than sitting).

Table 12-6.

WORK SIMPLIFICATION

1. *Organize storage.* Have similar items placed together. For example, have canisters of flour and sugar near the mixer. Have heavy items located on lower shelves to minimize lifting. Keep items used frequently at waist height.
2. *Plan ahead.* Schedule the week so that more strenuous tasks are spread throughout the week. Alternate hard with easy tasks. Make out a grocery list prior to shopping, which will also make meal preparation easier since all ingredients will be available. Shop during non-peak times to avoid crowds and a rushed, noisy environment.
3. *Have an easy flow of work.* An analogy is often an assembly line but comparing this objective to one's automobile is also useful. For example, when you drive your car on a highway at a constant rate, there is less wear and tear on mechanical parts and you get good gas mileage. Contrast this to city driving where there is much more stop and go driving, more wear and tear on engine parts, and less gas mileage. A functional task can acquire an easy flow of work by laying out all parts or ingredients in the order in which they are used.
4. *Eliminate steps and jobs.* Eliminate jobs or steps in a process that are not essential. For example, purchasing permanent press shirts eliminates the need for ironing. Let dishes drip dry in a drainer rather than hand drying them. Leave a tie knotted. Use premeasured laundry detergent and bleach.
5. *Use efficient methods.* This could include sitting while ironing or cutting vegetables for a salad. Use both arms whenever possible and slide objects rather than lifting them. Using a wheeled cart eliminates the need to transport hot or heavy objects. Move smoothly. Use electric appliances if they will be more efficient. For example, using a microwave oven or toaster oven may be more efficient than a conventional oven. Line a laundry hamper with a plastic bag with handles to be lifted out and taken to washer.
6. *Consider the environment.* Try to avoid loud, crowded, poorly lit, or smoky rooms, as these are factors that lead to fatigue.

---

result in additional performance impairments or may prevent proper use of the device (Marrelli & Krulish, 1999). A proper fit between the needs of the individual and the functions and options of the device must be made. Included in the decision is the cost and availability of the device, what adaptations may be needed, and what is involved in maintaining and repairing the device.

Adaptive equipment may radically change the way things are done. For example, a long-handled hairbrush may be recommended to a client to enable independent grooming. Use of the long-handled hairbrush minimizes the amount of ROM of the shoulder that is required to brush the hair, but the device still requires isometric contraction of the wrist and hand muscles with enough strength to hold the brush. In addition, coordination and arm strength is needed to control the longer lever created by the extended handle.

If the equipment or device is complex, the client will need higher levels of cognition to use the devices effectively and safely. It is easy to see that a reacher will compensate for decreased ROM, but judgment is needed when getting a heavy soup can down from a high cupboard. Not only might the soup can fall on the person, but there are additional stresses on the wrist and fingers and well as on the cardiovascular system with overhead movements.

Many items of adaptive equipment do not change the way the activity is done but makes the task easier. This is seen with Velcro shoe closures and adding foam to utensils to build up the handles. The fork with a foam handle is used the same way as a fork without foam; the difference is that the person can hold the fork more easily since less hand closure is required.

Another difference is that the foam makes the fork look different, which is one disadvantage to adapting the task objects for some people. Consideration of the psychological impact of adaptive equipment on the person is important in the consistent use of the devices by the client. By using tools or devices that look different, unwanted attention may be drawn to the person using them, which may be a constant reminder of loss of function. Sometimes a client would rather have assistance than use adaptive equipment. Some orthotic devices (e.g., mobile arm supports) may be bulky and unattractive, which may be another disadvantage for some clients.

Use of adaptive devices and orthotics have three advantages according to Dutton (1995):
1. Good face validity.
2. Offers a concrete, immediate solution.
3. Often inexpensive.

Specific pieces of equipment or adaptations to objects are numerous for each of the areas where compensation occurs.

The use of a sliding board in a depression transfer is a specific example of using an adaptive device that compensates for loss of LE function. Impediments to successful sliding board transfers would be poor trunk balance that cannot be compensated, excessive spasticity, excessive body weight, joint tightness, and cognitive deficits. A transfer board is used as a bridge from one surface to another. Transfer boards can be wooden or plastic; plastic boards are more lightweight. For a person with decreased grasp, there must be cutout areas on the board or loops attached so the client can maneuver the board during the transfer and secure or store the board after the transfer. Sliding board transfers can be done independently by the client or with assistance, if needed. Assistance can be provided by holding the client around the ribs, waist, or waistband or by using a transfer belt and maneuvering the client's legs if necessary. Transfer surfaces optimally should be at the same level for an even transfer.

Technique for Sliding Board Transfer

- Position wheelchair.
- Lock wheelchair brakes.
- Move footrest/legrest out of the way on the slide towards the destination surface; remove armrest on destination side.
- Client shifts body weight to side opposite the direction of movement and places the board under the buttocks.
- Client places one hand on the board and the other on the wheelchair seat and leans forward.
- Client then moves the upper body weight in direction opposite to that in which he or she is going.
- Client scoots along board by flexing/extending elbow or by externally rotating the humerus and locking the elbows to compensate for lack of triceps.
- Therapist assists by ensuring balance as needed and by helping the client move the lower extremities across the transfer surface.

Changing the Context

Contextual variables are an important consideration when implementing intervention. Context includes the physical environment, cultural and social aspects of the individual, virtual or realistic simulation of an environment, and spiritual aspects. Cultural and social changes in context may occur within this construct as a part of the teaching/learning process experienced by the client and caregivers and in the emphasis on the client as the primary person responsible for his or her own care. The contextual areas most obviously focused on in the rehabilitation construct are those that change the physical environment by providing mobility devices or in adapting the environment.

Changing the Physical Environment

Changes in the physical environment will enable greater access to public and private facilities and will promote independence that otherwise may not have been possible.

Environmental adaptation ranges from architectural design and new construction to slight modifications (Moyers, 1999). Environmental modifications are advantageous when problems cannot be solved any other way. By making these changes, valued roles may be regained.

One disadvantage to environmental adaptations is expense. Ramps, chair glides, elevators, and modified vans are all very expensive solutions to environmental problems. Another disadvantage is that often the changes are not portable. If a ramp is installed at one home, it often is not easily transported to another.

If the deficit is temporary, then the cost is not justified so the person may be without sufficient modifications to ensure independence.

Not all adaptations need to be complex or expensive, though. The President's Committee on Employment of People with Disabilities developed a sample list of adaptations to home and worksites particularly in reference to reasonable accommodation and the ADA. There are often simple solutions to problems of accessibility. A person who is unable to work because the wheelchair will not fit under the desk or a person who cannot transfer to a sofa because the sofa is lower than the wheelchair will benefit from raising these surfaces with wooden blocks. Changing the way a task is done can also provide simple solutions to accessibility problems. Using a tape recorder or transcriber rather than writing is helpful for people who need to write reports, and altering schedules to permit frequent rests is a helpful solution for people with poor endurance.

Specific Appliance Suggestions

Specific appliances that are preferred for household tasks might include a refrigerator with double doors. Turntables on the refrigerator shelves enable easy access to all items. Heaviest items should be placed at lapboard height for clients in wheelchairs. A built-in wall oven located 30 inches from the floor is very useful. Heat resistant countertops make placement of hot items easier and safer and a wheeled cart facilitates transport of items for functional ambulators. A 15 inch flat stick is useful in pushing and pulling the oven rack and oven mitts are easily obtained. A self-cleaning oven is the optimal choice. An electric stove with push buttons located on the front is easier for clients in a wheelchair but safety is a consideration for those with poor coordination and for those with small children in the home. A mirror can be placed on the stove to help one see into pots and pans on the stove. A disadvantage to the mirror is that it frequently will get splattered, greasy, and fogged by steam.

A sink that is 5.5 inches deep and open underneath enables a person in a wheelchair to get closer to it. Pipes under the sink need to be covered with foam to prevent burns in insensate areas. Single lever handles are easier for those with poor grasp. By placing a rubber mat in the sink, breakage might be reduced. For one-handed cleaning, use of suction bottle brushes and scrub brushes is helpful. A front loading dishwasher is preferred with controls on the front.

For clients who can ambulate, a top loading washing machine is best and a raised dryer would minimize bending. Having a waist high table for folding clothes nearby would enable a smooth, efficient sequence. For clients in a wheelchair, a front loading washer is preferred with a dryer with side-hinged doors (which is hard to find). If a top loading washer is used, use of an overhead mirror will enable the person to load the machine.

Having a clip mounted on the wall will allow one end of a sheet to be held while folding. Mounting an ironing board on a wall at 28 to 32 inches may provide a more appropriate height for this activity.

Childcare Suggestions and Modifications

Childcare presents several challenges to the disabled client. If the client is ambulatory but bending over is difficult, cribs can be raised by raising the crib legs, adjusting the mattress, or even by using two mattresses. For the client in a wheelchair, the typical drop-side crib can be adapted by cutting the middle of the crib side and attaching two hinges at each end with a latch in the center. Another alternative might be to make the crib side slide along horizontal rather than vertical channels. Bathing an infant may be easiest in a modified kitchen sink for both the wheelchair and ambulatory client. Although a plastic tub or small baby pool can be used to bathe a baby, emptying the tub may be difficult without assistance. Playpens are very useful in confining the child safely. Raising the legs of a playpen or using a portable crib will minimize bending. Adapting a playpen so that a person in a wheelchair can use it with his or her children would be similar to adapting the crib. While the safest place to handle a baby is on the floor, a changing table at a height of 31 inches is appropriate for most wheelchair users. Carrying a baby can be done by using a bassinet on wheels or a reclining stroller if one is ambulatory. Cloth infant carriers can also be used but be alert that the front styles require back muscle contraction against a load, while back styles compress the vertebrae. For those in a wheelchair, transporting the child on the lap with a seatbelt is appropriate.

Community Mobility

Accessibility in the community is enhanced by public transportation systems. Information about these options and modifications that can be made to private automobiles and drivers training for the disabled is a valuable resource to share with the client and family. Parking spaces for the disabled should be clearly marked, located near entrances, and need to be 16 feet wide for side-exit vans.

In general, doorways need to be a minimum of 32 inches wide and adaptations for narrow doorways include removal of the doorframe, offset or fold-back hinges or inset doors.

Ramps should follow a 1:12 ratio, i.e., for every rise in the slope, there needs to be 12 inches of ramp. Steeper ramps are possible for those clients in wheelchairs with good upper extremity strength. Since ramps that follow this ratio may become very long, switchback ramps are a good alternative with at least a 5 x 5 foot platform between rises for adequate turning. Curbs on ramps prevent wheelchair wheels from moving off the ramp and anti-skid material applied to the ramp surface increases traction for the wheelchair user. This can be commercially available non-skid strips or simply mixing sand in with paint to eliminate slippage.

Don't forget items like telephone height, light switch location, smoke alarms, elevator call button accessibility, thermostat, and water fountain heights when evaluating accessibility. Remember, too, that accessibility applies not only to those in wheelchairs but also for ambulators, persons with low vision, decreased endurance, and many other limitations.

DISABILITY PREVENTION

Family, client, and caregiver education involves teaching the family or caregiver about the ways in which the disorder or injury affects the client's performance in work, play, and self-care. Often the ramifications of a chronic disability are not realized by the family who, like the client, are adjusting to the medical and psychosocial aspects of the injury while being only minimally aware of the changes that will be needed in daily activities. The client with chronic disabilities needs to relearn how to move, dress, and perform daily tasks with an altered body and capabilities. The client and the family need help coping with the changes and the family needs help in learning how to help the client.

Teaching the family the specific ways to provide assistance in dressing, transfers, positioning, as well as provision of the appropriate level and type of cueing is important for successful return to home and for safety. Recommending adaptive equipment or assistive technology and available resources to aid the family/caregiver in providing assistance is an important aspect of caregiver training. Home programs, initiated with the therapist, are taught to the family so that functional gains can be continued or maintained.

Education to Ensure Safe Mobility and Transfers

Mobility issues and transfers are essential skills to teach the family. If possible, the client should also be taught how to instruct others in his or her own care if unable to perform the tasks alone. This acceptance of responsibility for oneself is an important intervention aspect of the rehabilitation approach. Management of wheelchair parts is important to review with the family prior to initiation of transfer skills.

Moving the client is the next consideration in teaching. Is the client totally unable to assist in any way with the transfer? Is the client able to come to a sitting position? Can the client weight bear or partially weight bear? Is there weakness in all four extremities or weakness in the lower extremities and trunk?

Transfers

Prior to beginning any type of transfer, it is important to know the client's strengths and limitations in all areas of function, including physical, cognitive, and levels of assistance required with current mobility. You also need to be aware of your own strengths and limitations and freely ask for help with transfers when needed. Use proper body mechanics when assisting with transfers and train caregivers to use these as well.

If the client is unable to assist with the transfer, then a dependent transfer will be done that requires the assistance of one or more persons to move the client from one surface to another. One-person transfers can be done with clients who need assistance as well as those with and without the ability to flex at the hip (Table 12-7). To help a person roll from side to side or to transfer a recumbent person, a draw sheet, mattress pad, or bed liner can be used, which may also help with transfers. For persons requiring more assistance, a two-person transfer or carry can be done where one

Table 12-7.

ONE PERSON TRANSFER TECHNIQUES

One Person Technique (Clients Without Limited Hip Flexion)

- Stand in front of client.
- Place client in forward flexed position with chest lying on the thighs.
- Shifts body weight over knees and ankles rather than on buttocks so allows buttocks to be more easily moved.
- Helper can control movement.

One Person Technique (Clients with Limited Hip Flexion)

- Slide buttocks toward edge of wheelchair.
- Place client's knees between the helper's knees.
- Rock client forward slightly and simultaneously pull client's transfer belt and rotate hips to surface to be moved to.

Reprinted with permission from Trombly, C. A. (Ed.). (1995). *Occupational therapy for physical dysfunction* (4th ed.). Baltimore: Williams & Wilkins.

---

person stands behind the client and moves the trunk while the other person assists with lower extremity management as they both move simultaneously from one surface to another. An alternative for dependent clients would be use of a hydraulic lift (i. e., Hoyer lift), which is a good choice for very large, dependent clients and/or small caregivers. Other mechanically assisted transfers have been made from adapted battery operated winches or garage door openers.

A logroll transfer can be done by one person. Starting with a locked wheelchair, and facing the foot of bed, be sure that the seat is located near the client's hips. Remove the armrest and place a pillow over the wheel to facilitate the transfer and minimize skin breakdown. The client is rolled onto his side with his back toward the chair. His hips are near the chair seat at edge of the bed with arms and legs flexed to distribute the weight. Move the hips onto the chair seat, keeping the trunk and upper body on the bed. Then the upper trunk is moved to an upright position in the chair and finally the feet are placed on the footrests (Trombly, 1995, p. 295).

Assisted swivel trapeze transfers can be done by having the client hook an extended wrist around the bar and pull himself to a sitting position. With forearms across the bar, the client would then contract his elbow flexors while the helper holds onto the legs and pulls off the bed and swings the lower body over to the chair (Trombly, 1995).

If there is weakness in all four extremities, then the assisted depression or sliding board transfer would be a good choice. Assistance is provided by helping to place the transfer board, then by holding onto the client's waist, waistband, or transfer belt to guard against loss of balance. Do not hold onto the belt loops of

pants since these rarely remain secure when pulled on strenuously. Further assistance can be provided in helping the person slide across the transfer board and then to maneuver and position the person's feet.

If the client can partially weight bear or has loss of function on one side of the body, an assisted pivot transfer can be used. Assistance can be provided by giving physical and/or verbal cues; by helping the client scoot forward in the chair; by holding the client by a transfer belt, belt loop, or waistband during the transfer; stabilizing the client in standing; maneuvering the client's feet during the pivot and when sitting; and easing the client into the chair.

It may be necessary to assist in repositioning the client once in the wheelchair. The helper stands behind the wheelchair, which is locked and tipped back to point of balance. Gently shake the chair, which assists gravity in sliding the client's hips back into the seat. A precaution is if the client has spasticity, which would necessitate a different method. In that case, have the client flex the elbows so the forearms go across the body. The helper puts his/her arms in between the client's folded arms and the chest wall, under the axilla from behind to grasp each forearm just distal to the forearm. The helper applies an upward force to reposition the client (Trombly, 1995).

Helping a client in a wheelchair navigate over curbs and stairs is a valuable skill in which to train a caregiver. To assist with ascending a curb, the easiest and safest method is to ascend the curb with the chair facing forward or toward the curb. This gives the greatest control of the chair and requires the least effort by the caregiver (Pierson, 1994, p. 169).

The helper approaches the curb with the front of the wheelchair and depresses the foot projection on the back of the frame. Next, the helper will push down on push handles and tipping lever to push casters over the curb. The client can assist by leaning forward and pushing on the tire rims as the wheelchair is elevated. Roll the wheelchair forward so all four wheels are on the elevated surface (Figure 12-1A-D).

To ascend a curb backwards, the rear wheels are placed close to the edge of the curb. The helper stands behind the chair and tips the chair so that the casters are elevated. Pull the push handles so that the rear wheels come over the curb. Turn the wheelchair 90 degrees and gently place the casters down.

Helping a client in a wheelchair descend a curb backwards is the easiest, safest method, and requires the least effort by the caregiver. The helper approaches the curb backwards with the back wheels of the wheelchair eased down first. The helper can use his or her hip or thigh to slow the downward movement. Turn the wheelchair 90 degrees and then ease the casters down. Descending a curb in a forward position is done by tipping the wheelchair back to a point of balance with the center of gravity over rear axle. Then push large wheels down gently over the curb (Turner, Foster, & Johnson, 1996).

Two people are needed to assist a client in a wheelchair going up stairs. Approach the stairs backwards with one helper behind the wheelchair. This person tips the wheelchair backward into a balanced position. The second person is in front and holds onto the leg rest upright (onto the frame, not removable parts). The

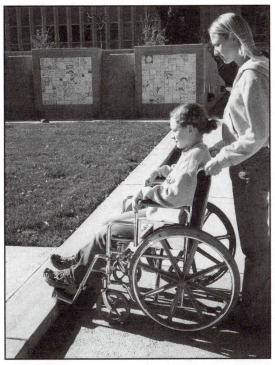

Figure 12-1A. Approach curb with casters facing the curb.

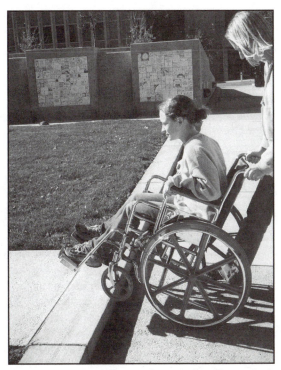

Figure 12-1B. Assistant pushes on handles and tilts wheelchair back while patient leans forward if possible.

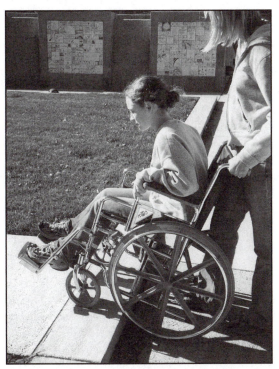

Figure 12-1C. Assistant rolls wheelchair and pushes casters over curb.

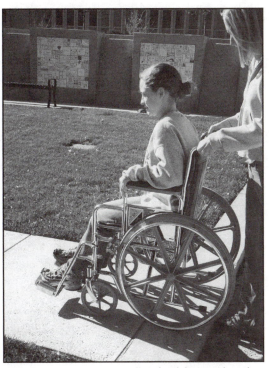

Figure 12-1D. Assistant rolls wheelchair and pushes back wheels over curb.

second person helps to maintain the point of balance while pulling the wheelchair up each step, while the person at the foot assists with lifting and maintaining point of balance (Pierson, 1994, p. 294). Going down the stairs, the stairs are approached in a forward position. The wheelchair is tipped in balanced positions and the process above is reversed.

Placing a wheelchair into a car is also a skill that can be taught to the caregivers. The wheelchair can fit either into the trunk or into the back seat of the car, especially if a two-door car is used and the client is loading the wheelchair into the car.

Teaching Caregivers the Proper Use of Equipment

Teaching the family and caregiver how to use any pieces of adaptive equipment, devices, or orthotics is also important for continued and proper use of these items. Studies document that over 50% of the adaptive devices that have been vended to clients during hospitalizations are not used when the client is at home (Pierson, 1994). Education about adapted techniques used in dressing, feeding, and daily living skills as well as adaptations for work and play need to be clearly explained and demonstrated to the family.

Preventing further structural damage is often achieved by orthotic devices or positioning in bed or in the wheelchair. It is important for both the client and the family to know how to apply the devices, minimize potential harm (i. e., skin breakdown, duration of use), and achieve maximal benefit from the devices. Devices may be used to protect a specific vulnerable body part during activities, to relieve pain, or to promote rest for healing structures. Wrist cock-up splints are useful for clients following a CVA, slings are often used following an upper extremity injury, and arm troughs are placed on wheelchairs to position a dependent extremity. Other examples are seen in prosthetic devices for clients with amputations or with the use of an ankle-foot orthosis (AFO) or knee-ankle-foot orthosis (KAFO). These devices not only position the parts but protect them from further structural damage. Positioning a client with loss of movement on one side of the body provides support for weakened parts, which maintains normal symmetry with additional goals of inhibition of abnormal tone, provision of normal sensory input, and increased awareness of the affected side (NDT goals). In supine, pillows are placed under the knees to maintain knee flexion and a folded sheet is placed under the pelvis on affected side to maintain symmetrical pelvic alignment. A rolled towel under the head will maintain head in midline with slight flexion.

Safety Education

In addition to skills that the client and caregiver need, safety education is vital to successful reintegration of the family and client in the home and community. It is important to prevent further disability related to the condition or as a result of it. This is known as *tertiary prevention* and has been defined as applicable "for those with activity limitations, impairments, or participation restrictions" with the intent "to maximize function and minimize the detrimental effects of illness or injury". Primary prevention programs are aimed toward those who have no limitations or impairments and secondary prevention efforts are directed toward those considered to be "at risk" for injury or impairment (Moyers, 1999).

An advantage to safety education for the client is that the client may be able to live in a less restrictive environment in order to maintain valued roles and interests. Clients and their families may not always see the need for safety education since often safety awareness and precautions require vigilant application of abstract concepts. Clients with cognitive impairments may not be able to visualize safety problems or be able to view their own body while performing a task, and many techniques require changes in habit. In these cases, the obligation of safety will fall to the caregivers.

Maintaining ROM may be indicated for those individuals who are unable to actively move or who are not permitted to move through full, partial, or any amount of motion. This may include a client on extended bed rest (e. g., in a coma) or may be a client with the potential for scar development due to surgery. ROM is performed to prevent deformities, contractures, and shortening of soft tissues, as well as prevent adhesions and mold collagen into orderly chains. If ROM exercises and activities are not done in healing tissues, collagen fibers would bind into tangles and adhere adjacent structures together (Dutton, 1995).

The focus of this intervention is on prevention of further impairments, activity limitations and participation restrictions and is a form of tertiary prevention. Maintenance of ROM is motion through the range that is currently available. No attempt is made to move the part past the currently available ROM. Whether the movement occurs passively, active assisted, or actively depends upon the capabilities of the client and safety issues. For example, if the client has sensory losses or cognitive/judgment deficits, active motion controlled by the client may progress too far or too fast and harm healing structures. In these cases, therapist intervention in providing passive or active assisted range via activities or exercise may be indicated.

Some of the benefits of passive range of motion (PROM) are:
- Maintenance of joint and soft tissue integrity.
- Minimize contracture formation.
- Maintain the mechanical elasticity of muscle fibers.
- Assist circulatory and vascular functions.
- Enhance synovial movement for cartilage nutrition.
- May decrease pain.
- Assist in healing after surgery or trauma.
- Helps to maintain an awareness of movement.

PROM will not prevent muscle atrophy, increase strength or endurance since there is no active muscle contraction. While PROM assists circulation and vascular functions, more value is gained by active or active-assisted motion than by passive movement. In addition to the benefits of PROM, when the client actively contracts muscle fibers, additional benefits are gained, such as maintenance of physiologic elasticity and contractility of participating muscles, provision of sensory feedback, increased stimulation for bone integrity, and increased circulation, which also helps prevent thrombosis formation.

The principle of maintaining ROM is that movement needs to go through the full available ROM in order to be effective. This can be accomplished by activities such as overhead checkers, macrame, putting dishes into a cupboard, placing clothes in a side loading dryer or making a bed. ROM can also be maintained by movement in anatomical planes, in muscle range of elongation, or in combined patterns of movement. Self range exercises are particularly beneficial for the client to enable independence and elicit responsibility in this aspect of care. Activities likely to be found in the clinic might be the use of a finger ladder, shoulder wheel, overhead pulley, or a suspension device (i.e., suspension sling). The most valuable activities, though, are those that the client needs to perform in daily life and those performed with active motion.

A special case in maintaining ROM might be the client who has sustained an SCI and is still in a halo device. ROM should not go past 90 degrees (nor will it likely be possible) in shoulder flexion and abduction. Above these levels, the humerus will likely have contact with the halo. In addition, the finger flexors of a client with an SCI should have ROM maintained, not increased, if natural teneodesis is to develop. Assisted motion may be required for the client with burned hands and gentle active motion can be performed by a client with rheumatoid arthritis, even in an acute flare-up, provided clients respect their pain limits.

Scar prevention devices, which use compression, may slow collagen synthesis. Devices such as pressure dressings, elastomer molds, transparent face masks, and pressure garments apply a uniform pressure gradient to promote healing and minimize heterotrophic scar formation. Orthosis, like a foot drop splint, and positioning are also used to prevent deformities while maintaining joints and soft tissues in functional positions.

Active movement also can be used to maintain strength by using currently intact muscles and joints, preventing disuse atrophy, pain and stiffness. Daily activities, such as activities of daily living and wheelchair propulsion, can be used to maintain the strength of the muscles. The goal is conservation and preservation, not increasing, the muscle strength.

Preventing further disability may involve ensuring joint protection. Instruction to the family and client about joint protection techniques is useful for many clients, especially those with fragile joints, as in rheumatoid arthritis. Joint protection techniques involve seven different principles. The first is to encourage the client to avoid positions of possible deformity. Usually this would be static, flexed positions. Examples would be to avoid leaning the head on the back of the hand or avoid pushing up in a chair with the back of the fingers bent at the knuckles. Instead, push up by leaning on the palm. Avoiding movements in an ulnar direction also would be an example of avoiding a position of possible deformity. Most objects and fasteners are designed for use by right-handed people, using ulnar movements. Consider opening a pickle jar lid: one turns the lid to the ulnar side. An alternative way to open the jar would be to press down on the jar with the palm and use the

shoulder, not wrist, to open the lid. Using a knife with a pulling motion is another example. Avoid activities that require a tight grip by enlarging handles or gripping items between the palms of both hands. Avoid wringing out a washcloth; instead, press down to remove excess moisture.

The second major idea behind joint protection techniques is to avoid holding joints or using muscles in one position for a long time. Specific examples include:

1. Don't stand too long.
2. Use a book rest or prop it up.
3. Substitute typing for writing.
4. Avoid unnecessary jobs.
5. Activities requiring repetitive actions should be done for short periods of time only (i.e., wash windows, vacuuming).

Using the strongest joints available helps to protect joints. This principle is obvious in body mechanics principles that stress using the legs rather than the back to lift. Carrying the purse on the forearm rather than by the hand can decrease stress to joints and even using the crook of the elbow to stabilize a bowl when stirring rather than using the hands can be protective of the joints.

This is related to another joint protection principle, that of using each joint to its best mechanical advantage. Using both arms and legs to stand up and maintaining a good posture while working at comfortable work heights enables joints to work at their best capacity.

Being able to stop an activity is an important consideration in joint protection. Clients should be encouraged to organize their days so that activities are sequenced based on alternating strenuous activities with rest, using knowledge of fatiguing situations and times of day as guides. The client should conscientiously conserve energy and respect pain when it occurs (Table 12-8).

Safety education can be very specific to postsurgical conditions or particular diagnostic categories. Precautions for clients with total hip replacement are designed to reduce the possibility of hip dislocation during the first 10 to 14 days following surgery. While individual orthopaedic surgeons may have slightly different preferences, the following are guidelines generally accepted for clients following total hip replacement surgery (Dutton, 1995).

Clients who have recently had shoulder surgery or have unstable shoulder girdles should not be pulled up in bed or repositioned using their arms. During transfers, support these clients around their trunk rather than under the axilla to avoid structural damage or further instability. This advice is actually true for all clients. Safer transfer mechanisms have been described and pulling on a client's shoulder girdle is not a recommended practice for any type of transfer.

After heart surgery, sternal precautions are in effect. Tell clients and their families to avoid activities where there is pushing or pulling with the arms, which includes using the arms to push oneself out of bed or a chair. No one should pull on the client's arms during activities or transfers because this applies too much pressure on the sternal area. Precautions for cardiac clients would include monitoring of heart rate and blood pressure and often rely on MET levels for choice of activities. If the heart rate goes up more than 20 beats per minute from the resting pulse or above 120 beats per

---

Table 12-8.

JOINT PROTECTION TECHNIQUES

1. Avoid positions of possible deformity.
2. Avoid holding joints or using muscles in one position for a long time.
3. Use the strongest joints available.
4. Do not start an activity you cannot stop.
5. Use each joint to its mechanical advantage.
6. Respect pain.
7. Regular rest periods.

---

minute or below 60, a physician should be consulted. If resting systolic blood pressure goes above 150 or below 90 and/or if diastolic blood pressure goes above 90 or below 50, consult a physician. Normal blood pressure is 120/80.

Body mechanics should be taught to the family to ensure safe movement of the client and prevent injuries to the caregiver. Sliding, pushing, pulling, or rolling objects rather than lifting uses better body mechanics. Lifting with the legs and not the back by bending the knees uses the strongest muscles to their best advantage. Working at a proper and comfortable work height will prevent repetitive motion injuries. Allowing adequate space for using the proper body alignments is a consideration as well. The following principles should be incorporated into all activities and especially those in which assistance is provided to a client.

A general rule cited by Gench, Hinson, and Harvey (1995) is: "if the head is kept erect while lifting, pushing and pulling, muscular involvement will tend to keep hips low and force the larger, stronger muscles of hip and knee to carry out the task" (p. 184).

Back pain can occur as a result of strains of muscle and ligaments due to improper lifting or trauma, muscular imbalance, poor posture, sedentary habits, and overeating. When standing, better body mechanics can be achieved by positioning one foot ahead of other and by bending the knees slightly (Gench et al., 1995, p. 184).

Clients with somatosensory losses will need to be aware of the areas that are insensate to prevent skin breakdown or damage. Pressure relief is a very important area of disability prevention for clients with lack of sensation. Clients are taught methods to inspect their skin daily. Pressure relief techniques, such as push-ups in the wheelchair or leaning to one side in a wheelchair, are essential to teach to clients with SCI to prevent decubiti ulcers (pressure sores). Clients are taught to relieve pressure at regular intervals, are able to differentiate pressure marks from pressure sores, and are provided with seating devices and special mattresses to minimize skin breakdown due to prolonged pressure.

Awareness of areas lacking sensation is important in compensatory practices. For example, a person with no thermal sensation will need to use alternative methods to prevent burns to the hand when checking water temperature. Decreasing the temperature of the hot water tank and using a thermometer are easily implement-

ed protective adaptations. Clients are taught to compensate for decreased sensation by relying more on vision.

Fall prevention is an important consideration in educating the client and family about safety. Teach the client and family to avoid using unsafe objects like a wheeled cart for support rather than a walker and to avoid using objects in an incorrect way. Poor lighting is also a variable to be considered when attempting to prevent falls. This is especially true in congested areas, halls, and entranceways. Furniture in poor repair is a danger as are loose scatter rugs. Instruct the client to be particularly diligent and attentive when using stairs. Be sure the family or caregiver is aware of transfer precautions and the level of assistance required by the client and why the assistance is needed. Falls in the bathroom are common and serious due to the small space, wet surfaces, lack of maneuverability, and hard surfaces. For children, playground equipment is a potential source of falls and many playgrounds being built now have reduced the fall impact by being covered with shredded rubber or mulch rather than concrete.

The family and client need to learn about environmental hazards in the home. Removal of small area rugs is important to consider for those who are ambulatory, in a wheelchair, have incoordination or ataxia or low vision. Railings on stairs that are brightly colored or of contrasting colors from the surrounding floor are helpful. Portable or cordless phones are very helpful because a person in a wheelchair may be unable to reach a wall-mounted telephone in an emergency. Checking the location of light switches, thermostats, and door locks may reveal that these are inaccessible for some clients. Buzzers, intercom systems, or environmental control units are commercially available as means of contacting others in the home or in independently controlling the environment. Use of adaptive equipment, such as tub seats, elevated commodes, and grab bars promote safety in bathrooms. Many of these concerns can be addressed in a home visit with the therapist, family, and client or by detailed descriptions of the home provided by the family and client.

General items in the home that are safety hazards include frayed cords, sharp kitchen implements, use of machinery, repetitive trauma, fires, and exposure to toxic substances. Often a home visit will identify potential safety hazards that may be overlooked by the family since they see the objects daily and may not see the danger as clearly. It is important to reinforce use of smoke and carbon dioxide detectors, which can be wired into the electrical circuits of the home. This would eliminate the need for batteries. Smoke detectors should be on every level of the home. The pitch of the alarm should be low enough to be heard easily by the elderly. Cordless utensils (including phones) are excellent devices that diminish the possibility of entanglement in the cord or inadvertently cutting the cord. Appliances that turn off automatically are excellent choices, especially if the client has decreased attention or short-term memory deficits. Devices that turn on automatically (outside lights with timers, coffee pots, etc.) are also good choices.

Education for the family and client may also include strategies for coping and stress management. This would be an important aspect of the rehabilitation frame of reference in enabling the client to become independent and responsible for his or her own care. Management of stress and coping techniques will prevent further disability and can contribute to the client's health promotion and wellness.

CASE STUDY

The following case study is provided to demonstrate how theory influences intervention. This case study has elements that are more appropriately considered within a compensatory/adaptation or rehabilitation intervention approach, while other aspects are better served using a remediation or biomechanical construct. This same case study is used in Chapter 11 so that the elements appropriate to each theory can be seen as they relate to this case. Other theories not covered in this text may also be appropriate and it is important to consider whether the all of the approaches selected can be implemented concurrently with others or if the design of the intervention needs to be sequential in nature.

Maggie

Maggie is a 61-year-old female referred to home health occupational therapy on October 29th with a diagnosis of right Colles fracture. Maggie fell while shopping at her neighborhood department store on October 27th. The physician has ordered occupational therapy to evaluate and treat.

On your first visit to see Maggie, you interview her and find out the following information. Maggie was in excellent health prior to this injury. Maggie's son, Fred, lives in the next town. She works part-time in her son's accounting office. A widow, she lives alone with her cat and her dog. Maggie is concerned that since she lives alone she needs to be able to do all of the cooking, cleaning, and care for her dog and cat. Her son is only able to come to her home every other day or every 3 days to assist with some of these activities.

Maggie is concerned about her present situation. She is right-handed and states that although she tries her best, she is not able to do very much for herself. Maggie has been very active in her local church organization. Maggie always heads up the Christmas crafts bazaar. Part of her responsibilities for the bazaar include organizing and teaching at craft nights. Maggie also has been one of the primary cooks for the annual fish dinner held just before Easter. She states that the church especially needs her this year because the other primary cook is moving to another state. She doesn't want to let the church organization down.

In the emergency room on October 27th, the emergency room physician performed a closed reduction and applied a plaster cast from mid-humeral level to the metacarpophalangeal (MCP) joints of the right hand. The elbow is casted in approximately 90 degrees of elbow flexion and the wrist is casted in approximately 30 degrees of wrist flexion. Maggie states that the physician has instructed her to stay home for the next 2 weeks and not to drive or do any housework. This is confirmed when you speak to the physician. A summary of information about Maggie as well as analysis of additional information that is needed and ideas about the next steps are as follows:

Facts

- 61-year-old female
- Enjoys shopping
- Right Colles fracture
- Fractures are immobilized, cause pain and edema
- Fractures may limit the use of the UE
- Lives alone
- Was independent in ADL, IADL
- Cares for dog and cat
- Active in church craft bazaar and fish dinner
- Anxious about present situation
- Immobilized in plaster case
- Physician restricted activities for 2 weeks

Additional Information Needed

- How did Maggie fall?
- Precautions
- Medical management of Colles fracture
- Possible complications
- Prognosis to return to prior level of function
- Tasks that Maggie will need to do to resume roles

Actions

- Continue dialogue with Maggie
- Review medical record
- Consult with physician
- Consult orthopedic textbooks and OT texts
- Perform OT assessments

From this information, an evaluation plan can be developed. Several assessments have been listed but these are not the only assessments that can be used to address the concerns about Maggie.

Evaluation Plan

Concerns

1. Maggie's perception of her strengths and weaknesses and her priorities for therapy.
2. Decreased ADL performance due to right (dominant) UE in cast.
3. Unable to carry out worker and volunteer roles.
4. Unable to participate in leisure pursuits.
5. Sensorimotor concerns (sensory): possible sensory loss or altered sensation due to pressure on nerves from swelling or tight cast.
6. Sensorimotor concerns (motor): potential for edema, stiffness and CRPS (complex regional pain syndrome previously known as RSD or reflex sympathetic dystrophy) in right hand; potential for frozen right shoulder.
7. Psychological and cognitive concerns: potential for depression due to loss of role performance and feelings of helplessness.

Assessments

1. Canadian Occupational Therapy Performance Measure (COPM) or other client centered informal interview tool.

2. Observe Maggie attempting to perform ADL tasks; Klein-Bell ADL assessment; self report; Functional Independence Measure (FIM).

3. Interview Maggie to determine specific worker and volunteer tasks and activities.

4. Interest checklist; formal or informal interview.

5. Sensory evaluation to exposed areas; observe cast for fit, look for areas of redness where cast is pressing against the skin.

6. AROM and PROM of PIP and DIP joints of the right hand; circumferential edema measurements of the digits; pain assessment; AROM and PROM of right shoulder.

7. Formal and informal interview; observe Maggie during evaluation; speak with family members and other team member.

How Assessment Results Will Be Used

1. Set client-centered goals for therapy; establish rapport; gain better understanding of Maggie's occupational context.

2. Assess potential for teaching compensatory techniques or use of adaptive equipment; determine components of ADL task causing difficulty; determine baseline for therapy.

3. Determine readiness for return to work and volunteer duties; assess potential for adapting tasks and activities.

4. Determine realistic leisure interest; assess potential for adapting leisure activities.

5. Set baseline for therapy; make suggestions for alterations of cast if necessary; determine need to teach compensatory techniques or sensory reeducation program if sensation is impaired or absent.

6. Set baseline for therapy; develop treatment plan which includes management of edema and home exercise program (HEP) to maintain ROM and prevent complications.

7. Determine Maggie's motivation for therapy; assess ability to follow directions and carry out HEP, set realistic goals appropriate for Maggie's cognitive and emotional status.

You evaluated Maggie and found the following.

Maggie is cognitively intact and motivated to be independent. Maggie is proud as she describes her success at figuring out how to open the foil packet of cat food with her left hand so that she could feed her cat. She is unable to don some types of blouses and dresses over the cast and is not able to don pants or skirts with closures. She requires minimal assistance to don a house dress, underpants, and socks. She is unable to don her bra or panty hose, or tie her shoes. Because of the inability to use her dominant right hand, Maggie is unable to manage buttons, has difficulty feeding herself with her nondominant left hand (spills food on herself frequently),

requires minimal assist with person hygiene after toileting, sponge bathing and brushing her teeth. She requires maximal assistance in simple meal preparation. Maggie states she is able to get herself some simple food items, such as prepared foods (prepared by her son's wife) from plastic containers. She is dependent in household chores such as cleaning.

Through further interview, you learn that much of Maggie's work at her son's office involves working with Excel, a spreadsheet computer program. She has a computer at home and is an avid Internet user. She tells you that it is difficult to use the computer now because she cannot use her right hand.

Tasks associated with her responsibilities as chairperson of the Christmas craft bazaar include phoning church members to inform them of meeting times and craft supplies they will be required to bring, and delegation of other responsibilities such as making refreshments, teaching certain crafts, and clean-up duties. She is having difficulty using her rotary dial telephone to keep in touch with other church volunteers.

Maggie complains of (c/o) moderate pain in her right upper extremity, mainly the wrist and fingers. She rates her pain an 8 on a scale of 1 to 10. She describes it as a burning, throbbing type of pain. Severe edema is noted in all of the digits of the right hand (approximately two times the size of the left hand). She has a great deal of difficulty flexing her fingers to make a fist (the cast restricts the MP motion). She is unable to oppose her thumb to her index or any other finger. She is unable to hold any objects in her right hand because of the cast. She states that at times her hand feels numb and other times she has paresthesia. The fingers are discolored, a dusky reddish color.

In your conversation with the home health coordinator and the social worker, you find out that Maggie's insurance will cover home health occupational therapy for up to 3 months for the purpose of improving independence in ADL. Table 12-9 would be an example of the intervention that would address compensatory, adaptation, or rehabilitation concerns in this case. This is not a complete intervention plan in that many areas that can be addressed in treatment by an occupational therapist are not included. By combining the treatment plan for the biomechanical remediation treatment plan with this, a more complete intervention for Maggie can be realized.

In Table 12-9, deficits as identified previously are related directed to long- and short-term outcomes. Specific principles or rationales are provided so that the reason for the specific intervention is clear.

Table 12-9.

TREATMENT PLAN: REHABILITATION/COMPENSATION AND ADAPTATION APPROACH

Deficits	Stage-Specific Cause	Short-Term Goals	Methods	Principle	Specific Activity/Modality
1. Spills food when eating with left hand.	1-7: Unable to use right dominant hand as it is nonfunctional due to immobilization and pain. Using left, nondominant hand for activities.	1. Client will use adapted utensil to feed self with non-dominant hand without spilling.	1. Provide textured built-up handle to compensate for de-creased manipulation of nondominant hand. Provide adapt-ive aids and educate in use of compensatory techniques for cutting, scooping, and spearing foods with one hand.	1. Textured handle will enable better manipulation of utensil. Compensate for lost RUE function.	1. Client will be provided with textured handle for utensils (plastizote) and instructed how to hold and use them. Client will practice using adapted spoon with left hand.
2. Minimal assist with personal hygiene (toilet hygiene, brushing teeth).		2. Independent personal hygiene using one-handed techniques and adaptive equipment.		2, 3, 4, 5, 6: Comp-ensate for lost RUE-function.	2. Client will be educated in and practice one-handed technique of opening toothpaste and applying to brush.
3. Minimal assist with sponge bathing.		3. Independent sponge bathing using one-handed techniques and adaptive aids.	2, 3, 4, 5, 6: Educate client in use of comp-ensatory techniques and adaptive aids, which compensate for lost UE function.		3. Client will be provided with "octopus" suction cup to hold soap and educated how to soap wash cloth using left hand only. Client will learn to wring out wash cloth by pressing against sink and will practice one-handed techniques with assistance and verbal cues from therapist.
4. Minimal assist with donning/doffing house dress, under-pants, socks.		4. Independent in donning/doffing house dress, under-pants, socks using compensatory techniques.			4. Client will be educated in and helped to select type of clothing that will fit easily over cast. Client will be educated in one-handed dressing techniques and will practice these tech-niques with assistance and verbal cues by the thera-pist.
5. Dependent in donning bra, panty hose, shoes.		5. Minimal assist donning/doffing bra, pantyhose, shoes using adaptive aids and compensatory techniques.			5. Client will be provided with elastic laces and/or taught one handed shoe tying. Client will practice donning/doffing shoes with assistance and verbal cues from therapist. Client will be educated in and will practice one-handed bra donning.

Table 12-9, continued.

Deficits	Stage-Specific Cause	Short-Term Goals	Methods	Principle	Specific Activity/Modality
6. Maximal assist with meal preparation.		6. Minimal assistance in simple meal preparation using adaptive aids and compensatory techniques.			6. Client will be educated in use of prepackaged food, compensatory techniques for opening packages; cutting board will be adapted with stainless steel nails, etc. Client will be educated in energy conservation and work simplification techniques and will practice simple meal preparation with assistance and verbal cues from the therapist.
7. Unable to perform volunteer role of chairperson of craft bazaar.		7. Independent in using phone to contact volunteers to organize bazaar using adaptive aids and compensatory techniques.	7. Educate client in use of compensatory techniques and adaptive aids which compensate for lost RUE function.	7. Compensate for lost RUE function.	7. Client will be assisted in obtaining a speaker phone with large numbers for dialing. Phone will be positioned in easily accessible place and in an area where other volunteer work supplies are placed. Client will be educated in using the phone with one-handed techniques. Client will delegate some duties to other volunteers.
8. Unable to perform worker role/tasks; using computer to manage accounting files.	8. Unable to use RUE functionally and unable to travel to workplace.	8. Independent in using home computer to perform work tasks using adaptive aids and compensatory techniques.	8. Educate client in use of compensatory techniques and adaptive aids which compensate for lost RUE function and restricted ability to travel to work.	8. Compensate for lost function of RUE and restricted ability to travel to work.	8. Home computer will be adapted for left hand use (eg, mouse function changed, etc.). Client will be educated in sending and receiving files via email.

SUMMARY

- The rehabilitation frame of reference is a compensatory and adaptation approach used when there is little or no expectation for change and where there are residual impairments. It may also be used when there is limited time for intervention and when the client or family prefers more immediate resolution of functional problems.

- This intervention approach focuses on the areas of occupation, which includes work, play, leisure, education instrumental ADL, and social participation rather than on the underlying performance skills. This is known as a "top-down" approach where intervention starts by identifying the environmental demands and resources with the client.

- Intervention methods include changing the task or changing the context.

- Changing the task can be accomplished by adapting how the task is done or by changing the task objects or using adaptive equipment.

- Changing the context would include environmental modification and training the client and caregivers.

- Disability prevention is accomplished by client and caregiver education. This is especially true of those who already have activity or participation limitations as well as those who may be a member of an at-risk population.

REFERENCES

American Occupational Therapy Association. (1995). Position paper: Occupation. *Amer J Occup Ther*, 49(10), 1015-1018.

Beaver, K., & Mann, W. C. (1995). Overview of technology for low vision. *Amer J Occup Ther*, 49(9), 913-921.

Colenbrander, A., & Fletcher, D. C. (1995). Basic concepts and terms for low vision rehabilitation. *Amer J Occup Ther*, 49(9), 865-869.

Cooper, B. A. (1985). A model for implementing color contrast in the environment of the elderly. *Amer J Occup Ther*, 39(4), 253-314.

Cristarella, M. (1977). Visual functions of the elderly. *Am J Occup Ther*, 31(7), 432-440.

Dutton, R. (1995). *Clinical reasoning in physical disabilities*. Baltimore: Williams & Wilkins.

Gench, B. E., Hinson, M M., & Harvey, P. T. (1995). *Anatomical kinesiology*. Dubuque, IA: Eddie Bowers Publishing Co.

Lempert, J., & Lapolice, D. J. (1995). Functional considerations in evaluation and treatment of the client with low vision. *Am J Occup Ther*, 49(9), 885-889.

Marrelli, T. M., & Krulish, L. H. (1999). *Home care therapy: Quality, documentation and reimbursement*. Boca Grande, FL: Marrelli and Associates, Inc.

Moyers, P. A. (1999). The guide to occupational therapy practice. *Amer J Occup Ther*, 53(3), 247-321.

Palmer, M. L., & Toms, J. E. (1992). *Manual for functional training*. Philadelphia: F. A. Davis Co.

Pierson, F. M. (1994). *Principles and techniques of patient care*. Philadelphia: W. B. Saunders Co.

Turner, A., Foster, M., & Johnson, S. E. (1996). *Occupational therapy and physical dysfunction: Principles, skills and practice* (4th ed.). New York: Churchill Livingstone.

Trombly, C. A. (Ed.). (1995). *Occupational therapy for physical dysfunction* (4th ed.). Baltimore: Williams & Wilkins.

BIBLIOGRAPHY

American Occupational Therapy Association. (1994). Uniform terminology for occupational therapy, third edition. *Amer J Occup Ther*, 48(11), 1047-1054.

Andersen, L. T. (2002). *Adult physical disabilities: Case studies for learning*. Thorofare, NJ: SLACK Incorporated.

Bowen, J. E. (1999). Health promotion in the new millennium: Opening the lens, adjusting the focus. *OT Practice*, 14-18.

Christiansen, C., & Baum, C. (1997). *Occupational therapy: Enabling function and well-being* (2nd ed.). Thorofare, NJ: SLACK Incorporated.

Collins, L. F. (1996). Understanding visual impairments. *OT Practice*, Jan. 1996, 27-33.

Cook, A. M., Hussey, S. M. (1995). *Assistive technologies: Principles and practice*. St. Louis, MO: C. V. Mosby.

Greene, D. P., & Roberts, S. L. (1999). *Kinesiology: Movement in the context of activity*. St. Louis, MO: C. V. Mosby.

Kielhofner, G. (1992). *Conceptual foundations of occupational therapy*. Philadelphia: F. A. Davis Co.

Kisner, C., & Colby, L. A. (1990). *Therapeutic exercise: Foundations and techniques* (2nd ed.). Philadelphia: F. A. Davis

Pedretti, L. W. (1996). *Occupational therapy: Practice skills for physical dysfunction* (4th ed.). St. Louis, MO: C. V. Mosby.

Sine, R., Liss, S. E., Rousch, R. E., Holcomb, J. D., & Wilson, G. (2000). *Basic rehabilitation techniques: A self instructional guide* (4th ed.). Gaithersburg, MD: Aspen Publishers.

Toth-Riddering, A. (1998). Living with age-related macular degeneration. *OT Practice*, Jan 1998, 18-23.

Appendices

Appendix A

MEASUREMENT OF GRIP STRENGTH STUDIES

Author	Instrument	Population	Sex	Age	Height/ Weight	Hand Dominance
An et al. (1980)	Strain gauge					
Balogun et al. (1991)	Harpenden dynamometer	f=26; m=35 healthy; 16-18 years	M>F	Positive correlation	Positive correlation	Dominant only tested
Balogun et al. (1991)	Harpenden dynamometer	f=480; m=480 healthy, 7-84 years	M>F	Positive correlation up to 3rd decade; thereafter a negative correlation	Positive correlation.	R>L
Balogun et al. (1991)	Harpenden dynamometer MS	f=6; m=31 healthy; 16-28 years				R only tested
Desrosiers et al. (1995)	Jamar dynamometer Martin vigorometer	f=179; m=181 mean age 73.9 healthy	M>F	Negative correlation with age		
Downie et al. (1978)	VAS	7 healthy				
Fransson and Winkel (1991)	Strain gauged pliers	f=8; m=8 healthy 18-60 years	M>F			R only tested
Fraser and Benten (1983)	Vigorometer	f=60; m=60 healthy; 20-80 years	M>F	Increase to 30 years then deterioration with age especially after 50 years		No significant differences between R and L
Gilbert and Knowlton (1984)	Load cell	f=16; m=20 healthy; 20-26 years	M>F			Dominant only
Goldman et al. (1991)	Jamar	f=16; m=10 healthy; 23-29 years; f=11, m=10 hand patients 23-84 years				Both hands tested Injured less than noninjured
Jarit (1991)	Jamar	44 controls; 44 baseball players				Nondominant 89.7% of dominant in baseball players; 86.5% in control group
Kellor et al. (1971)	Jamar	f=126; m=126 healthy; 18-84 years	M>F	Negative correlation		R>L
Lunde et al. (1971)	Kny-sheer dynamometer	f=57; healthy			Positively correlated with height and weight	Dominant 13% stronger than nondominant hand
Lusardi and Bohannon (1991)	Jamar MS	f=34; healthy 19-64 years				

Appendix A, continued.

Author	Instrument	Population	Sex	Age	Height Weight	Hand Dominance
Mathiowetz et al. (1985)	Jamar	f=328; m=310 healthy; 20-94 years	M>F	Peaked 25-39 years, gradual decline		R>L
Masaki et al. (1999)	Smedle dynamometer	3,218 men; 45-48 years; initially healthy				
Mawdsley et al. (2000)	Jamar dynamometer	f=6; m=12; healthy; mean age 20.4 years				Dominant > than nondominant
Mathiowetz et al. (1985)	Jamar	f=29; healthy 20-34 years				R>L
Mathiowetz et al. (1990)	Jamar	49 controls 49 rehabilitation patients				
Marion and Niebuhr (1992)	Jamar	f=30; healthy 21-45 years				R only tested
Newman et al. (1984)	Strain gauged system	1417 healthy children; 5-18 years	M>F	Boys-linear increase; girls increase to 13 then plateau	Positive correlation with height and weight	Dominant hand > strength
Shifman (1992)	Jamar	f=20; m=20 healthy; 24-87 years		Negative correlation with age		R>L
Solgaard et al. (1984)	Vigorometer my-gripper steel spring dynamometer	f=5; m=45; healthy; 20-87 years		Negative correlation with age	Positive correlation with height and weight	Dominant > nondominant
Somedeepti et al. (1990)	Jamar	f=30; m=30 unilaterally injured; mean age 28 years	M>F			
Speigal et al. (1987)	Sphygomoman-ometer	92 rheumatoid patients with mean age 58 years				R and L measured; results not specified
Teraoka (1979)	Smedley dynamometer	9543 healthy 15-58 year olds	M>F	Negative correlation with age		R>L
Unsworth et al. (1990)	Inflatable cuffs					

Reprinted with permission from Durward B., Back, G., & Rowe, P. *Functional Human Movement*. Oxford: Butterworth Heinemann.

Appendix B

SUMMARY OF SHOULDER MOVEMENTS

Articulation	Plane/Axis	Normal Limiting Factors	End Feel	Muscles
Scapular motions: Elevation: scapulothoracic acromioclavicular sternoclavicular	Frontal/sagittal	Tension in the costoclavicular ligament, inferior sternoclavicular joint capsule, low fibers of trapezius, pectoralis minor, and subclavius.	Firm	Upper trapezius, levator scapulae, rhomboids
Depression scapulothoracic acromioclavicular sternoclavicular	Frontal/sagittal	Tension in the interclavicular ligament, sternoclavicular ligament, articular disk, upper fibers of trapezius, and levator scapulae; bony contact between the clavicle and the superior aspect of the first rib.	Firm	Pectoralis minor Lower trapezius (pectoralis major) (latissimus dorsi) (these act on humerus)
Abduction/ Protraction scapulothoracic acromioclavicular sternoclavicular	Horizontal/ vertical	Tension in the trapezoid ligament, anterior sternoclavicular ligament, posterior laminal of costoclavicular ligament, trapezius, and rhomboids.	Firm	Abduction: serratus anterior Protraction: serratus anterior pectoralis minor pectoralis major
Adduction/ Retraction scapulothoracic acromioclavicular sternoclavicular	Horizontal/ vertical	Tension in the conoid ligament, anterior lamina of the costoclavicular ligament, posterior sternoclavicular ligament, pectoralis minor and serratus anterior.	Firm	Trapezius rhomboids
Medial Rotation/ Downward Rotation scapulothoracic acromioclavicular sternoclavicular	Frontal/ sagittal	Tension in the conoid ligament and serratus anterior.	Firm	Levator scapula rhomboid
Lateral Rotation/ Upward Rotation scapulothoracic acromioclavicular sternoclavicular	Frontal/ sagittal	Tension in the trapezoid ligament, the rhomboid muscles and the levator scapula.	Firm	Middle trapezius serratus anterior
glenohumeral Motions: Flexion glenohumeral	Sagittal/ frontal	Pain at ends of range; capsular stretch if capsule damaged.	Firm if coraco-clavicular or coracohumeral ligaments soft	Pectoralis major (clavicular head) anterior deltoid coracobrachialis biceps brachii

Appendix B, continued.

Articulation	Plane/Axis	Normal Limiting Factors	End Feel	Muscles
Extension glenohumeral	Sagittal/ frontal	Tension in anterior band of the coracohumeral ligament, anterior joint capsule and clavicular fibers of pectoralis major.	Firm due to biceps with elbow extended; hard with greater tuberosity hitting the acromion posteriorly	Latissimus dorsi teres major triceps brachii (long head) posterior deltoid
External Rotation glenohumeral	Horizontal/ vertical	Tension in all bands of the glenohumeral ligament, coraco-humeral ligament, the anterior joint capsule, subscapularis, pectoralis major, teres major, and latissimus dorsi.	Firm	Infraspinatus teres minor posterior deltoid
Internal Rotation glenohumeral	Horizontal/ vertical	Tension in the posterior joint capsule, infraspinatus, teres minor.	Firm	Subscapularis pectoralis minor teres major anterior deltoid latissimus dorsi
Horizontal Abduction glenohumeral	Horizontal/ vertical	Tension in the anterior joint capsule, the glenohumeral ligament, and the pectoralis major.	Firm	Posterior deltoid teres major teres minor infraspinatus
Horizontal Adduction glenohumeral	Horizontal/ vertical	Tension in the posterior joint capsule.	Firm	Pectoralis major anterior deltoid
Adduction glenohumeral			Soft since arm contacts trunk; firm if tension in serratus anterior and pectoralis minor	Pectoralis major latissimus dorsi teres major subscapularis
Abduction glenohumeral				Middle deltoid supraspinatus infraspinatus subscapularis teres minor (long head biceps)

Appendix C

SUMMARY OF ELBOW MOVEMENTS

Articulation	Plane/Axis	Normal Limiting Factors	End Feel	Muscles
Flexion humeroulnar humeroradial	Sagittal/frontal	Soft tissue apposition of the anterior forearm and upper arm, posterior capsule and extensor muscles; coronoid process contacting the coronoid fossa.	Soft tissue approximation due to compression of forearm against upper arm; if muscle bulk is small, end feel may be hard because contact of radius and radial fossa of humerus and contact of coronoid process with coronoid fossa	Biceps brachii brachialis brachioradialis pronator teres flexor carpi ulnaris ECRL and ECRB
Extension humeroulnar humeroradial	Sagittal/ frontal	Olecranon process contacting the olecranon fossa.	Hard due to olecranon process in olecranon fossa, sometimes firm because anterior joint capsule and collateral ligaments and tension in biceps and brachialis muscles	Triceps Anconeus
Supination humeroulnar humeroradial superior radioulnar inferior radioulnar interosseous membrane	Horizontal/ longitudinal	Tension in the pronator muscles, palmar radial ligament of the inferior radioulnar joint, oblique chord and interosseous membrane.	Firm due to radioulnar ligaments and interosseous membrane, pronator quadratus, and pronator teres	Supinator biceps brachioradialis APL, EPB, EIP
Pronation humeroulnar humeroradial superior radioulnar inferior radioulnar interosseous membrane	Horizontal/ longitudinal	Contact of the radius on the ulna; tension in the dorsal radioulnar ligament of the inferior radioulnar joint, interosseous membrane and biceps muscle.	Firm if due to tension in ligament	Pronator teres pronator quadratus palmaris longus flexor carpi radialis brachioradialis ECRL

Appendix D

SUMMARY OF WRIST MOVEMENTS

Wrist motion	*Articulation*	*Plane/Axis*	*Normal Limiting Factor Muscles*	*End Feel*
Flexion	Midcarpal Radiocarpal	Sagittal plane/ frontal axis	Tension in the posterior radiocarpal ligament and posterior joint capsule.	Firm
Extension	Radiocarpal Midcarpal	Sagittal plane/ frontal axis	Tension in the anterior radiocarpal ligament and anterior joint capsule; Contact between the radial and carpal bones.	Firm
Radial deviation (radial flexion or radial abduction)	Midcarpal Radiocarpal	Frontal plane/ sagittal axis	Tension in the ulnar collateral ligament, ulnocarpal ligament and ulnar portion of the joint capsule; Contact between the radial styloid process and the scaphoid bone.	Firm
Ulnar deviation (adduction, ulnar flexion, ulnar abduction)	Radiocarpal	Frontal plane/ sagittal axis	Tension in the radial collateral ligament and the radial portion of the joint capsule.	Firm

Appendix E

SUMMARY OF HAND MOVEMENTS

Flexion

Metacarpophalangeal (MCP)	Sagittal plane/ frontal axis	MCP: tension in the posterior joint capsule collateral ligaments; contact between the proximal phalanx and the metacarpal.	MCP: firm	FDMB FDS FDP FDM
Proximal Interphalangeal (PIP)	Sagittal plane/ frontal axis	PIP: contact between the middle and proximal phalanx; soft tissue apposition of the middle and proximal phalanges; tension in the posterior joint capsule, collateral ligaments.	PIP: hard	
Distal Interphalangeal (DIP)	Sagittal plane/ frontal axis	DIP: tension in the posterior joint capsule, collateral ligaments and oblique retinacular ligament.	DIP: firm	

Extension

Metacarpophalangeal (MCP)	Sagittal plane/ frontal axis	MCP: tension in the anterior joint capsule, palmar fibrocartilagenous plate (palmar ligament).	MCP: firm	
Proximal interphalangeal (PIP)	Sagittal plane/ frontal axis	PIP: tension in the anterior joint capsule, palmar ligament.	PIP: firm	
Distal interphalangeal (DIP)	Sagittal plane/ frontal axis	DIP: tension in the anterior joint capsule, palmar ligament.	DIP: firm	

Abduction

Metacarpophalangeal (MCP)	Frontal plane/ sagittal axis	Tension in the collateral ligaments, fascia and skin of the web spaces and palmar interosseus muscle.	Firm	

Adduction

(of fingers)	Frontal plane/ sagittal axis			

Opposition

(of little finger)

Appendix E, continued.

Flexion

Carpometacarpal (CMC)	CM: oblique frontal plan/oblique sagittal axis	CM: soft tissue apposition between the thenar eminence and the palm; tension in the posterior joint capsule, EPB and APB.	CM: soft	OP FPB FPL APB* DI*
Metacarpophalangeal (MCP)	MCP: frontal plane/ sagittal axis	MCP: contact between the first metacarpal and the proximal phalanx; tension in the posterior joint capsule, collateral ligaments, EPB.	MCP: hard	
Interphalangeal (IP)	IP: frontal plane/ sagittal axis	IP: tension in the collateral ligaments, posterior joint capsule; contact between the distal phalanx, fibrocartilogenous plate and the proximal phalanx.	IP: firm	

Extension

Carpometacarpal (CMC)	CMC: frontal plane/ oblique sagittal axis	CMC: tension in the anterior joint capsule, FPB and first dorsal interosseus.	CM: firm	EPB EPL APL
Metacarpophalangeal (MCP)	MCP: frontal plane/ sagittal axis	MCP: tension in the anterior joint capsule, palmar ligaments and FPB.	MCP: firm	
Interphalangeal (IP)	IP: frontal plane/ sagittal axis	IP: tension in the anterior joint capsule, palmar ligament.	IP: firm	

Abduction

Carpometacarpal (CMC)	Oblique sagittal plane/oblique frontal plane	Tension in the fascia and skin of the first web space, first dorsal interosseus and APL.	Firm	APL OP** APB
Metacarpophalangeal (MCP)				

Adduction

Carpometacarpal (CMC) Metacarpophalangeal (MCP)	Oblique sagittal plane/oblique frontal plane	Soft tissue apposition between the thumb and index finger.	Soft	FPB AP FPL** EPL**

*Assist

**No agreement between sources

Reprinted with permission from Baxter, R. *Pocket Guide to Musculoskeletal Assessment.* Philadelphia: W.B. Saunders Co; 1998.

Appendix F

OVERVIEW OF SHOULDER PATHOLOGY

Pain

Location: May be referred from many parts of the body including the heart, lungs, diaphragm, gallbladder, spleen, pancreas, cervical or thoracic spine, ribs, wrist, hand, elbow, temporomandibular joint.

Type:

Sharp   May suggest injury to:
- superficial muscles or tendon
- acute bursitis
- injury to the periosteum

Dull   May suggest injury to:
- tendon sheath
- deep muscle (serratus anterior or subscapularis)
- bone

Ache   May suggest injury to:
- deep muscle (subscapularis, teres minor)
- deep ligament (glenohumeral, coracoclavicular)
- tendon sheath or fibrous capsule
- chronic bursitis

Pins and needles   May suggest injury to:
- peripheral nerve
- dorsal root of a cervical nerve

Tingling   May suggest injury to:
- A circulatory or neural structure (thoracic outlet, brachial plexus, brachial artery, etc.)

Numbness   May suggest injury to:
- cervical nerve root
- peripheral cutaneous nerves

Twinges   May suggest injury to:
- subluxation
- muscle strain
- ligamentous sprain

Stiffness   May suggest injury to:
- capsular swelling
- arthritic changes
- muscle spasms

Severity   Varies according to emotional state, cultural background, previous injuries.

Timing of pain
- night pain may suggest inflamed bursa, vascular disease, metastatic disease, or RSD.
- sleeping postures can affect shoulder pain.
- pain with specific movements suggests musculoskeletal problem, possible capsular problem or an impingement problem.

Sensations

Clicking   May be due to glenoid labrum tear or due to glenohumeral subluxation.

Snapping   May be caused by biceps tendon, or catching of thickened bursa under the acromion during abduction.

	Appendix F, continued.

Sensations

Grating	May be due to osteoarthritic changes, calcium in the joint, thickened bursa.
Locking or catching	May be due to calcium in the joint, piece of articular cartilage fractured off of the humerus or labrum.
Warmth	May indicate inflammation or infection.

Contusion

Acromioclavicular joint most frequent.

Frequent deltoid contusions if shoulder pad not worn in sports activities.

Contusions on upper arm over biceps and triceps common because these are below shoulder pads.

Deltoid midbelly contusions in hockey and lacrosse where sticks are used.

Coracoid process can be contused when marksmen gun recoils.

Fracture

Clavicle: greenstick of shaft frequent in children and preadolescents.

Distal end of clavicle when acromion hits downward in relation to clavicle.

Fractures occur when one falls on shoulder or outstretched arm as in contact sports.

Acromion can fracture when there is a fracture of the distal end of clavicle or due to a direct blow down over acromion.

Scapula: rare.

Humerus due to a fall on outstretched arm but can be direct blow.

May hold arm to side.

Sprain, Subluxation, Dislocation:

Glenohumeral	Anterior dislocation frequent; indirect force such as fall on outstretched arm or elbow.

Subscapularis: primary rotator cuff responsible for prevention of anterior displacement of humeral head.

Usually damage to anterior portion capsule and subscapularis.

Prevention via strengthening activities and bracing/splinting for chronic instabilities.

Subluxation often due to trauma to joint where there is excessive ER and abduction.

Damage can be to anterior glenohumeral capsule or ligamental sprain or tear.

Coracohumeral ligament sprain.

Tear of labrum.

Bankcard lesion/labral lesion where there is injury to the glenoid rim and anterior capsule.

ligaments detach and do not stabilize humeral head when anterior joint capsule becomes stretched and loose from the humerus.

Ambri dislocations – hyperlaxity of connective tissue.

> a = atraumatic
>
> m = multidirectional
>
> b = bilateral
>
> r = rehabilitation, not surgery
>
> I = instability

Hill-sachs lesion, which is a compression fracture or defect in posterolateral humeral head due to repeated trauma.

Brachial plexis or axillary nerve damage may occur.

Humeral neck fracture or avulsion of greater tuberosity.

Appendix F, continued.

Sprain, Subluxation,
Dislocation:

Glenohumeral   Posterior dislocation occasional; usually subluxation.

                         Inferior dislocation rare.

Sternoclavicular   Most common injury is anterior or superior displacement.

                         Posterior or inferior displacement less common.

                         Rarely dislocated due to position in body; if dislocation occurs, there is very little discomfort
                         or dysfunction.

                         Ligaments can be sprained or torn with displacement. If acute posterior dislocation occurs,
                         requires emergency reduction due to proximity to trachea, subclavian artery and vein,

                         aortic arch and esophagus, respiratory status and circulatory system must be monitored.

Acromioclavicular   Sprains:

                              Degenerative and traumatic injuries, especially sports Level I intra-articular trauma without
                              disruption of joint capsule or coracoclavicular ligaments; Level II disruption of acromio-
                              clavicular joint capsule and acromioclavicular ligament but without disruption of coraco-
                              clavicular ligament; Level III acromion dislocation, disruption of capsule, acromioclavic-
                              ular ligaments, and coracoclavicular ligament.

                         Can be sprained by:

                              Fall on point of shoulder with arm adducted.

                              Fall on outstretched arm.

                              Fall on olecranon of elbow.

                              Blow from behind with ipsilateral arm fixed on ground.

                              Traction of humerus pulling acromion away from clavicle.

                              Direct blow over acromion.

Overstretch Injuries

                         Often involve nerve damage or injuries.

                         Overly forceful muscle contractions.

                         Most common strains are to:

                              Internal rotators: subscapularis, latissimus dorsi, teres major, pectoralis major.

                              External rotators: infraspinatus, supraspinatus teres minor.

                              Long head of biceps at superior tip of labrum.

Overuse Injuries

                         Impingement syndromes as seen in overhand tennis stroke, front crawl and butterfly swimming
                         strokes, and side arm and overhand throwing actions.

                         Overuse.

                         Microtrauma and inflammation.

                         Instability.

                         Subluxation.

                         Impingement (repetitive trauma without repair).

                         Rotator cuff tear.

Tendinitis

                         Supraspinatus, infraspinatus, or subscapularis often affected.

                         Tendon of the long head of biceps in bicipital groove, infraspinatus tendon and supraspinatus
                         tendon.

                         Young people: overuse syndrome in infraspinatus and long biceps; others may include pec-
                         toralis minor, short biceps, coracobrachialis.

Appendix F, continued.

Tendinitis

Older: supraspinatus especially vulnerable to impingement or overuse leading to degenerative changes, calcification, and eventual rupture; possible explanations are chronic ischemia and decreased healing.

Symptom: acute pain that can disturb sleep or chronic pain with low grade irritation.

Referred pain in c5 and c6 dermatome.

Painful arc with ROM, when isometric resistance, and when muscle is stretched.

Muscle contraction strong unless there is a tear.

Tenderness over tendon when palpated.

Immediate care: ice, rest, then anti-inflammatory medication, physical agent modalities.

Prevention via stretching, strengthening, and activity modification.

Bursitis

Due to trauma or overuse so that the bursae become inflamed.

Subacromial or bicipital bursitis or subdeltoid or subacromial bursa.

Similar to acute tendinitis.

Acute Conditions

Rheumatoid arthritis.

Osteoarthritis.

Trauma.

Diabetes mellitus.

Microtrauma from poor posture.

Immobilization.

Ischemic heart disease or stroke.

Subacute and Chronic Conditions

Osteoarthritis.

Metastasis in acromion.

Frozen Shoulder

Capsular pattern/
Adhesive capsulitis

Age 40-60, unknown cause.

Freezing = intense pain even at rest and limitation of motion 2 to 3 weeks following onset.

Frozen = pain only with movement; substitute patterns to achieve motions of the scapula. Atrophy of the deltoid, rotator cuff, biceps, and triceps muscles occurs.

Thawing = no pain but significant capsular restrictions.

Spontaneous recovery occurs in an average of 2 years after onset.

Inappropriately aggressive treatment will prolong this condition and treatment at the wrong time may prolong symptoms.

Severe = if there is no ER, and abduction is limited to 75 degrees, and flexion to 100 degrees. Moderate = if there is 30 degrees external rotation, abduction to 100 degrees, flexion to 120 degrees.

Types:

Primary: idiopathic, spontaneous onset of painful shoulder; insidious for no reason; progressive; women more than men; symptom is pain, nontrauma, and the condition runs its course; steroids help a little but doesn't change rate of recovery; maintaining range of motion and not exacerbating the pain are effective with codman exercises.

Secondary/traumatic: Other injury→immobilize→stiff shoulder; pain is not the issue, but joint tissues shortened.

Appendix F, continued.

Shoulder Impingement

Biceps tendon and rotator cuff often affected as these pass through the acromial space.

May be due to an insufficiently stabilized humeral head (due to weakened rotator cuff or biceps, which allows more movement; weak supraspinatus or infraspinatus).

May be inflammation, tendon damage, bony malformations, poor posture.

Shoulder-Hand Syndrome

Symptom:

Pain or hyperesthesia in shoulder, wrist or hand.

Limitation in shoulder ER and abduct; wrist extension; hand MCP and PIP flexion.

Edema with circulatory impairment of venous and lymphatic systems -> stiffness.

Vasomotor instability.

Trophic changes in skin.

Then...

Pain subsides but limitations remain.

Skin cyanotic and shiny.

Intrinsic hand atrophy.

Subcutaneous tissues in fingers and palmar fascia thicken.

Nail changes.

Can develop in association with CVA, MI, cervical osteoarthritis, trauma such as fracture of humerus; progressive unless vigorous intervention.

Appendix G

OVERVIEW OF ELBOW PATHOLOGY

Type	*Location/Description*
Pain	
Location	If easily localized, more likely to be a superficial structure; deeper structures elicit pain that is more difficult to localize or radiates.
	Local tenderness may occur with olecranon bursitis, epicondylitis, muscle strains, or ligamental sprains.
	Diffuse pain may be due to referred pain from dermatomes or cutaneous nerves, joint subluxations, severe hematoma, fractures.
Onset	Immediate pain suggests acute injuries such as hemarthroses, fractures, subluxations, or severe sprains or tears.
	Gradual onset suggests overuse injuries or epicondylitis, ulnar neuritis.
	Pain 6 to 24 hours after an activity may suggest a more chronic condition.
Sharp pain	May suggest injury to skin, fascia, superficial muscle or ligaments, inflammation of bursa or periosteum.
Dull ache	May suggest injury to subchondral bone, fibrous capsule, or chronic olecranon bursitis.
Tingling	May suggest injury to peripheral nerve damage, irritation of nerve roots of C5-8, or a circulatory problem.
Numbness	May suggest injury to peripheral nerves or dorsal nerve roots affecting C6-T1 dermatomes.
Time of pain	*Morning*: rest does not alleviate the pain and may suggest that the injury is still acute, that there is an infection or is systemic in nature, or that rheumatoid arthritis may be present.
	Evening: suggests that activities aggravate the pain.
	At night: may indicate bone neoplasm, local or systemic disorders.
Swelling	
Type	*Local*: may be due to bursae, muscle strains or contusions to tendons, muscle bellies; or may be due to intracapsular effusion.
	Diffuse: may be due to severe hematoma, dislocations, or fractures.
Time	*Immediate to within first 2 hours*: damage to a structure with rich blood supply.
	6 to 24 hours: suggests synovial irritation as may occur with bone chips, capsular sprains, ligament sprain, or joint subluxation.
	after activity: chronic bursitis or repeated trauma to bursae.
Sensations	
Locking warmth	May occur if loose body is in the joint; may suggest inflammation or infection.
Tingling, numbness	May suggest C5-8 nerve root compression, thoracic outlet syndrome, injury to peripheral nerves or neuritis or neuropathy.
Grating	Osteoarthritic changes or damage to articular surface (chondromalacia, osteochondritis, osteoarthritis).
Contusions	
	Olecranon contusion when fall on tip of elbow.
	Lateral epicondyle and radial head frequently contused.
	Biceps and triceps often contused, especially in contact sports; can lead to myositis ossificans.

Appendix G, continued.

Fractures

Especially in children and adolescents due to epiphyseal plates are not closed and ligamental structures are stronger than cartilaginous plates; condylar and epicondylar fractures, especially on the medial aspect.

Medial epicondylar fractures, usually avulsion fractures due to excessive force on ulnar collateral ligaments.

Lateral epicondylar fracture, often avulsion through growth center due to excessive force through the common extensor origin.

With all fractures of the elbow, disruption of arterial supply may cause Volkman's ischemic contractures, which is a medical emergency.

Supracondylar fracture, usually in children, is very serious due to nearness of brachial artery and median nerve. Occurs often due to a fall on an outstretched hand or forced elbow hyper-extension without dislocation.

Monteggia fracture-dislocation is a fracture of the ulna just distal to the olecranon due to fall on the outstretched hand.

Head of radius may fracture.

Osteochondritis of the capitulum (panner disease) may occur due to direct trauma or inade-quate circulation through the elbow joint.

Bursitis

Olecranon bursitis due to fall on tip of elbow or direct blow causing swelling into the bursa.

Radiohumeral bursa can occur due to a direct blow or extensor muscle overuse; not to be con-fused with lateral epicondylitis.

Overstretch Injuries

Hyperextension due to falls on outstretched arm with elbow extended and forearm supinated potentially causing damage to: biceps, brachialis, brachioradialis, anterior portion of medial and/or lateral collateral ligaments, or elbow capsule.

In child or young adolescent, hyperextension usually causes a supracondylar fracture.

In older athletes, fractures occur in ulna or radius.

Very common in gymnasts and in wrestling.

Sprain/Strain

Valgus force causing medial collateral ligament sprain or tear and damage to anterior capsule; these are often associated with ulnar nerve paresthesias.

Forced pronation can cause posterior subluxation of ulnar head.

Forced supination can sprain the annular ligament or lateral collateral ligament.

Swelling, pain.

Overcontraction: Acute Muscle Strain

Common extensor tendon (lateral epicondyle).

Common flexor tendon (medial epicondyle).

Overuse

Wrist extensor-supinator overuse results in:

    lateral epicondylitis

    tendonitis

    radiohumeral bursitis

    radial head fibrillation

Appendix G, continued.

Overuse

radial tunnel syndrome

annual ligament inflammation

Entrapment of posterior interosseous nerve.

Lateral epicondylitis, especially with sports such as tennis and racquetball due to forceful contraction involving wrist extensors.

Wrist flexion with a valgus force at extending the elbow and incorrect biomechanics.

Medial epicondylitis or "little league elbow".

Repeated elbow extension with a valgus force.

Repeated wrist flexion (i. e., golfers at medial epicondyle; tennis players and athletes who are in throwing sports).

Repeated elbow flexion.

Joint Problems

Humeroulnar   Passive flexion is more limited than extension; capsular end feel.

Humeroradial   Flexion and extension limited only in prolonged immobilization or arthritis and then pronation and supination will also be limited.

Proximal Subluxation of the Radial Head

May be limited flexion or extension, limited wrist flexion or limited pronation.

Distal Subluxation of the Radial Head (pulled elbow)

Limited supination with pain following forceful traction to forearm; "tennis elbow".

Proximal Radioulnar Joint

Limited pronation and supination with pain when overpressure applied.

Distal Radioulnar Joint

May be limited pronation or supination and pain in distal forearm with overpressure.

Myositis Ossificans

Brachialis muscle may be affected following trauma to the elbow; most often seen with supracondylar fracture and posterior dislocation or tear of the brachialis tendon. Resisted elbow flexion causes pain; flexion is limited and palpation of distal brachialis muscle is tender.

Tendinitis

Pain and swelling in elbow region and pain and weakness of wrist muscles with forceful movements of wrist and fingers; due to repeated or excessive use of the muscle or incorrect biomechanics.

Common extensor tendons = lateral epicondylitis or tennis elbow (ECRB).

Common flexor tendon = medial epicondylitis or golfers elbow.

Surgical Interventions:

Elbow synovectomy and   Total elbow arthroplasty.
resection of the radial head

Appendix H

OVERVIEW OF WRIST PATHOLOGY

Pain

May be localized, which would be indicative of more superficial structures.

Muscles like EDL, PL, opponens.

Ligaments such as radial and ulnar collateral ligaments.

Periosteum (pisiform, styloid process or metacarpal heads).

Deeper pain may be due to referred pain and may occur in more deeply located muscles, ligaments, bursae, or bones (scaphoid or radius).

Sharp	May suggest injury to skin, fascia, tendon (deQuervain's disease), ligaments, muscles, bursitis.
Dull	May suggest injury to neural problem, bony injury, chronic capsular problem, deep muscle injury, or tendon sheath problem.
Ache	May suggest injury to tendon sheath, deep ligaments, fibrous capsules, or deep muscles; may signify RSD or rheumatoid arthritis.
Pins and needles	May suggest injury to peripheral or dorsal nerve root damage; systemic condition or vascular occlusion (Raynaud's disease).
Onset	*Immediate*: usually more severe than pain occurring gradually.
	6 to 12 hours after activity: synovitis or irritation to joint synovium, secondary to subluxation of capitate or lunate, disk lesion, ligamental sprain or capsular sprain.
	Gradual: may indicate overuse syndromes, neural lesions, arthritic problems.

Swelling

May be localized as in ganglions (synovial hernia in tendinous sheath or joint capsule), may be inflammation of a tendon or its synovial sheath.

Diffuse swelling difficult to observe but likely to limit motion.

May occur due to fractures, tenosynovitis or direct trauma to carpal area.

Immediate swelling suggests more severe injury.

Gradual swelling suggests ligamental or capsular sprains or subluxation.

Sensations

Warm	May indicate inflammation or infection.
Numbness	May be carpal tunnel syndrome at the elbow or wrist; radial nerve palsy or injury, cervical nerve root problems, thoracic outlet syndrome, local cutaneous nerve injury, or cubital tunnel syndrome at the elbow.
Clicking	There may be a lesion on the disk between the lunate and radius and triquetral; may be a sign of carpal bone subluxation (lunate or capitate).
Popping	May occur with ligament or muscle tears, with carpal subluxation or joint dislocation.
Grating	Osteoarthritic changes, cartilage deterioration.
Crepitus	Tenosynovitis of tendons in tendon sheaths as the fingers move.
Tingling	Neural or circulatory involvement may be suspected; C7-8 dermatome or peripheral nerve involvement.

Fracture

Scaphoid may be impinged between capitate and radius causing a fracture.

Particularly high incidence in young athletes in contact sports.

Point tenderness in the anatomical snuff box and history of hyperextension.

Fracture often misdiagnosed so bone heals poorly due to poor blood supply.

Appendix H, continued.

Rheumatoid Arthritis

Commonly affects the wrists bilaterally.

In advanced stages, there may be subluxation or deformities that may include:

Volar subluxation of the triquetrum with relation to the ulna; this can lead to ECU tendon displacing volarly causing a flexor force at the joint ulnar subluxation of the carpals, which would result in radial deviation.

Strains

FCR and FCU most commonly strained.

Inflammation can irritate the tendon sheath, causing tenosynovitis, which may lead to carpal tunnel syndrome.

Dislocation

Distal ulna

Dislocation of distal ulna can occur often with ulnar styloid fracture.

Distal radioulnar ligaments and triangular fibrocartilage complex must occur before dislocation can occur.

Radiocarpal or midcarpal joints

Extremely rare due to protection by ligaments.

Carpals

With hyperextension, lunate dislocates anteriorly then remains stationary while the rest of the carpals dislocate anteriorly.

Lunate dislocation is the most common and can result in carpal tunnel syndrome, median nerve palsy, flexor tendon constriction, progressive avascular necrosis of the lunate, or a scaphoid fracture.

Deviation

Forced radial deviation can sprain or tear the medial ligament of the radiocarpal joint at the ulnar styloid process, the anterior band into the pisiform or the posterior band into the triquetrum; may fracture the scaphoid or distal end of the radius or avulse the ulnar styloid process.

Forced wrist ulnar deviation can sprain or tear the lateral ligament of the radiocarpal joint at the radial styloid process, the anterior band into the scaphoid or the posterior band into the scaphoid tubercle, strain the ECRL or APL tendons, or avulse the radial styloid process.

Hyperpronation and Hypersupination

Hyperpronation can cause dorsal subluxations or dislocations of the distal radioulnar joint.

Hypersupination is less common but can result in volar radioulnar subluxations or dislocations.

Rotational forces usually are what injure the distal radioulnar joint when the hand is fixed and can result in subluxation or dislocation of the distal ulna causing damage to the disk, radioulnar ligaments, and ulnar collateral ligaments.

Overuse

Carpal tunnel syndrome, which can occur in baseball, rowing, weight lifting, and wheelchair athletes.

Carpal tunnel can become constricted due to many conditions and the pressure causes numbness or tingling in the hand and fingers that are supplied by the median nerve. Motor weakness can develop from prolonged or severe constriction.

Extensor Intersection syndrome is caused by overuse of thumb or wrist causing inflammation of APL and EPL in upper forearm where they cross each other; common in weightlifters and paddlers.

Ulnar nerve entrapment as it passes around the hook of hamate or can be damaged with scaphoid or pisiform fractures causing tingling and paresthesia of the hand and fingers in ulnar distribution. Can be seen from trauma from handle of baseball bat or hockey stick, karate blows or prolonged wrist extension that occurs with long-distance cycling.

Appendix I

OVERVIEW OF HAND PATHOLOGY

Pain

Synovitis, degenerative joint diseases, RSD often present with complaints of pain.

Differentiate pain from stiffness.

Differentiate articular from periarticular pain (as in subcutaneous nodules, synovial cysts, osteophytes, or muscular conditions).

Local tenderness: likely more superficial structures affected blisters, lacerations of the fascia.

Disruption of superficial ligaments.

Disruption of superficial muscles (e.g., EDL, PL, or opponens).

Disruption in periosteum.

Deep pain may be due to impairments in deep muscles, ligaments, or bursae.

Sharp	May indicate injury to skin, fascia, tendons, superficial ligaments and muscles; acute bursitis.
Dull	May indicate injury to neural problem, bony injury, chronic capsular problems, deep muscle injury, or tendon sheath problem.
Ache	May indicate injury to tendon sheath, deep ligaments, fibrous capsule, or deep muscles.
Pins and needles	May indicate injury to peripheral nerve conditions, dorsal nerve root problems, systemic conditions (e.g., diabetes), vascular occlusion.
Onset	Immediate is indicative of more severe pain.
	Gradual onset may indicate overuse syndromes, neural lesions, or arthritis.

Contusions

Repeated direct blows can cause vascular damage; blows to palmar surface can also cause dorsal hand swelling.

Subungual hematoma = accumulation of blood under fingernail.

Thenar and hypothenar eminences can be contused via direct blow, especially in racquet sports or those involving catching a ball.

Contusions to MCP common in boxing and football.

Extensor Intersection Syndrome

Overuse of thumb or wrist leading to inflammation of abductor pollicis longus and extensor pollicis brevis in upper forearm; often seen in paddlers or weightlifters.

Joint Pathology: Fractures and Dislocations

Fractures of the metacarpals more common than phalangeal fracture caused by direct blow to the shaft or metacarpal head.

Proximal phalange fractures more than middle or distal, which cause damage to flexor or extensor tendons.

Subluxations: most common at radiocarpal, radioulnar, and MCP joints.

Sensory: Radial Nerve

Least commonly injured.

Innervates extensor muscles of arm and forearm and skin covering them (triceps, anconeus, brachioradialis, extensor carpi radialis, part of brachialis).

Innervation to skin on dorsum of wrist and hand to lateral dorsal surface of thumb and index and middle fingers.

Injuries: cervical cord—dermatome sensory and brachial plexus lesions, PNI, dislocation of the shoulder, fractured humerus and radius.

Appendix I, continued.

Sensory: Radial Nerve

Severance: extensor paralysis, inability to extend thumb, PIP, wrist drop (inability to extend wrist), possibly loss of elbow/loss of grip since lacks stabilizing function of wrist/hand; could not pick up large objects from flat surface.

Compression (also called entrapment neuropathies): Radial Tunnel Syndrome: ECRB adheres to supinator; pain in extensor muscles below the elbow, which is increased and imitated by pronation or pronation and wrist flexion; grasp due to pain, may or may not be motor sensory.

Thoracic Outlet Syndrome (C8T Syndrome): compression due to bone, muscle, or fascia; numbness when hand held overhead, pain, entire UE may then get numb, painful.

Posterior Interossei Syndrome: rare; no sensory impairment; pain anterior to elbow = weakness in fingers and inability to extend MCP. Injury often as nerve crosses humerus secondary to trauma, fracture. Triceps usually escapes injury, paralysis of extensors of wrist and digits = wrist drop.

Sensory: Median Nerve

Most commonly injured.

Innervates radial side of flexor portion of forearm and hand (pronator teres and quadratus, flexor carpi radialis, palmaris longus, flexor digitorum superficiales and profundus, flexor pollices longus, abductor pollices, opponens pollices, flexor pollices brevis, 1st and 2nd lumbricales).

Injuries: cervical cord and brachial plexus, PNI, prolonged compression, dislocated ulna, fractured elbow or lower radius.

Severance: weak wrist flexors; inability to flex and abduct thumb; inability to flex index and middle finger; tendency for thumb and index to hyperextend due to unopposed finger extension force of EDC; loss of thumb opposition.

Simian, Ape Hand: wasting of thenar eminence; median nerve palsy; thumb in line with fingers; unable to oppose or flex thumb.

Bishops or benediction hand: wasting of hypothenar muscles and interosseus muscles and two medial lumbricals; due to ulnar nerve palsy.

Compression: Carpal tunnel syndrome. Compression commonly under transverse carpal ligament. Symptoms: numbness, tingling, burning sensations of wrist, first three fingers; symptoms occur at night accompanied by weakness, clumsiness.

Pronator Teres Syndrome: due to compression of median nerve at the forearm, less common than CTS. Symptoms: paresthesia of median fingers can be injured in the forearm by deep cuts with resultant loss of flexion at all IP joints except DIP of ring and little fingers. MCP joints can still be flexed by lumbricales and interossei but pronation restricted. Thumb in extension and adduction so loss of opposition (called Ape or Priest's hand). Serious in combination with sensory loss.

More commonly nerve compressed (carpal tunnel syndrome) where only thenar, 2 lumbricals and sensation will be affected.

Pain in proximal forearm (especially pro teres)

Anterior Interosseus N. Syndrome: usually characterized by nonspecific pain in forearm, elbow and weakness in FPL to index and middle finger.

Sensory: Ulnar Nerve

Innervates muscles and skin of ulnar side of forearm and hand (flexor carpi ulnaris, flexor digitorum profundus, palmaris brevis, muscles of little finger, 3rd and 4th lumbricales, all interossei, adductor pollices, flexor pollices brevis).

Appendix I, continued.

Sensory: Ulnar Nerve

Lesions: cervical cord and brachial plexus, PNI, fracture and dislocation of humeral head and elbow, pressure during sleep, inability to flex ring and little fingers, loss of hypothenar muscles and interossei, hyperextension of ring and little fingers, radial deviation, loss of thumb adductor

Claw hand/claw fingers: hyperextension of MCP, palmar arch is flattened, PIP and DIP; loss intrinsic muscle action and overaction of extrinsic extensor muscles on proximal phalanges of fingers; intrinsic minus → loss of normal cupping; arches of hands disappear; intrinsic muscle wasting.

Damaged by trauma or entrapment in groove behind medial epicondyle leading to partial or complete loss of muscular and sensory innervation.

At the wrist, nerve can easily be cut or lacerated because of superficial position. Can lead to "claw hand" = loss intrinsics, inability to abduct fingers or adduct thumb; 2 ulnar fingers hyperextend at MP, flex at PIP.

deQuervain's Disease

(constrictive tenosynovitis)

Overuse of thumb or wrist leading to tendinitis of abductor pollicis longus and extensor pollicis brevis as pass through first compartment.

Thumb is overused or fixed and wrist is overstressed (paddling, baseball, javelin, hockey).

Tendon Pathology

Tendons can shorten 2 degrees to immobilization, soft tissue contractures and/or spasticity.

Disease process often tenosynovitis, which is inflammation of tendon and synovial which leads to fluid trapped in synovial sheath, proliferation of tissue, gliding.

Rupture is caused by strength and integrity of the tendon and attrition over rough subluxed bones or spurs.

Rupture of extensor tendons is more common than flexors since extensor tendons go over the carpal bones.

Open EDQ ruptures first.

Mallet finger: when extensor tendon torn from insertion DIP drops into flexion; rupture of extensor tendons as inserts in DIP; DIP flexed position; can also be caused by a forceful flexion injury to DIP when extensor tendon is taut (e.g., catching a baseball); treatment: DIP in hyperextension.

Trigger Thumb: thumb snaps as it flexes or it may become locked in flexion or extension.

Trigger Finger/Digital tenovaginitis stenosis: thickening of flexor tendon sheath; tendons stick; low grade inflammation of proximal fold of flexor tendon leads to swelling, constriction (stenosis).

Usually occurs in middle or ring fingers due to direct, severe, or multiple trauma.

Extensor Mechanism Pathology

Boutonniére Deformity: extension of MCP and DIP; flexion of PIP; rupture central tendinous slip of extensor hood; common with RA, trauma.

Called buttonhole because the lateral bands of extensor tendons separate to allow joint to protrude between.

When the lateral bands slip, the intrinsics move to the flexor side and act as flexors.

The resultant position: PIP flexion.

The persistent flexion of the PIP with compensatory hyperextension of DIP is caused by weak ED and the slippage and laxity of the lateral bands.

Treatment: splint PIP in extension and DIP moves freely; often requires surgical intervention.

Appendix I, continued.

Extensor Mechanism Pathology

Ulnar Drift: probably due to laxity of capsule and laxity of collateral ligaments disease dislocation of extensor tendons to ulnar side of the joint.

Often encouraged by mechanical stresses placed on the unstable hand during normal use.

Flexor Apparatus Pathology

Swan Neck Deformity: flexion MCP and DIP; extension PIP, contracture of intrinsic muscles; often RA or trauma.

Usually synovitis but can be trauma.

When there is synovitis of the flexor tendon sheath, IP flexion is prevented.

Then the flexor power is concentrated on the MCP joint, which increases the pull on the intrinsics to the central tendon.

Position: PIP hyperextension, DIP flexion (caused by flexor profundus), MCP flexion.

If flexor tendons are severed, they are difficult to treat because suturing in no man's land has poor prognosis, lots of swelling but no room to swell.

Usually wait or repair one tendon at a time (usually profundus first), then immobilized 3 weeks in slight wrist flexion and flexion of involved fingers.

If flexor tendons are ruptured, mostly due to disease.

Wrist drop: extensor muscle paralysis result due to radial nerve; wrist and fingers cannot be extended.

Z deformity of thumb.

Thumb flexes at MCP, extends at IP; heredity or associated with RA.

Dupuytren's contracture of palmar fascia; fixed flexion deformity of MCP and PIP; usually ring and little fingers; skin often adherent to fascia; men more than women aged 50 to 70 years.

Sprains

Thumb

Skiers thumb: forceful hyperextension often combined with abduction of first MCP joint; also seen in baseball, basketball, volleyball. Can lead to sprain of ulnar collateral ligament; base of proximal phalange on ulnar side can be fractured, displaced; the adductor aponeurosis can become trapped under torn ulnar collateral ligament and prevent ligament from healing.

Thumb may become dislocated posteriorly.

Fingers

Second to fifth MCP commonly injured through hyperextension usually resulting in ligamental damage.

With PIP hypertension, the joint capsule, transverse retinacular ligaments, or volar plate can be injured.

Hyperextension of the DIP common in basketball and volleyball; sprained with anterior capsular damage, ligament and sometimes volar plate damage.

A flexed finger that is violently extended can cause the flexor digitorum profundus to rupture from insertion on distal phalange, as in football or rugby.

With forced ulnar deviation of the PIP joint, radial collateral ligaments can be injured, volar plate can be ruptured, or complete dislocation can occur.

Muscular

Hypothenar wasting: C8 nerve root problem.

Thenar wasting: C6 nerve root problem.

Wasting of hypothenar, interossei, and medial lumbricals = median nerve palsy and ape hand appearance (thumb in line with fingers; thumb cannot be flexed).

Intrinsic loss: clawed position; overpowered by extrinsic extensor muscles acting on PIP.

Appendix I, continued.

Muscular

Radial nerve palsy = wrist drop

Dupuytren's contracture of palmar aponeurosis pulling fingers into flexion

If intrinsic tightness, will not be able to fully flex PIP while MCP in extension or you will have quarter PIP flexion when MCP flexed than when MCP is extended.

Intrinsic tightness can be a causal factor of swan neck deformity. Can also lead to flexion deformities of MCP.

To test for extrinsic tightness, you want to see if the patient can simultaneously flex PIP and MCP:

1.   Put MCP into flexion and try PIP flexion passively

2.   Put MCP into less flexion and try PIP flexion passively

If PIP can be flexed when the MCP is extended but not when the MCP is flexed, there is extrinsic tightness. If PIP cannot be flexed irregardless of MCP position, problem is probably articular.

Vasomotor Changes

Redness, blanching—suspect circulatory problem.

Raynaud's disease: idiopathic vascular disorder where blood vessels spasm causing the finger(s) to become pale and numb followed by vasodilation and red and hot sensations.

Rheumatoid disease can cause warm, wet hand; joint swelling; ulnar deviation.

Causalgia can produce swollen, hot hand.

Acromegaly can enlarge the entire skeleton of the hand.

Joint Pathology

Ligamental

Incomplete injuries at PIP most common but usually no dislocation of PIP joint due to capsular support.

MCP - hyperextension injuries to radial collateral ligament immobilize (splint).

Thumb - collateral ligament on ulnar side often require surgery.

Appendix J

OVERVIEW OF HIP PATHOLOGY

Joint and Capsule Restrictions

Initially internal rotation is painful or restricted; hip may be fixed in adduction and have no IR or extension past neutral, be limited to 90 degrees of flexion or full ER.

DJD/osteoarthritis/hip joint arthrosis due to aging, result from trauma or injury, deformity or disease; pain on weight bearing during gait or at end of day with much activity often L3 along anterior thigh or knee; limitation in hip extension often leads to backache because attempted extension will rotate the pelvis anteriorly and cause hyperextension of lumbar spine; equilibrium and balance are also impaired due do changes in mechanoreceptor system; 50% idiopathic; 10 to 15% in those over 55 years of age equally distributed between men and women.

RA and asceptic necrosis.

Bursitis

Trochanteric bursitis: pain over lateral hip and possibly down the lateral thigh to knee, especially if standing asymmetrically for prolonged time with affected hip elevated and adducted and pelvis dropped on opposite side.

Psoas bursitis: pain in groin or anterior thigh and possibly into patellar area.

Ischiogluteal bursitis (tailor's or weaver's bottom): pain around ischial tuberosities, especially when sitting.

Referred Pain

Nerve roots and tissues from L1-3 and S1-2.

Lumbar vertebral joints.

Sacroiliac joints.

Surgical Management

Open reduction and internal fixation of hip fractures: often for elderly; actually fracture of very proximal portion of the femur; osteoporosis weakens the bone and neck of femur very susceptible to osteoporosis. Hip fracture pain in groin or hip region with shortening and ER of affected extremity.

Total hip replacement indicated for those with severe hip pain with motion and weight bearing due to RA or osteoarthritis, ankylosing spondylitis or aseptic necrosis; often history of previous failed hip surgery.

Hemireplacement of the hip: indicated when subcapital fractures of the femur in the elderly; pain deformity and instability of hip; head of femur is replaced.

Strain

Rectus femoris.

Hamstrings.

Iliopsoas.

Piriformis.

Fractures

Stress fractures to ASIS.

Pubic rami.

Ischial tuberosities.

Trochanters.

Femoral neck.

Appendix J, continued.

Short Leg

May be due to flat foot, genu valgum, coxa vara, tight hip muscles, anterior rotated innominate bone, poor standing posture, asymmetry in bone growth.

May cause lateral pelvic tilting (drop on short side) and side bending of trunk.

May lead to scoliosis.

Tendinitis

Gluteus medius.

Childhood Diseases

Congenital hip dislocation.

Legg-Calve-Perthes disease.

Juvenile rheumatoid arthritis.

Appendix K

GOOD VERSUS FAULTY POSTURE

Good Posture	Part	Faulty Posture
Head is held erect in a position of good balance.	Head	Chin up too high. Head protruding forward. Head tilted or rotated to one side.
Arms hang relaxed at the sides with palms of the hands facing toward the body. Elbows are slightly bent, so forearms hang slightly forward. Shoulders are level, and neither one is more forward than the other when seen from the side. Scapulae lie flat against the rib cage. They are neither too close together nor too wide apart. In adults, a separation of approximately 4 inches is average.	Arms and shoulders	Holding the arms stiffly in any position forward, backward, or out from the body. Arms turned so that palms of hands face backward. One shoulder higher than the other. Both shoulders hiked up. One or both shoulders drooping forward or sloping. Shoulders rotated either clockwise or counterclockwise. Scapulae pulled back too hard. Scapulae too far apart. Scapulae too prominent, standing out from the rib cage ("winged scapulae").
A good position of the chest is one in which it is slightly up and slightly forward (while the back remains in good alignment). The chest appears to be in a position about halfway between that of a full inspiration and a forced expiration.	Chest	Depressed, or "hollow-chest" position. Lifted and held up too high, brought about by arching the back. Ribs more prominent on one side than on the other. Lower ribs flaring out or protruding.
In young children up to about the age of 10, the abdomen normally protrudes somewhat. In older children and adults, it should be flat.	Abdomen	Entire abdomen protrudes. Lower part of the abdomen protrudes while the upper part is pulled in.
The front of the pelvis and the thighs are in a straight line. The buttocks are not prominent in back but instead slope slightly downward. The spine has four natural curves. In the neck and lower back, the curve is forward, and in the upper back and lowest part of the spine (sacral region), it is backward. The sacral curve is a fixed curve, whereas the other three are flexible.	Spine and pelvis (side view)	The low back arches forward too much (lordosis). The pelvis tilts forward too much. The front of the thigh forms an angle with the pelvis when this tilt is present. The normal forward curve in the low back has straightened out. The pelvis tips backward and there is a slightly backward slant to the line of the pelvis in relation to the front of the hips (flat back). Increased backward curve in the upper back (kyphosis or round upper back). Increased forward curve in the neck. Almost always accompanied by round upper back and seen as a forward head. Lateral curve of the spine (scoliosis); toward one side (C-curve), toward both sides (S-curve).

Appendix K, continued.

Good Posture	Part	Faulty Posture
Ideally, the body weight is borne evenly on both feet, and the hips are level. One side is not more prominent than the other as seen from front or back, nor is one hip more forward or backward than the other as seen from the side. The spine does not curve to the left or the right side. (A slight deviation to the left in right-handed individuals and to the right in left-handed individuals should not be considered abnormal. Also, because a tendency toward a slightly low right shoulder and slightly high right hip is frequently found in right-handed people, and vice versa for left-handed, such deviations should not be considered abnormal.)	Hips, pelvis, and spine (back view)	One hip is higher than the other (lateral pelvic tilt). Sometimes it is not really much higher but appears so because a sideways sway of the body has made it more prominent. (Tailors and dressmakers often notice a lateral tilt because the hemline of skirts or length of trousers must be adjusted to the difference.) The hips are rotated so that one is farther forward than the other (clockwise or counterclockwise rotation).
Legs are straight up and down. Patellae face straight ahead when feet are in good position. Looking at the knees from the side, the knees are straight (i.e., neither bent forward nor "locked" backward).	Knees and legs	Knees touch when feet are apart (genu valgum). Knees are apart when feet touch (genu varum). Knee curves slightly backward (hyperextended knee) (genu recurvatum). Knee bends slightly forward, i.e., it is not as straight as it should be (flexed knee). Patellae face slightly toward each other (medially rotated femurs). Patellae face slightly outward (laterally rotated femurs).
Toes should be straight, i.e., neither curled downward nor bent upward. They should extend forward in line with the foot and not be squeezed together or overlap.	Toes	Toes bend up at the first joint and down at middle and end joints so that the weight rests on the tips of the toes (hammer toes). This fault is often associated with wearing shoes that are too short. Big toe slants inward toward the midline of the foot (hallus valgus). This fault is often associated with wearing shoes that are too narrow and pointed at the toes.
In standing, the longitudinal arch has the shape of a half dome. Barefoot or in shoes without heels, the feet toe-out slightly. In shoes with heels, the feet are parallel. In walking with or without heels, the feet are parallel, and the weight is transferred from the heel along the outer border to the ball of the foot. In running, the feet are parallel or toe-in slightly. The weight is on the balls of the feet and toes because the heels do not come in contact with the ground.	Foot	Low longitudinal arch or flatfoot. Low metatarsal arch, usually indicated by calluses under the ball of the foot. Weight borne on the inner side of the foot (pronation). "Ankle rolls in." Weight borne on the outer border of the foot (supination). "Ankle rolls out." Toeing-out while walking or while standing in shoes with heels ("outflared or slue-footed"). Toeing-in while walking or standing ("pigeon toed").

Appendix L

OVERVIEW OF KNEE JOINT PATHOLOGY

Menisci

Especially medial, are common result of sudden rotation of femur on fixed tibia when knee is in flexion.

Medial meniscus most commonly injured when foot is fixed and femur rotated internally as when pivoting (getting out of a car or a clipping injury).

ACL often accompanies medial meniscal tear.

Ligaments and Sprains

Forces that cause joint to exceed normal range of motion:

• Blow to lateral aspect of knee.

• Forced hyperextension.

Usually people 20 to 40 years of age as result of sports injuries:

ACL when knee is forcefully hyperextended.

MCL valgus strain and external rotation of tibia with foot planted (injures ACL too).

Posterior cruciate ligament forceful blow to anterior portion of tibia with knee flexed.

Ligaments and Menisci

Tendinitis, iliotibial band syndrome.

Bony and Cartilaginous Structures

Application of direct force or indirect; knee joint instability as seen in ACL injury can lead to progressive changes in cartilage, menisci, and other ligaments.

Patellar subluxation, dislocation, chondromalacia patella (degeneration of cartilage of patella with multiple causes; c/o anterior knee pain, crepitation, and tenderness along medial part of articular surface of patella).

Bursae and Tendons at Knee

Direct blow or prolonged compressive or tensile stresses; bursitis in prepatellar bursa or superficial infrapatellar bursa (housemaid's knee).

Patellar Plica/Plica Synovialis/Medial Shelf Syndrome/Suprapatellar Plica Synovitis/Medial Plica Synovitis

Pain with prolonged sitting, stair climbing, and during resisted extension exercise; often, too, a snapping sensation.

Muscle Strains

Quadriceps femoris, hamstrings.

Rheumatoid Arthritis

Early, hands and feet first then knees; warm, swollen with more loss in flexion than extension; near 25 degrees flexion; genu valgum deformity commonly develops in advanced stages; knees should be protected during weight bearing with an assistive device.

Degenerative Joint Disease (DJD)/Osteoarthritis

Pain, muscle weakness, joint limitations progressively worsen; genu varum commonly develops; replacement surgery often in advanced stages.

Appendix L, continued.
Referred Pain
Nerve roots from L3 referring to anterior aspect and S1-2 to posterior aspect of knee; hip joint which is primarily L3.
Surgical Repair
Meniscectomy, ligamental repair or reconstruction, synovectomy of the knee, total knee replacement.

Appendix M

OVERVIEW OF FOOT AND ANKLE PATHOLOGY

Nerve Pressure and Trauma

      Common peroneal, posterior tibial nerve, plantar and calcaneal nerve.

Rheumatoid Arthritis

      Subtalar and other joints of foot; joint swelling and increased warmth; common deformities:
- Pronated foot
- Hallux valgus (shifts laterally)
- Dorsal dislocation of proximal phalanges on MT heads
- Claw toe (MT hyperextension and intertarsal flexion)

Other Types of Arthritis Affecting the Feet

      Traumatic arthritis; osteoarthritis; gout, commonly affecting big toe.

Sprains and Minor Tears of Ligaments

      Inversion stress sprain most common resulting in tear of anterior talofibular ligament.

Overuse Syndromes

      Tendinitis or teneosynovitis, plantar facitis, shin splints.

Referred Pain

      Lumbosacral spine between L4-5 and L5-S1 or nerve roots.

      Peripheral nerve cutaneous sensation in foot from common peroneal, superficial, and deep peroneal nerves; branches of tibial nerve, medial or lateral plantar nerves; surar nerve or terminal branch of femoral nerve; saphenous nerve.

Surgical Intervention

      Total ankle replacement.

      Arthrodesis at the ankle and foot.

      Arthroplasty for metatarsalgia.

      Repair of tendon ruptures and ligamental tears.

Foot Deformities

      Pes planus (flat or pronated foot).

      Pes cavus (supinated foot); less common but more serious.

Appendix N

REHABILITATION INTERVENTION

Part A: Adapted Task Method or Procedure

Goal	Method	Principle	Example
Client will be (I/modified I) (require maximal/moderate/ minimal/standby/verbal cue/ physical cue) to perform tasks (specify which tasks) in _____ weeks/days using...	Adapted task procedures and methods which...	Substitute for lost range of motion.	Loss of one side/weakness one side: Wheelchair mobility–unaffected arm and leg for propulsion Bed mobility changes Pivot transfers Adapted dressing: affected extremity in first Rheumatoid arthritis: Stand and then change the position of the feet rather than twisting at the knees when transferring. UE amputee using shoulder flexion to open the terminal device.
Client will be (I/modified I) (require maximal/moderate/ minimal/standby/verbal cue/ physical cue) to perform tasks (specify which tasks) in _____ weeks/days using...	Adapted task procedures and methods which...	Substitute for loss of strength.	General principles: Let gravity assist. Utilize principles of levers (force arm > resistance arm). Apply force closer or farther from fulcrum to change length of lever arms. Increased friction decreases power required for pinch or grasp. Use two hands. Weave utensils through fingers. SCI: ER/abduction replaces supination. Hook elbow around wheelchair upright to increase reach. Extrinsic tightness for selective tight- ening for hook grasp. Elbow-walk. Lock elbow. Tenodesis action with wrist extension. Adapted bed mobility. Transfers: independent depression. Adapted dressing.
Client will be (I/modified I) (require maximal/moderate/ minimal/ standby/ verbal cue/ physical cue) to perform tasks (specify which tasks) in _____ weeks/days using...	Adapted task procedures and methods which...	Provide stability (ataxic and uncoordinated movements).	PNF patterns (chop and lift, surface contact, move and stop). Teach to stabilize objects being used. Stabilize proximal part. Use body in as stable a position as possible.

			Use larger and/or less precise

Appendix N, continued.

Goal	Method	Principle	Example
			Use larger and/or less precise fasteners, tools, objects.
			Increase friction.
Client will be (I/modified I) (require maximal/moderate/ minimal/standby/verbal cue/ physical cue) to perform tasks (specify which tasks) in _____ weeks/days using...	Adapted task procedures and methods which...	Minimize the effect of spasticity.	Use "distal key points of control" (NDT technique). Use placing, lowering, and weight-bearing (NDT technique). Use affected arm as stabilization.
Client will be (I/modified I) (require maximal/moderate/ minimal/standby/verbal cue/ physical cue) to perform tasks (specify which tasks) in _____ weeks/days using...	Adapted task procedures and methods which...	Substitute for limited vision.	Organize—there is a place for everything. Plate organized like a clock. Adapted cutting by means of food placement. Pour liquid based on weight of cup when full. French knots in labels to identify colors. Store all colored clothes in one part of closet. Fold money for each denomination differently.
Client will be (I/modified I) (require maximal/moderate/ minimal/standby/verbal cue/ physical cue) to perform tasks (specify which tasks) in _____ weeks/days using...	Adapted task procedures and methods which...	Substitute for decreased endurance.	Have grocery list. Frequent rests. Shop during nonpeak times.
Client will (be independent/ modified I) (Require maximal/ moderate/minimal/standby assist/ verbal or physical cues) to perform (specify) tasks in _____ weeks/ days using... or Client will consistently use work simplification techniques to _____ (specify task)	Adapted methods which...	Simplify work.	Organize storage. Plan ahead. Have an easy flow of work. Eliminate steps and jobs. Use efficient methods. Consider the environment.

Appendix N, continued.

Goal	Method	Principle	Example
Client will (be independent/ modified I) (Require maximal/ moderate/minimal/standby assist/ verbal or physical cues) to perform (specify) tasks in _____ weeks/days using...	Adapted methods which...	Conserve energy.	Respect pain. Rest frequently. Prioritize activities. Avoid stressful positions.
or Client will demonstrate consistent use of energy conservation techniques when _____ (specify task)			

Part B: Adapting the Task Objects, Devices, or Orthotics

Goal	Method	Principle	Example
Client will (be independent/ modified I) (Require maximal/ moderate/minimal/standby assist/verbal or physical cues) to perform ADL (specify) tasks in _____weeks/days using...	Adapted task objects or adaptive devices or orthotics which...	Compensates for lack of full reach/ range of motion.	Bathing: long-handled sponge. Dressing: dressing stick, stocking aid, elastic shoelaces, long-handled shoe horn. Environmental control: long-handled reacher for lightswitches, etc. Feeding: long-handled utensils; long straw with clip. Grooming: long-handled comb, aerosol deodorant. Toileting: wiping tongs, suppository inserter, raised toilet seat. Cooking: reacher tongs for light-weight objects. Cleaning: vacuum cleaner wand attachments; long-handled dustpan, sponge mop with squeeze handle on side; long-handled dusters. Adjustable office chairs; electric or spring loaded lift for chairs to assist with standing, additional cushions. MAS or suspension sling.
Client will (be independent/ modified I) (Require maximal/ moderate/minimal/standby assist/verbal or physical cues) to perform ADL (specify) tasks in _____weeks/days using...	Adaptive devices or orthotics which...	Compensate for lack of UE strength.	Communication: mouthstick for typing, speaker phone. Feeding: mobile arm support, overhead suspension, sling, lapboard rocker knife, table elevated to axilla height support for arm and eliminates gravity. Cleaning: vacuum cleaner wand attachments, dolly with large casters for carrying a pail of water when mopping, self-propelled vacuum

Appendix N, continued.

Goal	Method	Principle	Example
			with automatic cord rewinder (except when balance is a problem), lightweight carpet sweeper requires no outlet but has to be pushed for longer time to cover same distance; cordless, handheld vacuum; lightweight brooms with angle cut. Bed mobility: rope ladder, trapeze bars. Transfers: sliding board for transfer. General: use powered tools and utensils; wheeled cart to transport items.
Client will (be independent/ modified I) (Require maximal/ moderate/minimal/standby assist/verbal or physical cues) to perform ADL (specify) tasks in ____weeks/days using...	Adapted task objects or adaptive devices or orthotics which...	Compensate for loss of LE strength/ function.	Tubseat. Grab bars. Sliding board.
Client will (be independent/ modified I) (Require maximal/ moderate/minimal/standby assist/ verbal or physical cues) to perform ADL (specify) tasks in ____weeks/days using...	Adapting task objects or adaptive devices or orthotics which...	Compensate for lack of full hand closure.	Communication: lightweight built-up handle on pencil, flexor hinge splint, writing devices, phone cuffs. Feeding: lightweight built-up handles on utensils, universal cuff with utensils inserted, open-bottomed handle, t-shaped handle; foam insulator can be used to provide friction to assist with weak grasp; use plexiglass or plastic straws; Grooming: lightweight built-up handles on comb, toothbrush; wash mitt; universal cuff with utensils inserted; cuff to hold electric razor. Hygiene: digit stimulators; suppository inserters, adapted faucet handles, soap on a rope; liquid soap; bath mitts; dry off with terry cloth bathrobe rather than towel. Dressing: button hook device Cooking: built-up handles on pots and pans. Cleaning: built-up handles on brooms, irons, bottle brush on suction base for glasses; mop with

Appendix N, continued.			
Goal	*Method*	*Principle*	*Example*
			mechanism to wring sponge one-handed.
			General: Use of a flexor hinge splint; adding friction material (dycem, plastisol).
			Recreation/work: book holder; electric page turner.
Client will (be independent/ modified I) (Require maximal/ moderate/minimal/standby assist/ verbal or physical cues) to perform ADL (specify) tasks in ____weeks/ days using...	Adapting task objects or adaptive devices or orthotics which...	Compensate for lack of vision.	Communication: page magnifier, prism glasses for reading in bed.
			Bathing: long-handled skin inspection mirror.
			Braille labels.
			Magnify type or images.
			Devices to provide auditory, tactile or kinesthetic feedback.
			Different shaped containers (e.g., square for pepper, round for salt).
			Computerized optical scanning devices.
			"Talking" or voice activated computers, watches, kitchen scales, clocks.
			Well-illuminated crosswalks and outdoor stairs.
			Double handrails.
			Guiderails in halls.
			Paint the first and last step a different color.
			Avoid open stairwells, low balcony rails, doors opening directly to steps.
			Remove low hanging objects such as fire extinguishers, metal signs.
			Minimize clutter and pattern designs on floors.
			Avoid highly polished surfaces.
			Contrast colors on thermostats, wall outlets, locks on windows, light switch, drawstring on draperies, stove and oven dials, measuring cups.
			Oversized phone dial, watches.
			Large print cookbooks.

Appendix N, continued.

Part C: Wheelchair Modifications and Mobility Devices

Goal	*Method*	*Principle*	*Example*
Client will be (independent/ modified I) (Require maximal/ moderate/minimal/standby assist/verbal or physical cues) to perform ADL (specify) tasks in _____weeks/days using...	Wheelchair modifications which...	Permit self-propulsion of the wheelchair.	Seat: narrow adult (requires less UE abduction, which is tiring), low hemi-seat (so propelling foot easily reaches the floor). Wheels: 8 inch diameter (more stable on rocks, curbs, etc.), 5 inch diameter (tighter turns). Rims: spoke extensions (clients with quadriplegia can push with palm or webspace; often use bicycle gloves for better traction); double rims (hemiplegic can push chair with one hand); flat rim (lighter weight). Electric wheelchair. One arm drive wheelchair for some clients with CVA.
Client will (be independent/ modified I) (Require maximal/ moderate/minimal/standby assist/ verbal or physical cues) to perform ADL (specify) tasks in...	Wheelchair modifications which...	Permit transport-ation of objects.	Pouches attached to wheelchair with Velcro straps. Wheelchair laptray/lapboard. Crutch holders attached to wheel-chair. Loop over back of wheelchair (for hooking elbow while reaching for objects).
Client will (be independent/ modified I) (Require maximal/ moderate/minimal/standby assist/ verbal or physical cues) to perform ADL (specify) tasks in _____ weeks/days using...	Wheelchair modifications which...	Facilitate proper positioning.	Back: reclining back (better trunk stability), reclines for low blood pressure head extension (for poor head control). Arm rest: adjustable height)to ensure proper arm and trunk support) Arm troughs/lapboards (UE position-ing). Offset arms (increases inside width between uprights for wider hips). Overhead sling (UE positioning for hand use in gravity-eliminated plane). Legrest: elevating (for edema or problems with blood pressure). Calf pad (prevents leg from sliding off footrest). Footrest: heelstrap (prevents foot from sliding off footrest).

Appendix N, continued.

Goal	Method	Principle	Example
			Seat: narrow adult (sides are from sliding off footrest).
			Lateral supports (for better and lateral stability).
			Seatbelt (keeps hips back so pelvis and trunk can rest against backrest and trunk is erect); hard seat (inhibits LE spasticity; promotes neutral pelvic tilt and symmetrical weightbearing).
			ROHO seat cushion (for pressure relief); Jay seat cushion (for pressure relief and lateral support).
			Numerous abductor devices (inhibits leg scissoring and extension which cause patient to slide out of wheel chair).
Client will (be independent/ modified I) (Require maximal/ moderate/minimal/ standby assist/ verbal or physical cues) to perform ADL (specify) tasks in _____weeks/days using...	Wheelchair modifications which...	Overcome architectural barrier.	Seat: narrow adult (for narrow doorways, navigating congested areas).
			Legrest: detachable reduces turning space for wheelchair.
			Armrest: wrap around is 2 inches less in overall width; desk arms; detachable armrests to get closer to tables; lapboard when wheelchair will not fit under table, sink, etc.
Client will (be independent/ modified I) (Require maximal/ moderate/minimal/standby assist/verbal or physical cues) to perform ADL (specify) tasks in _____weeks/days using...	Ambulatory aids which...	Protect the upper extremity.	Arm sling when walking. Wheelchair arm trough. Lapboard.
Client will (be independent/ modified I) (Require maximal/ moderate/minimal/ standby assist/ verbal or physical cues) to perform ADL (specify) tasks in _____weeks/days using...	Ambulatory aids which...	Permit transport-ation of objects.	Walker pouch. Backpack while crutch-walking.
Client will (be independent/ modified I) (Require maximal/ moderate/minimal/ standby assist/ verbal or physical cues) to perform ADL (specify) tasks in _____weeks/days using...	Change the context by modifying the environment which...	Provides access to housing, public and private facilities, recreation and transportation.	Disabled transport system: Paratransit will not take you out of the house; kneeling bus, buses with lifts, tie-downs in buses/trains.
			Private transportation: modified driver controls, vans with lifts.
			Parking spaces: located near entrances, 16 feet wide for side-exit vans.

Appendix N, continued.

Goal	Method	Principle	Example
			Doorways: Minimum 32 inches wide, electric doors with 13-second closure delay.
			Elevator: call button 36 inches from floor.
			Signage: use of symbols and Braille.
			Use of offset or fold-back hinges, inset doors or remove door frame.
			Ramps: 1:12 ratio of rise of ground with inches of ramp needed.
Client will (be independent/ modified I) (Require maximal/ moderate/minimal/standby assist/verbal or physical cues) to perform ADL (specify) tasks in _____weeks/days using...	Change the context by modifying the environment which...	Promote independence.	Lever faucet handles.
			Grab bars.
			Custom-made shower stall: raised slope to prevent water from running out but allow entrance (303T)
			Environment hardware: between one and a half and four and a half feet from floor for wheelchairs.
			Public bathrooms: wide stalls/high toilet seats/low sinks with 5 feet depth clearance for wheelchairs/low towel dispensers.
			Private bathrooms: roll-in shower stall; tub clearance 5 feet long and 4 feet out from tub; low sink with 5 feet depth clearance for wheelchairs; 6 feet between walls or 5 x 5 feet clear floor space; mirror and towel rack 40 inches or less.
			Water fountains: 36 inches high.
			Telephones: 48 inch mounting height enclosure is adapted or 36 inches wide.
			Adapted kitchens: lower counter height and overhead cabinets; cut out in countertop to accommodate wheelchairs; front controls on stove; counter 30-32 inches high, floor space 60 inches across.
			High contrast floor surfaces, low glare.
			Increased illumination.
			Well-lit entrances.
			Minimize clutter.

Appendix N, continued.

Part D: Disability Prevention—Client and Caregiver Education

Goal	Method	Principle	Example
Client/Caregiver will (be independent/ modified I) (Require maximal/moderate/ minimal/ standby assist/verbal or physical cues) to perform (specify) tasks in _____ weeks/days using...	Client and caregiver education which...	Ensures safe mobility.	Wheelchair parts and maneuverability. Assisted transfers: hoyer lift, 2 person carry logroll, assisted swivel transfer, assisted sliding board, assisted pivot transfer. Assistance in repositioning in wheelchair. Assistance in ascending/descending curbs and stairs.
Client /caregiver will (be independent/ modified I) (Require maximal/moderate/ minimal/standby assist/verbal or physical cues) to perform (specify) tasks in _____weeks/days using...	Safety education which...	Ensures safe transfers.	Gets wheelchair as close as possible, removes wheelchair parts if necessary. Equalizes heights as much as possible. Locks wheelchair brakes. Moves hips forward to get close to edge of chair/bed. Places feet flat on floor and directly under knees before standing. Identifies safe landing site for fall before standing up. Moves smoothly; doesn't thrust self out of chair.
Client/Caregiver will (be independent/ modified I) (Require maximal/moderate/ minimal/standby assist/verbal or physical cues) to perform (specify) tasks in _____weeks/days using...	Safety education to...	Prevent further structural damage by protecting a specific vulnerable body part during activities.	Cock up splint for client with hemiplegia. Sling for UE injury. Spinal board. Wheelchair arm trough with cone for client with hemiplegia.
Client/Caregiver will (be independent/ modified I) (Require maximal/moderate/ minimal/standby assist/verbal or physical cues) to perform (specify) tasks in _____weeks/days using...	Safety education which...	Maintains joint range of motion in the current range to prevent adhesions and mold collagen into orderly chains.	Functional patterns in occupational activities and tasks related to interests such as overhead checkers, macrame, putting dishes into a cupboard, placing clothes in a side loading dryer, making a bed. Range of motion in anatomical plane. Range of motion in muscle range of elongation Range of motion in combined patterns of movement (e.g., PNF). Self range of motion exercises. Range of motion dance. Finger ladder.

Appendix N, continued.

Goal	Method	Principle	Example
			Shoulder wheel. Overhead pulleys. Suspension devices (i.e., suspension sling).
Client/Caregiver will (be independent/modified I) (Require maximal/moderate/ minimal/standby assist/verbal/ or physical cues) to perform (specify) tasks in _____ weeks/days using...	Education to...	Prevent scar formation using devices that apply compression, which may slow collagen synthesis.	Pressure dressings. Elastomer molds. Transparent face mask. Pressure garments.
Client/Caregiver will (be independent/modified I) (Require maximal/moderate/ minimal/standby assist/verbal or physical cues) to perform (specify) tasks in ____ weeks/days using...	Orthoses and positioning which...	Maintains joints and soft tissue in functional positions and prevents deformities.	Foot-drop splint Client with rheumatoid arthritis should sleep in supine with as little flexion as possible.
Client/Caregiver will (be independent/modified I) (require maximal/moderate minimal/standby assist/verbal or physical cues) to perform (specify) tasks in ____ weeks/days using...	Safety education to provide...	Maintenance of strength by active use of currently intact muscles and joints, which prevents disuse atrophy and stiffness during periods of enforced rest.	AROM in anatomical planes. Diagonal PNF patterns. ADLs, which maintain strength. Wheelchair propulsion.
Client/Caregiver will (be independent/modified I) (Require maximal/moderate minimal/standby assist/verbal or physical cues) to perform (specify) tasks in ____weeks/days using...	Safety education which...	Ensures good body mechanics.	Keeps objects/people close to body. Keeps wide base of support, feet wide apart with no obstacles in the way. Slides/pushes/pulls/rolls objects/people rather than lifting if possible. Lifts with legs not back by bending knees to squat and then stand up. Uses good pacing; lifts smoothly; doesn't twist. Pivots whole body en bloc by moving feet instead of twisting torso. Maintain your center of gravity close to the object/person's center of gravity. Use short lever arms for better control.

Appendix N, continued.

Goal	Method	Principle	Example
Client/Caregiver will (be independent/modified I) (Require maximal/moderate minimal/standby assist/verbal or physical cues) to perform (specify) tasks in ____weeks/days using...	Safety education which...	Ensures safety for somatosensory loss.	Inspects skin daily. Differentiates between a pressure mark and pressure area. Relieves pressure at regular intervals. Wears protective splints and orthotics. Uses appropriate positioning. Moves desensate body part carefully using visual feedback.
Client/Caregiver will (be independent/modified I) (Require maximal/moderate/minimal/standby assist/verbal or physical cues) to perform (specify) tasks in ____weeks/days using...	Safety education which...	Ensures cardiac precautions.	Rest if heart rate goes up more than 20 bpm from resting pulse. Rest if heart rate goes above 120 bpm or below 60 bpm. Rest if systolic BP goes above 150 or below 90 (normally SBP=120). Rest if diastolic BP goes above 90 or below 50 (normally DBP 80) NOTE: consult physician for exceptions to these guidelines.

Goal	Method	Principle	Example
Client will (be independent/modified I) (Require maximal/moderate/minimal/standby assist/verbal or physical cues) to perform ADL (specify) tasks in ____ weeks/days using...	Safety education which...	Ensures that hip precautions are followed.	Avoid hip abduction (e.g., don't cross legs to roll in bed). Avoid hip internal rotation (e.g., don't line up foot with shoe by twisting leg into internal rotation). Avoid hip flexion past 90 degrees (e.g., stand up from chair by leaning back and sliding hips to edge of seat, then extend knee of operated leg, and push off from armrests). Use elevated commode to maintain hip flexion 90 degrees or less. Do not cross ankles or legs when sitting, laying or getting in/out of bed. When in bed, keep legs apart and toes pointed toward ceiling.
Client will (be independent/modified I) (Require maximal/moderate/minimal/ standby assist/verbal or physical cues) to perform ADL (specify) tasks in ____ weeks/days using...	Safety education which...	Ensures joint protection.	Avoid positions of possible deformity. Avoid holding joints or using muscles in one position for a long time. Use the strongest joints available. Don't start on an activity you cannot stop. Use each joint to its mechanical advantage. Respect pain. Regular rest periods.

		Appendix N, continued.	
Goal	*Method*	*Principle*	*Example*
Client/caregiver will (be independent/modified I) (Require maximal/moderate/minimal/standby assist/verbal or physical cues) to perform ADL (specify) tasks in _____ weeks/days using...	Safety education which...	Ensures shoulder precautions.	Never pull client up in bed using their arms; use a drawsheet. Do not support a client under their arms during transfers; support clients around their trunk.
Client/caregiver will (be independent/modified I) (Require maximal/moderate/minimal/standby assist/verbal or physical cues) to perform (specify) tasks in _____ weeks/days using...	Safety education which...	Ensures sternal precautions (after heart surgery).	Do not push/pull with arms. Do not use arms to push out of bed or pull on siderails. Do not allow others to pull on your arms.

Adapted from Dutton, R. (1995). *Clinical reasoning in physical disabilities*. Baltimore: Williams & Wilkins; and Marrelli, T. M., & Krulish, L. H. (1999). *Home care therapy: Quality, documentation and reimbursement*. Boca Grande, FL: Marrelli and Associates, Inc.

Index

Build Your Library

Along with this title, we publish numerous products on a variety of topics. We are sure that you will find the below titles to be an essential addition to your library. Order your copies today or contact us for a copy of our latest catalog for additional product information.

KINESIOLOGY FOR OCCUPATIONAL THERAPY

Melinda Rybski, MS, OTR/L

272 pp., Soft Cover with CD-ROM, 2004,
ISBN 1-55642-491-4, Order #34914, $45.95

Kinesiology for Occupational Therapy helps occupational therapists manage each step of the kinesiology continuum from problem identification of client musculoskeletal factors to the final stage of selecting appropriate intervention strategies. To help bridge the gap from classroom to clients, a comprehensive analysis of normal human movement is included.

VISION, PERCEPTION, AND COGNITION: A MANUAL FOR THE EVALUATION AND TREATMENT OF THE NEUROLOGICALLY IMPAIRED ADULT, THIRD EDITION

Barbara Zoltan, MA, OTR

232 pp., Soft Cover, 1996, ISBN 1-55642-265-2,
Order #32652, $32.95

This extraordinary book is an indispensable reference for outlining the theoretical basis for visual, perceptual, and cognitive deficits, as well as specific procedures for the evaluation and treatment of these deficits. The book clearly explains each deficit and provides step-by-step testing techniques along with complete treatment guidelines.

QUICK REFERENCE DICTIONARY FOR OCCUPATIONAL THERAPY, FOURTH EDITION

Karen Jacobs, EdD, OTR/L, CPE, FAOTA and Laela Jacobs, OTR/L

600 pp., Soft Cover, 2004, ISBN 1-55642-656-9, Order #36569, $25.95

This definitive companion provides quick access to words, their definitions, and important resources used in everyday practice and the classroom. Used by thousands of your peers and colleagues, the *Quick Reference Dictionary for Occupational Therapy, Fourth Edition* is one of a kind and needed by all in the profession.

Contact Us

SLACK Incorporated, Professional Book Division
6900 Grove Road, Thorofare, NJ 08086
1-800-257-8290/1-856-848-1000, Fax: 1-856-853-5991
orders@slackinc.com or www.slackbooks.com

- -

ORDER FORM

QUANTITY	TITLE	ORDER #	PRICE
	Kinesiology for Occupational Therapy	34914	$45.95
	Vision, Perception, and Cognition, 3E	32652	$32.95
	Quick Reference Dictionary for Occupational Therapy, 4E	36569	$25.95
		Subtotal	$
		Applicable state and local tax will be added to your purchase	$
		Handling	$5.00
		Total	$

Name: _____

Address: _____

City: _____ State:_____ Zip: _____

Phone:_____ Fax: _____

Email: _____

- Check enclosed (Payable to SLACK Incorporated)_____

- Charge my: ____ _____ ____ VISA ____ _____

    Account #: _____

    Exp. date: _____ Signature:_____

NOTE: *Prices are subject to change without notice.*
Shipping charges will apply.
Shipping and handling charges are non-refundable.

CODE: 328

Instructions for using *Goniometry: An Interactive Tutorial*

Suggestions

- It is best to close all programs before installing any software.
- For peak efficiency, disable screen savers while running this program.
- This program uses QuickTime 3 technology. If you are having problems with audio/video playback, reinstall QuickTime from this CD to ensure that the proper version is being used.

For Your PC

Windows 95/98/NT Installation

1. Insert the CD-ROM into the CD-ROM drive.
2. Click the "Start" button in the bottom left-hand corner of the screen.
3. Click "Run", then click "Browse".
4. Select your CD-ROM drive (most often drive D:) from the "Look in:" menu.
5. Select the file SETUP.EXE and click "Open".
6. Click "Next" to begin installation.
7. As the installer runs, it will ask you to select a directory to install the application, or to confirm the default location.
8. The installer asks if you would like to install QuickTime 3.02. Click yes if QuickTime 3.02 is not already installed on your computer. Follow the instructions that appear on your screen.
9. After installation, click the "Start" button in the bottom left-hand corner of the screen.
10. Select "Programs", then click the "Goniometry" folder, and select "Goniometry".

System Requirements

- Pentium-based PC or above
- Microsoft Windows 95 or later
- 16 MB of RAM (32 MB preferred)
- 15 MB of hard disk storage
- 1 MB (or higher) SVGA video card
- 8-bit Sound Blaster-compatible sound card

For Your Macintosh

Installation

1. Insert the CD-ROM into the CD-ROM drive.
2. If you do not have QuickTime 3.02 installed in your computer, double click on the " QuickTime 3.02 Installer" icon. You will need to restart your computer after this installation.
3. Follow the instructions that appear on the screen.
4. When QuickTime 3.02 installation is complete, double click the "StartGoniometry" icon.

System Requirements

- Power PC or above
- 16 MB of RAM (32 MB preferred)
- 15 MB of hard disk storage
- MAC OS version 7.1.2 or later